# BETTER FOOD FOR Kids

YOUR ESSENTIAL GUIDE TO NUTRITION FOR ALL CHILDREN FROM AGE 2 TO 6

# BETTER FOOD FOR Kids

**Your Essential Guide to Nutrition for all Children from age 2 to 6**

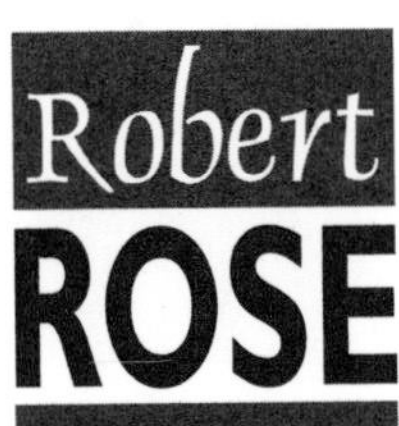

# Better Food for Kids



For complete cataloguing information, see page 6.

DESIGN, EDITORIAL AND PRODUCTION: MATTHEWS COMMUNICATIONS DESIGN INC.

COVER ILLUSTRATION: SHARON MATTHEWS

MANAGING EDITOR: PETER MATTHEWS

INDEXER: BARBARA SCHON

We acknowledge the financial support of the Government of Canada through the Book Publishing Industry Development Program (BPIDP) for our publishing activities.

Published by: Robert Rose Inc. • 120 Eglinton Ave. E, Suite 1000,

Toronto, Ontario, Canada M4P 1E2 Tel: (416) 322-6552

Printed in Canada

1234567 BP 05 04 03 02

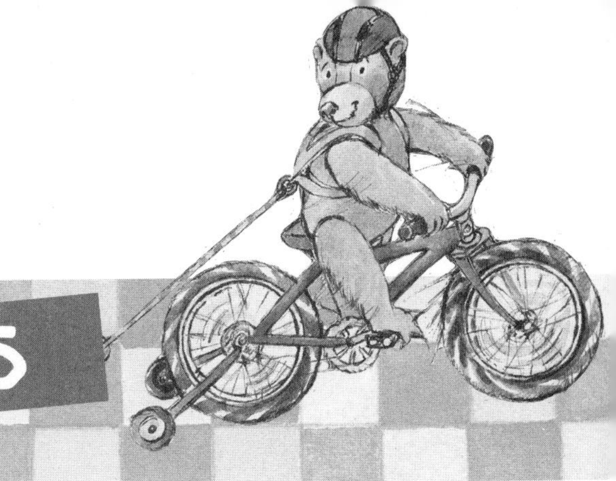

# Contents

**National Library of Canada Cataloguing in Publication Data**

Saab, Joanne

Better food for kids : your essential guide to nutrition for all children from age 2 to 6

Includes index.

ISBN 0-7788-0051-2 (bound : Canada).—ISBN 0-7788-0049-0 (bound : U.S.).—ISBN 0-7788-0045-8 (pbk. : Canada).—ISBN 0-7788-0048-2 (pbk. : U.S.)

1. Cookery. 2. Children – Nutrition. I. Kalnins, Daina. II. Title.

TX740.S15 2002 641.5'622 C2002-90032-3

# Introduction

*Better Food for Kids* is designed to give parents or caregivers what they need to know about feeding children 2 to 6 years of age. As such, it is a continuation of our gratifyingly successful first book, *Better Baby Food*, with a special focus on the nutritional needs of young children. The book is not a public health policy statement, but it does provide much-needed information and advice.

This book shares its predecessor's easy-to-read style, with a wealth of useful information about food and nutrition, as well as a wide selection of kid-pleasing recipes to help make meal planning easier.

Many *Better Baby Food* readers have told us how surprised they were to find that our "baby food" recipes were good enough for the whole family, not just for babies! Well, that was the point. As long as a food's texture is appropriate to the age of the child, its flavor can still be appealing to every member of the family.

In the first portion of the book, you'll find a broad range of topics covered, including advice on feeding children at specific ages and helping them to appreciate for themselves the value of good nutrition and a healthy lifestyle. In addition, we look at essential nutrients, vitamins and minerals, as well as common issues such as vegetarianism, food safety, food allergies, organic vs. conventional foods, disorders such as constipation and diarrhea, childhood obesity, feeding in daycare and school facilities, and many others.

The information in this book has been gathered through careful research, using current and established studies that have been reported in leading-edge professional journals. We also bring to this book our skills as registered dietitians with more than 20 years' combined experience in pediatric nutrition – involving both healthy and sick children – as well as the considerable knowledge we have gained in teaching programs for children, parents and health providers.

In addition to our professional roles at the Hospital for Sick Children, one of us (Daina) has personal experience as the mother of two young children who, as they did with *Better Baby Food*, provided valuable feedback (in a variety of ways!) for the recipes in this book.

We hope you will find the information in *Better Food for Kids* helpful, and that you'll find the recipes as delicious as they are nutritious. Remember to enjoy these precious, fleeting years with your children. By encouraging them to adopt good eating and lifestyle habits now, you will help them to enjoy a lifetime of good health.

*– DK and JS*

# Acknowledgements

Were it not for all the encouragement and support of many friends, family members and colleagues, *Better Food for Kids* would have been a much more difficult project to undertake. We were inspired, too, by the enthusiastic response to our previous book, *Better Baby Food,* which showed us the great demand that exists for more information on children and nutrition – and for more tasty and nutritious recipes! Our thanks to the many people who contributed so much to this book.

To the friends and colleagues who assisted us with reviewing and revising the information provided, heartfelt thanks to Dr. Deborah O'Connor, Dr. Paul Pencharz, Dr. Milton Gold, Dr. Sanjay Mahant, Leanne Falkner, Gloria Green, Jess Haines, Diana Mager, Sarah Farmer and Kellie Welch. For all the hard work and attention to detail in preparing the recipe analysis and calculations, thanks to Linda Chow, Gurvinder Sehra and Jessica Posthuma. And for their encouraging words and advice, we thank Randi Kirshenbaum, Wendy Lands, Terri Hawkes-Sackman, Jeff Sackman, Patrice Banton and Abbe Goldman Klores.

For the people who shared their recipes, and who tested ours, a special thank you to Leya Aronson, Joan Brennan, Christine Dunlop, Lucy Dardarian, Denise Hawman, Joyce Hawman, Inta Huns, Ilze Kalnins, Karen Kurilla, Jacqueline McKenzie, Lori Moreau, Erika Munro, Gisele Poulin, Maria Roso Rosa, Chantal Saab, Connie Saab, Jhana Shimizu and Jaye Shintani. Daina would also like to thank testers Matis, Natali and Blair for their honesty, and for those incredible facial expressions (MR)!

And to all those friends and colleagues at The Hospital for Sick Children, whom space does not allow us to name individually, our thanks for your professional support and encouragement.

To our publisher, Robert Rose Inc., thank you for your support of this project.

For the editorial, design and production work that made this book a reality, thanks to the team at Matthews Communications Design Inc.

From Daina, a special thank you to Blair, who supported and encouraged me along the way. And to Joanne: Thank you so much for your sincere and ever-growing friendship, knowledge and advice. Once again, I cannot express in words what an absolute pleasure it is to work with you. We share ideas, respect each other's opinions, and have a great team spirit.

From Joanne, thanks to David for always being there and supporting everything I do, and for cooking and cleaning when I didn't have time to. And to Daina: Thanks for always thinking of the bigger picture. You have more drive, commitment and focus than any person I know! Thank you for all your encouragement and advice, and most of all, your friendship. I truly value both our personal and professional relationships.

# Nutritional Advice in Brief

Here, in no particular order, we offer our top 10 recommendations for parents of young children. Each provides references for additional information within the book.

1. Whenever possible, serve your child homemade rather than prepared or convenience foods. Commercially prepared foods can add excess calories (including many derived from fat) and salt to the diet. They can also displace fresh foods such as vegetables and fruits (see pages 13 to 15).
2. Limit your child's intake of juice (see page 16). For quenching thirst, water should be the main beverage of choice.
3. Encourage consumption of fresh fruits and vegetables by having a constant supply readily available.
4. Eat meals with your children whenever possible (see pages 27 to 30). This time spent together as a family has many benefits, including the opportunity to demonstrate to your children your commitment to healthy eating practices which, in turn, will influence theirs.
5. Make sure you are knowledgeable about food and nutrition, and its overall effect on health and well-being (see pages 11 and 35 to 56).
6. Share your knowledge of nutrition with your children (see page 31). Use games or arts and crafts to teach kids about all the good things in the food they eat.
7. Make sure that iron-rich foods are part of your child's diet (see pages 49 to 51). Iron deficiency can have serious consequences on the health of young children.
8. Don't rely on vitamin supplements as a substitute for a healthy, balanced diet (see page 21).
9. Enjoy an active lifestyle together as a family (see pages 31 to 32). Exercise, along with healthy foods, can help decrease the incidence of obesity in children (see pages 100 to 103) – and adults!
10. Variety is the spice of life – and essential to healthy and enjoyable eating. Experiment with new foods and try new recipes (starting with those in this book!).

# About the recipes in this book

The recipes in *Better Food for Kids* are actually not just for kids, but are intended to be enjoyed by the entire family. We have made every effort to ensure that most of the recipes are quick and easy to prepare. We have tried to provide simple breakfast ideas that are well balanced. Lunches include soups that can be made ahead, as well as a number of alternatives to traditional sandwiches. Dinners range from simple pastas to more special evening meals that may require a little more time to prepare. Snacks and desserts include everything from healthy yogurt dips to more indulgent chocolate treats.

Many people might believe that our recipes – since they come from three registered dietitians – must necessarily be focused on serious, "healthy" foods, with little attention paid to foods that are fun to eat. But the opposite is actually true. Dietitians believe that healthy eating depends on enjoying a variety of foods, with a balanced diet that includes all 4 food groups, as well as moderate amounts of sugar and salt. Children should not be placed on restrictive "diets", and we have tried to reflect this message in *Better Foods for Kids*.

### Nutritional information

In keeping with the public demand for information about the nutrients in food, we have supplied with each recipe a detailed analysis that specifies the number of calories, as well as the amounts of protein, carbohydrate and fat per serving. In addition, we have included a "percent of children's daily value" (% CDV) for both calcium and iron. These figures are based on the dietary reference intakes (DRIs) for North American children 4 to 8 years old. (See pages 45 and 50 for more information.) All nutritional analysis data is calculated on metric measurements of ingredients in each recipe.

CHAPTER 1

# Feeding Your 2- to 4-year-old

*As your child passes the age of 2 years, the experience of eating becomes more rewarding – and challenging. Feeding skills continue to improve, which makes mealtimes less messy (although not exactly mess-free), and better chewing skills mean that choking is less of a worry. On the other hand, as children become more independent, they are less willing to accept the purely passive role in feeding that they had as infants. They are both more curious and more demanding about the food they eat. For parents, this provides an important opportunity to guide and educate their children in making healthy choices that will last them a lifetime.*

## Young minds want to know

Between the ages of 2 and 4 years, children absorb new information at an astonishing rate, and this is particularly true when it comes to food. A parent or caregiver should therefore be prepared with at least some basic information on food-related topics, such as where food comes from and why it is important for our well being, so that a child can begin to understand the importance of good nutrition.

Here it helps to provide information in a way that relates food to other aspects of a child's experience. For example, you might tell your child that eating is important because food contains energy, which is essential for play and learning. This may not always transform a finicky eater into a child with a healthy appetite, but it will encourage him or her to start thinking about food in a wider context. And as you are probably aware, children do not forget!

## FEEDING MILESTONES FOR CHILDREN BETWEEN 2 AND 4 YEARS

| Age | Motor skills | Social/Personal skills |
|---|---|---|
| 2 to 3 years | Holds cup in hand<br>Puts spoon straight into mouth<br>Spills a lot<br>Chews more thoroughly than at 18 to 24 months, but choking still a concern | Has definite likes and dislikes<br>Insists on doing things "by myself"<br>Ritualistic<br>Dawdles<br>Food jags<br>Demands food in certain shapes, whole foods<br>Likes to help in kitchen |
| 3 to 4 years | Holds handle on cup<br>Pours from small pitcher<br>Uses fork<br>Chews most food | Improved appetite and interest in food<br>Favorite foods requested<br>Likes shapes, colors, ABCs<br>Able to choose between 2 alternate foods<br>Influenced by TV commercials<br>Likes to imitate food preparer |

*Adapted from: Canadian Pediatric Society.* Little Well Beings. *1994*

NOTE: *This information is provided so parents and caregivers will understand what tasks most children should expect to have mastered by a certain age. It is important to remember that children grow and learn new skills at different rates.*

## Expanding food horizons

While young children become more curious about food as they get older, they still require encouragement to try new and unfamiliar foods. Toddlers will generally reject a new food when given for the first time. But with a little patience and persistence, they can often be tempted to try it. Here the key is to provide a variety of different foods, prepared in a variety of ways, on a consistent basis.

Also, as noted in the following chapter (see page 23), it is important that the child be given the choice of whether or not to eat a particular food. Research indicates that children's food habits are influenced by many factors, including availability of a variety of foods, and by the behavior of their parents at meal times.

See the box, below, for specific strategies that parents and caregivers can use to encourage children to accept new foods.

### Try it, you'll like it...

Seven tips for introducing unfamiliar foods to young children

1. Set an example. Young children are more enthusiastic about trying new foods when they see parents, family and friends enjoying them also.
2. Tempt the eye as well as the palate. Prepare food in a variety of appealing ways, combining different colors, textures and shapes.
3. Don't overload the plate. Try offering new foods in small amounts. Typically, a child-sized portion is one-quarter to one-half an adult portion.
4. Use a little peer pressure. Try serving a new food when children are with their friends.
5. Introduce foods before they reach the table. Let your children become familiar with different foods when you buy, prepare or even grow them.
6. Don't force, but persist. If your child rejects an unfamiliar food the first time, don't force him or her to eat it. Instead, simply offer it again later. The more often children are exposed to new foods, the more likely they will be to taste them and learn to accept them.
7. Don't use food as a bribe or a reward. Studies have shown that children are less likely to accept a food when it is used in this way. For example, making children eat their broccoli before they can go outside will not increase their love of vegetables. Respect your child's food preferences. Every child has different likes and dislikes, just as adults do.

SOURCE: Health Canada. Canada's Food Guide to Healthy Eating. Focus on Preschoolers, 1995.

## Balancing acts

The dietary needs of 2- to 4-year-olds (and for 4- to 6-year olds) vary from one child to another. Factors such as age, body size, growth rate, appetite and activity – all have an effect on food intake. With all these variables, parents often wonder if their children are getting a balance of the right amount of nutrients through their diet or, in some cases, worry that they are getting too many calories.

In most cases, such concerns are unfounded. If you provide your child with a variety of different foods – including breads or cereals, fruits and vegetables, milk and milk products, as well as protein foods such as meats, chicken, fish, soy or lentils – then chances are he or she will get all the energy and nutrition required. See pages 17 and 28 for examples of balanced menus.

### Consistency is the key

A consistent approach to feeding is usually best for children between the ages of 2 and 4 years. A variety of foods provided in three meals and two or three (or more) snacks every day will supply the energy and nutrients your child needs to meet the demands of continued growth and weight gain. A diet of balanced meals and snacks will also ensure that your child has the energy for learning, playing, and interacting with their peers.

## Dealing with dairy foods

For 2- to 4-year-olds, milk and milk products (such as cheese and yogurt) provide an adequate source of calories (energy) for growth and, in most cases, are the main source of vitamin D and calcium, both of which are essential for the normal development of bones and teeth. (See pages 45 to 49 for more information on these nutrients.)

That being said, however, it is important to recognize that consuming too much milk – for example, amounts greater than 24 oz (750 mL) per day – can lead to a deficiency of other nutrients. When milk intake is high, a child may have a diminished appetite for other foods. This is particularly true for younger children who are still on the bottle, which, research suggests, tends to encourage excessive consumption of milk. Because this may replace other important foods, and can lead to iron deficiency (which can affect appetite and behavior), children over the age of 2 should be given milk in a sippy cup or regular cup instead of a bottle.

### How much milk fat?

Whole milk contains the highest amount of fat and calories, and it is this type to which infants are usually introduced when they make the transition from breast milk or formula to cow's milk. After the age of 2 years, however, children do not necessarily require whole milk, and can be offered the 2% or 1% varieties. The exception is if a child is not gaining weight adequately, in which case whole milk is still recommended.

Although milk and milk products do contain some iron, these amounts are inadequate for a growing child's needs. Better sources of iron include meats, as well as some vegetables if taken in appreciable amounts and with a source of vitamin C. (See page 49 for more information on iron.)

Nutritious dairy foods also include cheese and yogurt. Slices or strips of Cheddar or mozzarella cheese are good for snacks. You can also choose from many flavors and varieties of commercially prepared yogurt, although many of these contain a substantial amount of added sugar. A better choice may be to buy plain yogurt and mix in your own fruit. Alternatively, you can buy a sweetened variety and dilute the sugar content with plain yogurt.

## Vegetables matter

If there is one type of food that children seem to resist almost universally, it is vegetables. In fact, one study of preschool children found that their daily consumption of vegetables was less than 25% of the recommended number of servings. Yet vegetables are an important part of a young child's diet, providing a rich source of different vitamins and minerals, as well as fiber, which helps maintain a normal bowel routine. (In many instances, the fiber in vegetables, along with adequate fluids, can help to prevent constipation; see page 39 for more information.)

So how do you encourage children to eat more vegetables? To make them more appealing, prepare vegetables in a variety of ways that can be enjoyed by your child as well as the whole family. For example, try adding a little low-sodium soy sauce to cooked spinach. Green beans or carrots can be perked up with a dip of ranch-style salad dressing. Corn on the cob is usually popular; by the age of 3 years, many children can eat whole corn on the cob.

The recipes in this book also include a number of tempting vegetable dishes, such as ZUCCHINI STICKS (page 168) and SWEDISH POTATOES (page 213). We think you'll discover (as we have) that it is possible to get young children excited about vegetables.

## The whole fruit

Many parents believe that fruit juice is an adequate substitute for whole fruit. But this is not the case. Whole fruits provide fiber, which juices do not, and are lower in sugar. For this reason, make a point of including seasonal fresh fruit in your child's diet. Experiment with different fruits, introducing your child (and perhaps yourself) to new and interesting varieties. Keep a supply of cut-up fruit on hand for snacking at any time.

What about canned fruit? While not as flavorful as fresh, canned fruit is an acceptable alternative. Just make sure that it is packed in fruit juice or water – not heavy syrup.

### *Your child's daily bread*

Breads and cereals provide important minerals and vitamins (such as iron and B vitamins), as well as carbohydrates (for energy) and fiber (which helps ensure regularity). Since children tend to enjoy these foods, it is usually not difficult to get them to eat the recommended number of servings per day. Good examples of breads and cereals include whole wheat bread or bagels, as well as pastas and rice. (Whole wheat varieties are higher in fiber.)

### *Chew chew*

As children get older and their feeding skills become more advanced, the risk of choking is reduced – but it does not disappear. For children under the age of 4, be sure to encourage thorough chewing, and avoid foods such as whole grapes, which can obstruct a child's airway if accidentally inhaled. See Chapter 10, page 95, for more information on avoiding choking hazards.

## Fruit juice abuse?

There are few things more popular with parents and young children than fruit juice. Parents like the fact that it contains important vitamins and minerals (such as vitamin C ), and they appreciate the convenience of juice boxes and straws, which are easy to pack for lunch boxes or traveling. Kids like juice simply because it's sweet and tastes great. Still, it's always possible to have too much of a good thing – and fruit juice is a perfect example of this.

In a recent study of preschoolers, fruit juice was found to account for over 50% of all fruit servings consumed. This means the children were not getting the fiber that comes from whole fruit. In addition, the high intake of juice was almost certainly displacing other foods that could provide a balance of various nutrients.

While the occasional juice served with a meal is perfectly acceptable, constant sipping of juice is not. This habit results not only in unbalanced nutrition, but can contribute to higher rates of tooth decay. (See Chapter 13, page 111, for more information.)

So what's the alternative? Encourage your children to choose water as their beverage of choice. It's refreshing, and essential to good health.

### Juice pretenders

Often sold side by side on supermarket shelves, fruit juices and fruit drinks may appear to be the same. But they're not. Fruit juices contain 100% juice, while fruit drinks typically contain a much smaller proportion of juice, which is supplemented by water, as well as excessive sugar and other ingredients. Although some fruit drinks are fortified with vitamins, they are still less desirable than real juice, and are generally not recommended for young children.

## Packing some protein

Meats and meat alternatives (such as beans, lentils and tofu) provide energy, protein and iron for a growing child. While these foods can be difficult to chew for a 2-year-old, this problem is usually overcome by the age of 4 years. In the meantime, serve your child more tender meats such as soft meatballs served with rice or pasta, or tender chicken served with a sauce or dip. Bite-size pieces of foods such as homemade chicken or fish fingers are also good, as are thinly sliced roast beef or chicken from the supermarket.

## KID CUISINE • Sample menu for a 2- to 4-year-old

| Breakfast | | |
|---|---|---|
| 1/2 cup | WEEKEND BREAKFAST QUICHE (see recipe, page 129) | 125 mL |
| Half | orange, sectioned and seeded | Half |
| 1/2 cup | whole milk | 125 mL |

| Snack | | |
|---|---|---|
| Half | banana | Half |
| Half | apple | Half |
| 1/4 cup | o-shaped cereal | 50 mL |
| 1/2 cup | water | 125 mL |

| Lunch | | |
|---|---|---|
| 1/2 cup | TASTY TOFU (see recipe, page 172) | 125 mL |
| 1/2 cup | rice, steamed | 125 mL |
| 1/2 cup | green beans (with 1 tsp [5 mL] butter) | 125 mL |
| 2 tbsp | ranch-style dressing | 25 mL |
| 1/2 cup | whole milk | 125 mL |
| 1/2 cup | water | 125 mL |

| Snack | | |
|---|---|---|
| 4 | unsalted soda crackers | 4 |
| 1 oz | Cheddar cheese | 25 g |
| Quarter | apple | Quarter |
| 1/2 cup | whole milk | 125 mL |
| 1/2 cup | water | 125 mL |

| Dinner | | |
|---|---|---|
| Half | serving MACARONI AND BEEF WITH CHEESE (see recipe, page 176) | Half |
| 1/2 cup | grated carrots | 125 mL |
| 1/2 cup | whole milk | 125 mL |
| 1 | piece CHOCOLATE CHIP AND BANANA CAKE (see recipe, page 260) | 1 |
| 1/2 cup | water | 125 mL |

Provides 1500 calories, 61 g protein, and meets 100% of CDV for calcium and iron.

## I'll eat it my way

Because young children tend to be curious about the foods around them, they generally look forward to eating. At the same time, however, their growing independence often manifests itself in clearly expressed likes and dislikes about food. Some of these may appear to be quite arbitrary – for example, your child may insist on having a piece of bread sliced diagonally instead of straight through the middle, or on eating the same food for lunch every day for a few weeks.

### Taking part

As they become more independent, young children like to feel that they are actively participating in family life, and this includes food preparation, selection and tasting. Foods that your child has helped to prepare or select at the store are much more interesting – and consequently more likely to be eaten with enthusiasm – than those with which he or she has not been involved.

Such preferences may often be difficult to understand. But it is important for parents to recognize that children are simply exploring their ability to make decisions in situations that they are able to control – specifically, at meal and snack times. Encourage this independence, and respect that your children have their likes and dislikes of food (as you do). This is not to say that you should not set limits, of course, but you should allow children some degree of latitude in requesting certain foods at meals, and understand that their appetite may not always be consistent from one day to the next.

When dealing with your child's likes and dislikes, remember that opinions formed at this age are changeable and subject to influence. Foods that are rejected outright today may be requested tomorrow. The brown rice that is spurned at your dinner table may suddenly become palatable when served at a friend's house. As you did with your children when they were infants, try not to let your own dislikes of food serve as a negative influence. Children love to imitate their parents or caregivers, so act accordingly.

Keep mealtime as calm and pleasant as possible, no matter how tiring or hectic your day has been. Children read cues and will not respond positively to your attempts to influence them unless they feel that at least some of their decisions are being respected. Social interactions and changes in appetite will influence the choices of food your child makes.

## Feeding frustrations

Does your child take forever to finish a meal? Does he or she seem abnormally fussy or difficult about eating? Well, you're not alone. In fact, behavioral research into children's eating habits reveals that over 30% of parents of toddlers describe some feeding-related problem, including slow eating, poor appetite, unhappiness during mealtimes, rigid food preferences, or other negative behavior. The important thing for parents to realize is that, in most instances, these behaviors are relatively short-lived. It is only in a minority of cases, where children have been slow feeders for a number of years, that a more detailed assessment of their feeding skills may have to be evaluated.

So what do you do until children grow out of their "picky eater" stage? Like most parents, you may be concerned that the child is not getting enough to eat. But you probably don't need to worry. As long as your child is growing normally, chances are that he or she is receiving an adequate supply of energy and nutrients.

Consider, for example, the sample menu shown on page 20. While the amount of food may seem quite minimal (at least, compared to the menu given on page 17), it still provide more then 70% of the child's nutritional requirements (except for iron). The occasional "picky" day will generally not affect your child's nutritional status. Children are very good at self-regulating their overall energy intake – at least, when we allow them to do so, and give them the freedom to indicate when they are hungry or full.

## MEALS AT A MINIMUM • Sample menu for a picky 3-year-old

| Breakfast | | |
|---|---|---|
| 1/4 cup | o-shaped cereal | 50 mL |
| 1/2 cup | whole milk | 125 mL |
| Quarter | banana | Quarter |
| **Snack** | | |
| 1 | unsalted soda cracker | 1 |
| Half | banana | Half |
| **Lunch** | | |
| Half | slice bread with 1 tbsp (15 mL) peanut butter | Half |
| Quarter | raw carrot | Quarter |
| 1 cup | whole milk | 250 mL |
| **Snack** | | |
| 2 | unsalted soda crackers | 2 |
| 1 oz | Cheddar cheese | 25 g |
| **Dinner** | | |
| 2 | fish sticks | 2 |
| Quarter | baked potato | Quarter |
| 1 tbsp | mayonnaise-type dressing (for potato) | 15 mL |
| **Snack** | | |
| 1/2 cup | whole milk | 125 mL |
| 1 | oatmeal cookie | 1 |

Provides: 1032 calories, 44 g protein, and meets 56% of iron requirements.

# Q&A *for feeding 2- to 4-year-olds*

**Q.** ***My daughter is 2 1/2 years old, and now eats some meals away from home – either at daycare or at a friend's house for play group. How can I be sure that she is eating enough?***

**A.** Normal growth and weight gain are the most important signs to watch for when assessing nutritional intake. Other indicators include your daughter's energy level and tolerance for exercise. At home, make every attempt to offer each of the 4 food groups at each meal to provide a balanced diet with a variety of vitamins and minerals. If you are really concerned, you could also ask your child's daytime caregiver(s) to make a note of your child's food intake over a 3-day period. This will help you to determine if there are any types of food lacking in her diet.

**Q.** ***My 3-year-old son seems to be much heavier than other children his age. Should I be putting him on a diet?***

**A.** Placing a child on a diet – at least, in the adult sense of the word – is not appropriate at this age. Keep in mind that being heavier than other children does not mean he is fat. If your son has always been larger than most kids his age, this may be normal for him. Children typically grow into their weight and need a constant supply of the appropriate amount of energy and other nutrients required for normal development. So continue to give him 3 meals and snacks daily, and do not restrict foods. Snack foods should be healthy, including fresh vegetables and fruits. Try to limit snacks such as chips or candy, which are high in fat or low in fiber and nutrients. (This recommendation applies to all children.) Also, keep an eye on your son's juice consumption, since these calories can add up. Encourage him to drink water.

**Q.** ***Should I give my 3-year-old a vitamin supplement? I think he is eating a balanced diet, but I would like to be sure that he is getting all the nutrients he needs.***

**A.** Vitamin supplements are costly and unnecessary for a young child who is growing normally and eating a variety of nutritious foods. In fact, these supplements often provide parents with a false sense of security, encouraging them to believe that less effort or attention is required to give their children a properly balanced diet. There are some exceptions, of course, such as those children who have iron-deficiency anemia and require a period of iron supplementation. Children with lactose intolerance may also require a supplement to provide the calcium and vitamin D that would otherwise be supplied by drinking milk (unless they are drinking a lactose-free fortified beverage). (See page 45 for more information on calcium.) Finally, keep in mind that children are especially vulnerable to vitamin toxicity when supplements are taken in excessive amounts. If your child requires a supplement, ask your doctor to recommend the appropriate type and dose.

**Q.** ***My 4-year-old daughter had a viral illness with diarrhea that lasted for a few days. I have read that the "BRAT diet" can help relieve diarrhea. What is this diet and how effective is it?***

**A.** BRAT (an acronym for Bananas, Rice, Applesauce and Toast [or Tea]) is not a balanced diet, since it is limited in protein, fat and calories – and may even promote more diarrhea. It has never been proven to help decrease diarrhea. Your child will be better off with her normal diet and adequate fluid. Check with your family doctor to see if a special electrolyte replacement fluid is necessary. (See page 92 for more information.)

**Q.** ***Should I be giving my 2-year-old son organic vegetables and fruits? Are they safer and more nutritious?***

**A.** Although organic foods are promoted as being free of any pesticides or preservatives, existing government regulations are designed to ensure that conventionally produced foods are safe for consumption. Generally speaking, there is no evidence to support the use of organic over non-organic produce. Their nutrient values do not differ, although their prices do: Organic produce can be 10 to 40% more expensive than conventional fruits and vegetables.

**Q.** ***I have a lot of difficulty getting my 3-year-old to drink plain milk – although she loves chocolate milk. Is it OK to give her this instead?***

**A.** Chocolate milk provides the same important nutrients (including calcium and vitamin D) as plain milk. It is higher in sugar, however, and contains caffeine (from the chocolate), so you may want to dilute these ingredients by mixing some of the chocolate milk with plain milk. You might also try compromising with your child by alternating plain and chocolate milk with each snack or mealtime.

**Q.** ***Getting my 3-year-old boy's teeth brushed each night is a constant battle. How often should we be brushing his teeth? Can we let him do it himself?***

**A.** Children should have their teeth brushed at least twice a day – once in the morning and once in the evening – using only a small amount of toothpaste (about the size of a pea). Ideally, you should also brush your son's teeth after he eats sugary foods such as raisins or sticky candy. (As well, drinking water [instead of juice] throughout the day helps to cleanse teeth.) You should encourage your son to brush his own teeth – preferably by the example of brushing your teeth at the same time. After he has been given the opportunity to brush his own teeth, quickly brush them again.

**Q.** ***My 4-year-old daughter seems to be eating less and less. Is there a safe appetite stimulant that I can give her?***

**A.** No. Children have different growth stages, and each is accompanied by increases and decreases in appetite. Provided your daughter's growth is normal (ask your family doctor or pediatrician if you're unsure), there should be no reason to worry. Children are usually quite good at regulating their own intake when given a varied supply of nutritious and healthy foods. Appetite stimulants are not safe in children.

**Q.** ***I hear so much about food allergies in young children. Should I eliminate high-risk foods from my child's diet to prevent allergies from occurring?***

**A.** There is no evidence to suggest that eliminating certain foods from a child's diet will prevent allergy. If there is a strong family history of allergy (parent or sibling with food allergy), you may wish to speak with your family doctor about allergy testing before introducing certain foods.

CHAPTER 2

# Feeding Your 4- to 6-year-old

*Between the ages of 4 and 6, a child's physical growth begins to slow down a little (although it probably won't seem that way!), while rapid changes continue in skill development and feeding behavior. It is at this stage that parents face a new set of challenges in educating their children, and helping them to understand the essentials of healthy food, good nutrition and an active lifestyle.*

## The preschooler's progress

As children make the transition from toddlers to school-age, they typically become a little leaner-looking, losing some of the baby fat that was apparent when they were younger. This reflects their higher activity levels which, in turn, means that the child will often have a greater need for higher-energy foods (see page 35).

Eating habits also change as children get older. Since they have been introduced to a wider variety of foods, they become less likely to reject anything that is new or unfamiliar. Meal routines and self-feeding skills also become well-established, so your children are able to assume a more active and independent role at the family dinner table.

Children between the ages of 4 and 6 will also gain new eating experiences outside the home – sometimes beginning in daycare and then, later, at school. The result is that children are often eating one or two meals, plus snacks, away from home each day. While this offers the benefit of exposing children to new foods and eating experiences, it also means that parents have a special responsibility to ensure that their child receives structured, nutritious meals and snacks, and develops the eating habits that will contribute to a lifetime of health.

## FEEDING MILESTONES FOR CHILDREN BETWEEN 4 AND 6 YEARS

| Age | Motor skills | Social/Personal skills |
|---|---|---|
| 4 to 5 years | Uses knife and fork<br>Good use of cup<br>Good self-feeder | Rather talk than eat<br>Likes to help with food preparation<br>Interested in the nature of food and where it comes from<br>Peer influence increasing |
| 5 to 6 years | Fully able to self-feed | Imitating<br>Less suspicious of mixtures, but still prefers plain foods<br>Social influence outside home increasing<br>Food important part of special occasions |

*Adapted from: Canadian Pediatric Society.* Little Well Beings. *1994*

NOTE: *This information is provided so parents and caregivers will understand what tasks most children should expect to have mastered by a certain age. It is important to remember that children grow and learn new skills at different rates.*

### Delegating mealtime authority

When children are very young, their role in the feeding process is essentially passive: It is their parents who decide what, when, where and how much they eat. As the child gets older and more independent, however, these roles change, and the child begins to assume greater responsibility for his or her eating decisions.

The concept of divided responsibility for childhood feeding has been put forth by Ellen Satter, a registered dietitian, social worker and author of several books on child behavior as it pertains to eating. The basic premise here is that both the child and the parent have certain responsibilities at mealtime, and that parents should be aware of the child's obligations as well as their own. This idea of delegating responsibility is more evolutionary than revolutionary, since the bulk of decision-making remains with parents, who continue to be responsible for determining what, when and where the child eats. It simply becomes the child's responsibility to decide whether or not he or she will eat and, if so, how much to eat.

For many parents who are accustomed to exercising control over every aspect of their children's lives, it may be difficult to accept the notion that a 4- to 6-year-old should be given any decision-making power at all – particularly with respect to eating. So let's look at the child's responsibilities first.

### Too young to diet

Some well-meaning parents attempt to restrict a child's food intake in an effort to control what they perceive as excessive weight gain. But research has shown that such restrictions can actually have the opposite effect, leading children to overeat and gain even more weight. When food is perceived as a carefully controlled commodity, children can become obsessed with it, eating more than they need to avoid the possibility of becoming hungry. (See Chapter 11, pages 97 to 106, for more information on childhood obesity.)

## To eat or not to eat...

If given the chance, children are remarkably good at determining whether or not, or how much, they need to eat. In fact, it is usually when parents interfere excessively with the child's eating decisions (or do not provide enough support for those decisions) that children end up consuming too much food or too little.

The important thing to remember is that between the ages of 4 and 6, a child's appetite does not remain consistent from day to day. It will increase during growth spurts or at times when your child is very active. Conversely, it will often decrease when a child is tired or over-excited. (Don't worry: these fluctuations become less frequent as children get older.)

Children should be allowed to eat as much food as they wish during mealtimes – but not between meals (see below) – until they are full. On the other hand, when children are not hungry at a given meal or snack time, they should not be forced to eat. Let them decide for themselves whether or not they are hungry. But make sure they understand the consequences of their decision – specifically, that if the child chooses not to eat now, he or she will not have another opportunity to do so until the next scheduled meal or snack. Do not feel guilty about saying this. It will encourage eating at designated meal and snack times, and will enable your child to trust his or her own sense of hunger and fullness.

## How much to serve...

While children should ultimately decide how much they will eat, it is still the parent's responsibility to provide the structure in which these decisions are made. For example, you will need to decide how much food to offer your child, recognizing that overly large portions can be intimidating.

As a rule, it's best to provide children with smaller amounts of food, giving them the option of seconds if they wish. To determine the serving size appropriate for your 4- to 6-year-old, use the table below as a guide. Keep in mind that there are a number of variables to consider, including the child's age (younger children will eat less) and individual eating patterns.

### Suggested serving sizes for 4- to 6-year-olds*

| Food group | Food item | Range of serving sizes |
|---|---|---|
| Grain products | Bread | Half to 1 whole slice |
| | Cold cereal | 1/2 to 1 cup (125 to 250 mL) |
| | Hot cereal | 1/3 to 3/4 cup (75 mL to 175 mL) |
| | Bagel, pita or bun | Quarter to half |
| | Muffin | Half to 1 whole |
| | Pasta or rice | 1/4 to 1/2 cup (50 to 125 mL) |
| | Crackers | 4 to 8 |
| Vegetables and fruit | Whole fruit or vegetable | Half to 1 medium |
| | Vegetables, fresh, frozen or canned | 1/4 to 1/2 cup (50 to 125 mL) |
| | Salad | 1/2 to 1 cup (125 to 250 mL) |
| | Fruit, fresh or canned | 1/4 to 1/2 cup (50 to 125 mL) |
| | Vegetable or fruit juice | 1/4 to 1/2 cup (50 to 125 mL) |
| Milk products | Milk | 1/2 to 1 cup (125 to 250 mL) |
| | Cheese | 1 to 2 oz (25 to 50 g) |
| | Yogurt | 1/3 to 3/4 cup (75 mL to 175 mL) |
| Meat and alternatives | Meat, fish or poultry | 1 to 2 oz (25 to 50 g) |
| | Egg | 1 whole |
| | Beans, legumes | 1/4 to 1/2 cup (50 to 125 mL) |
| | Tofu | 1/4 to 1/3 cup (50 to 75 mL) |
| | Peanut butter | 1 to 2 tbsp (15 to 25 mL) |

* NOTE: *For each range of serving sizes, the lesser amounts are appropriate for 2- to 4-year olds.*

## When to eat...

Providing toddlers and preschoolers with structured meal and snack times helps to establish hunger and facilitates eating at meal times. Snacks should be well-timed, and of appropriate size, so that children are hungry but not "starving" at mealtime. Snacking is an important source of energy and nutrients. However, if you find that you are having difficulty getting children to eat at the table, "grazing" should be limited between meals. When children are thirsty throughout the day, encourage them to drink water. If appetite at mealtime is a problem, you may wish to restrict consumption of milk, juice, or other nutritious beverages to meals and snacks only.

### No TV dinners here

Meals should be a time for enjoying food and conversation, not watching television. So turn off the set. You'll find that it enhances family togetherness. What's more, since research has shown that children who eat in front of the television often ignore satiety cues (that's dietitian-speak for "feelings of fullness"), there's less chance that your child (or you) will overeat.

## Where to eat...

Meals should be eaten in a designated spot. For most families this will be the kitchen table. Whenever possible, sit with your children and eat meals together as a family.

Keep in mind that eating with your child involves more than just sitting with your child while he or she eats. It is important to talk with children so that they appreciate mealtime as a time to interact with the family. The dinner table should not be a place for family arguments; instead, it should provide the kind of environment where your child can tell you about his or her day – or about anything at all. Try to establish the ritual of eating together when your children are young; it will be much more difficult to get into the habit once members of the family are older and have schedules of their own.

## What to eat

The final responsibility of parents is to provide their child with healthy meals and snacks. This task will be considerably easier if you have a basic understanding of the four food groups, the essential nutrients children need, and if you use the recipes in this book.

Remember that growing children require energy-dense foods (such as peanut butter, cheeses and whole milk), as well as lower-energy foods (such as vegetables and legumes), and you should try to provide a balance of both types at meals. A sample menu, providing a well-balanced diet, is shown below.

## JUNIOR CARTE DU JOUR • Sample menu for a 4- to 6-year-old

| Breakfast | | |
|---|---|---|
| 1 | slice whole wheat toast | 1 |
| 1 tsp | margarine | 5 mL |
| 3/4 cup | oatmeal | 175 mL |
| 1 cup | 2% milk | 250 mL |
| **Snack** | | |
| 1 | apple | 1 |
| 1 oz | cheese | 25 g |
| 1/2 cup | water | 125 mL |
| **Lunch** | | |
| 3/4 cup | TUSCAN BEAN SOUP (see recipe, page 142) | 175 mL |
| 1 | whole grain roll | 1 |
| 1/2 cup | 2% milk | 125 mL |
| 3/4 cup | strawberry yogurt | 175 mL |
| **Snack** | | |
| 2 | banana oatmeal cookies | 2 |
| 1/2 cup | apple juice | 125 mL |
| **Dinner** | | |
| 1 | serving BEEF SATAYS (see recipe, page 202) | 1 |
| 1/2 cup | steamed rice | 125 mL |
| 1/4 cup | broccoli | 50 mL |
| 1/4 cup | cauliflower | 50 mL |
| 1/2 cup | 2% milk | 125 mL |
| 1/2 cup | fruit cocktail | 125 mL |

Provides: 1530 calories, 65 g protein, and meets over 100% of calcium and iron requirements.

## Packing some punch in your child's lunch

Once children reach kindergarten, many parents provide them with a bag lunch to take to school each day – usually at the last minute and without giving its contents a lot of thought. Not surprisingly, children often complain that they "don't like what mom sends for lunch" or that they are "tired of peanut butter sandwiches." Here are a few healthy and nutritious suggestions that will add variety to your child's lunch bag.

- Purchase a small thermos and fill it with hot soups or leftover stews and pastas. It can also be used to help keep milk or other beverages cold.
- A small ice pack (or frozen juice or water container) is ideal for keeping cold foods cold and to protect them from spoilage (see Chapter 6, page 65, for more information on food safety). Use it with milk, cheese slices, yogurt or meat sandwiches.
- Liven up sandwiches by using different types of bread, such as pita pockets, small submarine buns, raisin bread or whole grain bread.
- Make sandwiches with a variety of fillings such as sliced deli meats, tuna, ham, and salmon or egg salad. Other ideas include: hummus; nut butters (where not prohibited; many schools have declared themselves "nut-free" zones because of allergy concerns); refried beans; leftovers, including roasted chicken or meatloaf; soy alternatives, such as textured vegetable protein slices; and various types of cheese, such as Cheddar, cream cheese, havarti, and Monterey Jack.
- Instead of ordinary sandwiches, try making one of the following alternatives: rice cakes with peanut butter; hummus with pita bread; Melba toast and cheese slices; bagel pieces with flavored cream cheese; muffins with cheese slices; leftover pizza slices; and crackers with cheese slices.
- Pack a combinations of fruits and vegetables, such as: baby carrots and celery slices; vegetable pieces with salad dressing dip; fresh fruit pieces with flavored yogurt for dipping; and individual fruit cups.

- When in season, provide whole fresh fruit, including apples, pears, plums, grapes, bananas, melon pieces, mango or kiwi slices (the list is endless).
- Good dessert choices can include: cookies, such as arrowroot, chocolate chip, oatmeal; granola or other cereal bars; small pudding cups; and flavored yogurt.
- See the lunch recipes in this book for other terrific ideas!

## Setting an example

Young children learn from what they see, and this is reflected by imitating the people around them. Between the ages of 4 and 6 years they especially love to copy their moms and dads. So it is parents who need to present a model of good eating habits to their children.

By eating with your children at the table during mealtimes, you can teach them to enjoy a variety of familiar foods, as well as the experience of trying out new ones. By making mealtime a pleasant place to be for your child, you can provide positive reinforcement for learning, and thereby contribute to his or her self-esteem.

### *Avoid weighty issues*

Research shows that, in recent years, children have started to develop adult-like preoccupations with weight and dieting at increasingly younger ages. Part of this is no doubt attributable to endless coverage of these issues in the media (to which children are exposed almost from infancy), but parents still need to ensure that they avoid contributing to the problem. So don't complain about your weight in front of your children.

## Developing feeding skills

Every child develops self-feeding skills at different rates. Nevertheless, it is reasonable for parents to expect that their children achieve certain basic abilities when eating with the family.

Typically, between the ages of 4 and 5 years, children make real progress in being able to feed themselves efficiently. They become proficient in using a knife and fork to cut foods (provided that utensils are small enough for them to use). They have good use of a cup and, although they may still dribble and spill milk out the sides, it happens less often than it did when they were 2 or 3. These skills should continue to develop between the ages of 5 and 6 years.

### *Table manners*

By the age of 4 years, a child should be capable of behaving pleasantly at the dinner table. You can encourage this by making the table a pleasant and privileged place to be. It should not be a place for punishment – for example, where children are made to stay until they finish their carrots.

## Steps to healthy eating and living

**Educate your children.** Studies have shown that children are quick to absorb health and safety information, and that their ability to be "health smart" begins at a young age – as early as 3 1/2 years, according to a study from the University of Texas – with much of this information being mastered by their sixth birthday. For example, by the age of 4 years, many children are able to identify that drinking milk is better for you than drinking soda pop. By 5 1/2 years, many children can evaluate the relative health benefits of different food choices – an apple versus a piece of cake, for example, or a chicken dinner versus a pizza dinner. As a parent, it is important to understand that your children are capable of learning a great deal about food and health, and that much of this will come from your teaching and the example you set as a role model.

**Explore the possibilities.** It is important for parents to explore a variety of foods for themselves and their children. Look for foods with different colors, flavors and textures. Preschoolers are naturally curious and eager to learn about food. Use new ingredients or try new dishes from different ethnicities or cooking styles. For example, if you usually eat white bread for dinner, try substituting something different, such as a whole wheat baguette, pita bread, bannock, chapati, or focaccia. When parents explore new types food, they encourage their children to do so as well.

**Be active.** An active lifestyle needn't involve strenuous exercise or punishing workouts at a gym. It can be something as simple as taking a stroll in the evening with your children or participating in recreational family sports, such as skiing or rollerblading. The key is to ensure that your children don't spend all their free time in front of the television or the computer screen.

**Encourage vitality.** Essentially this means living life to the fullest – enjoying good food, being active, feeling good about yourself and fostering these feelings in your children. Children enjoy eating and exploring food. Children like to feel good about themselves and need to have a positive body image fostered by their parents. It is important for parents to help build self-esteem by providing affection and attention. When parents feel good about themselves, they are more likely to have children who feel good about themselves as well.

# Q&A *for feeding 4- to 6-year-olds*

Q. ***My 5-year-old daughter won't eat any vegetables, what should I do?***

A. While having an aversion to one or two vegetables is common, it is unusual for a child to dislike *all* vegetables. Try preparing a vegetable with which your child is unfamiliar (and has yet to be identified as "bad"). Take your daughter shopping and ask her to pick out a vegetable that appeals to her. Try frozen instead of canned vegetables. Prepare vegetables with ingredients that change or embellish their flavor – adding a small amount of butter to green beans, for example, or low-sodium soy sauce to bok choy, maple syrup to carrots, or a cheese sauce to broccoli. Also, make sure that you are setting a good example by eating vegetables yourself. Regardless of whether or not these strategies are successful, do not force your child to eat her vegetables. Instead, continue to place a small quantity on her plate each day. It may take many exposures, but there's a good chance she'll eventually give in and sample the food.

Q. ***Is brown sugar or honey more nutritious than white sugar?***

A. White sugar is produced from sugar cane or sugar beets. Brown sugar is granulated sugar that contains some molasses (refiner's sugar), while honey is a sweet syrup produced by bees. Each type of sweetener is a simple sugar or carbohydrate. All provide some calories but none is more "nutritious" than the others, since they contain no vitamins or minerals. Regardless of their form, these sugars are best consumed in moderation.

Q. ***When is it okay to give my child soda pop?***

A. Nutritionally speaking, there is no reason ever to give soda pop to a child, since these sugary carbonated beverages offer nothing more than "empty" calories and an increased risk of tooth decay. As a practical matter, however, school-aged children enjoy the flavor of soda pop, which is why it is often served at birthday parties and other special occasions. Allowing your child a small amount of pop at these events is fine, although consumption on daily basis is not. While there are no specific recommendations on the subject, we suggest that soda pop not be given to children under the age of 5 years.

Q. ***My 5-year old son refuses to drink milk. How can I be sure he gets the nutrients he needs?***

A. Milk and dairy products are an important source of energy, calcium and vitamin D for children of all ages. While government food guides recommend that preschoolers have 2 to 3 servings of milk per day, there is nothing that says it has to be plain milk. Like many children, your son may enjoy chocolate milk instead of the white variety. Also, cheese or yogurt are healthy alternatives to milk. And if your son refuses to drink milk but puts it on his cereal (as many children do), keep in mind that this amount (typically 4 to 6 oz [125 to 175 mL]) represents half a serving of milk products.

**Q.** ***Every day I pack my son a lunch for school, but he often brings much of it home uneaten. What should I do?***

**A.** Young children often respond unenthusiastically to a bagged lunch. As a result, they may bring food home at the end of the day. But this does not mean they are not eating at all. Ask your son why he is not eating his lunch. Is he trading with friends? This is not unusual, although you may want to find out what he is eating instead. Another question to ask your son is whether his lunch is too large for his appetite. There is also the possibility that he simply doesn't like the food you've given him. If this is the case, see page 29 for packed lunch ideas.

**Q.** ***My 6-year-old daughter won't eat breakfast. How can I convince her?***

**A.** Breakfast is often referred to as the most important meal of the day. For many people who are rushed for time in the morning, it often consists of a granola bar, milk or juice, muffins, or fresh fruit. But there's no rule that says you have to restrict your breakfast to traditional choices. For example, a slice of leftover pizza and a glass of milk will provide your daughter with the calories and energy she needs to get through the morning. Another strategy is to take your daughter with you to the grocery store and encourage her to pick out foods that she would enjoy for breakfast. Above all, make sure that you are setting a good example for your daughter by eating breakfast yourself.

CHAPTER 3

# Essential

## *Foods and nutrients*

*What we eat provides us with the essential elements of life and health. It provides us with the raw materials that our bodies need to function and, particularly in the case of young children, to grow. In this chapter we look at the basic components of food and how each is important to your child's well being.*

### Food as fuel

For weight-conscious adults, calories (or kilocalories, to be technically accurate) are something to be controlled, mostly because we tend get more of them from our food than we require. This is generally not the case for young children, however. For children, calories are a measure of the energy their young bodies need to grow and develop normally.

Energy is required by the body for a variety of reasons. It is used for muscular work, to fuel the brain and nervous system, and to make and repair body tissues. The nutrients in food – specifically, carbohydrate, protein and fat – are metabolized by the body to release usable energy. We all need a constant supply of food to meet our body's energy needs for survival.

Compared to adults, children require more energy per unit of body weight. This is because energy is needed not only for basic body functions (as it is for adults), but for growth as well.

Factors that affect total energy needs include sex, age, overall body composition (relative proportions of fat and muscle in the body), nutritional status (for example, normal weight, underweight or overweight), levels of physical activity, hours of sleep, fever – even climate. All of these energy

### Measuring metabolism

How do we know how many calories a child requires daily? There are a variety of techniques for determining energy requirements, most of which involve measuring the process of metabolism itself. For example, we know that in order to metabolize a given quantity of energy, the body will take in a certain amount of oxygen and release a certain amount of carbon dioxide. By measuring the quantity of these gases inhale/exhaled over a specific time, and by performing these measurements on a number of subjects within a particular group (selected by age or sex, for example), the average energy requirements can be determined for that group.

needs must be met by the food we eat. If the supply of food energy matches the body's requirements, we achieve an energy balance. But if the food energy is greater than our needs, the excess is stored in the body as fat. This is why exercise is such an important factor in helping children to achieve an energy balance.

To calculate your child's energy requirements, use the table shown below. For example, an average 4-year-old child with a weight of 16.5 kg (36 lbs), requires about 16.5 kg X 100 kcal/kg, or 1600 calories to meet his or her daily energy needs. (Boys and girls have about the same energy needs per unit of body weight until they reach the age of 7 years.)

## How much energy does your child need?

**Daily energy requirements per unit of body weight**

| Age (years) | Energy (g/kg) | Energy (kcal/lb) |
|---|---|---|
| 0 to 2 | 101 | 46 |
| 2 to 3 | 94 | 43 |
| 4 to 6 | 100 | 45 |

## Powerful proteins

Proteins are part of the living tissue in the body. Built from long chains of amino acids, they serve as the building blocks from which components of cells are constructed, as well as for antibodies, enzymes and hormones.

Most protein is found in muscle tissue, with the remainder found in the soft tissues, bones, teeth, and blood. Certain components of protein can only be delivered to the body through the diet. The quality of the protein, then, is of great importance. Once proteins are broken down by the body's digestive system, they are absorbed as amino acids into the body and are used for many different body functions, including building and repair of tissues, fighting infections, providing a source of energy and transporting other substances.

During growth, protein needs per unit of body weight are high for infants and children. If protein intake is very low, fat and carbohydrate (assuming an adequate supply) can act to spare the need for protein as energy.

Generally, the typical diet of North American children provides about 3 to 4 times the amount of protein they actually require. Vegetarians are a possible exception, however, particularly in terms of the quality (if not quantity) of protein they consume to meet their needs. (See Chapter 5, page 57, for more information on vegetarian diets.)

To calculate your child's protein requirements, use the table shown below. For example, an average 4-year-old child with a weight of 16.5 kg (36 lbs), requires about 16.5 kg X 1.06 g/kg, or 17.5 grams of protein to meet his or her daily needs.

### Do athletic children need more protein?

Some people believe that athletic children need more protein than those who are less active. In fact, their protein needs are quite similar – although an athletic child's need for energy may be greater. More significant factors affecting protein needs include illness, fever, and chronic losses due to disease.

## How much protein does your child need?

**Daily protein requirements per unit of body weight**

| Age (years) | Protein (kcal/kg) | Protein (g/lb) |
|---|---|---|
| 0 to 2 | 1.21 | 0.55 |
| 2 to 3 | 1.16 | 0.53 |
| 4 to 6 | 1.06 | 0.48 |

## Essential fatty acids

The fats we get from our food include many compounds that are required for maintaining the structure and function of cells in the body. Fatty acids are the smallest part of fat. They are a vital source of energy and provide most of the calories from dietary fat.

Depending on their chemical structure, fatty acids are generally classified as either saturated or unsaturated. Most saturated fats come from animal products and are solid when they are at room temperature. Polyunsaturated fats are liquid at room temperature, and are derived from vegetable sources, as well as from fish.

Linolenic acid (or omega-3) and linoleic acid (or omega-6) are "essential" fatty acids, which means that they cannot be synthesized by the body and have to be provided in the diet. Both are unsaturated fatty acids.

Omega-3 fatty acid is relatively well known by most health-conscious adults, since it has the effect of lowering levels of blood cholesterol. But what about children? Can they benefit from more omega-3 or omega-6 fatty acids in their diet?

The fact is that cholesterol is generally not a concern for kids. Fat is an important source of energy for growing children, and should provide a minimum of 30 to 35% of their total calories. (See Chapter 11, page 100, for more information on fat requirements.) A diet that includes fish (such as salmon and tuna) and vegetable oils (such as soy and canola), as well as leafy vegetables, will meet all their requirements for omega-3 fatty acid. And while they may not need the cholesterol-lowering effects of omega-3 now, children may benefit later in life if they get in the habit of eating these omega-3-rich foods and following a healthier diet.

## Increasing dietary fiber

Dietary fiber is a component of plant-based food that is not completely broken down in the digestive tract. This happens because we do not have all of the enzymes necessary to digest fiber (as we do for other parts of the foods we eat, such as protein, fat and other carbohydrates). Fiber is contained in many foods, and includes compounds such as cellulose, pectin, lignins and other undigestible carbohydrates.

Dietary fiber is categorized as either soluble or insoluble.

SOLUBLE FIBER is found in fruits, some legumes, and grains such as oats, rye and barley. This type of fiber dissolves in water to form a gel. This gel helps to slow the rate at which food passes through the digestive system and helps to increase the absorption of certain nutrients in the foods we eat. Soluble fiber is also known to help lower blood cholesterol levels.

INSOLUBLE FIBER is found in vegetables and wheat bran. This type of fiber absorbs water and helps to increase the volume of stool. It also helps to increase the movement of material through the colon and makes stool easier to pass.

## Why kids need fiber

Most adults understand the need for fiber in their own diets, but dietary fiber has important health benefits for kids as well. A fiber-rich diet can help prevent constipation, which can be a problem in children. Studies have shown that children who consume sufficient quantities of fiber also have better intakes of vitamins and minerals, including vitamins A and E, folate, iron and magnesium. On the other hand, where their diet is low in fiber, children have been shown to have higher intakes of dietary fat and cholesterol. A low-fiber diet may also increase a child's risk of developing in later life chronic conditions such as obesity, hyperlipidemia (a risk factor for cardiovascular disease), and adult onset (type II) diabetes.

Yet the fact is that a great many North American children – about 50%, according to some studies – are not getting enough dietary fiber.

So how much fiber should your child be eating?

The American Health Foundation (AHF) suggests using the following formula to determine the minimal intake of dietary fiber for children between 3 and 20 years of age:

Age in years + 5 = required grams of fiber per day

In other words, a 3-year-old child should consume at least 8 grams of fiber per day, a 6 year old 11 grams of fiber per day, and so on. This rule of thumb is supported by pediatricians and other health care providers. It is also consistent with adult recommendations of 25 to 35 grams of fiber per day set by the AHF, the American Cancer Society, the National Cancer Institute, and others.

For children under the age of 3 years, the American and Canadian Pediatric Societies (as well as other authorities) suggest that as solid and table foods are started, parents should introduce foods such as whole grain cereals, breads, vegetables and fruits. They also point out, however, that a high-fiber diet should not exclude energy-dense foods (such as cheese or milk, which are low in fiber) or exclude any one particular food group.

### *Are there disadvantages to a high-fiber diet?*

High fiber intakes may decrease the amount of certain minerals available for absorption. This is because high-fiber foods often contain phytates – compounds that can bind with minerals such as iron or calcium and make them less available to the body. That being said, however, the risks of vitamin/mineral deficiency are vastly outweighed by the potential health benefits of eating a diet high in fiber. In fact, adults who live a vegetarian lifestyle (and who consume a diet very high in fiber) typically don't suffer from vitamin or mineral deficiencies.

### No quick fiber fix

A number of commercial products claim to provide a quick and easy way to add more fiber to your diet. But these supplements – whether pills or powders – are no substitute for the fiber contained in foods. This is particularly true for children.

## How to increase the fiber in your child's diet

In many cases, if your child isn't getting enough fiber, then neither is the rest of the family. So start taking steps to increase everyone's fiber consumption by serving more fiber-rich fruits and vegetables, as well as legumes, cereals and other grains.

As always, of course, be sure that you keep your diet in balance. Consult the USDA's Food Pyramid or Canada's Food Guide for Healthy Eating for suggestions about choosing the foods that will provide enough fiber to meet the "age + 5" recommendation without sacrificing calories or other nutrients. (See pages 42 and 43.) Remember that although milk, milk products and meats are low in dietary fiber, they remain an important source of other nutrients, including energy, protein, calcium, vitamin D, iron and zinc.

Start by adding one or more servings of fiber-rich foods per day. The key here is to increase the amount of fiber gradually. Keep in mind that while fresh fruits and vegetables are great sources of fiber, fruit and vegetable juices are not. Try switching from white breads and processed cereals to whole grains, breads and cereals. Legumes (such as dried peas and beans) are also a great source of fiber. See if you can include them in your family's diet at least once a week.

Finally, in order to avoid gas, bloating or the other complaints occasionally associated with high-fiber diets, be sure that your child consumes more water (or other fluids) as the amount of fiber in his or her diet increases.

### FIBER-FULL EATING

**Meeting a 6-year-old's fiber needs***

| | SERVING SIZE | FIBER (G) |
|---|---|---|
| Bran cereal with raisins | 3/4 cup (175 mL) | 5.0 |
| Carrot, raw | 1 medium | 2.3 |
| Peanut butter | 1 tbsp (15 mL) | 1.0 |
| Apple | 1 medium | 3.0 |
| Total | | 11.3 |

* Using the "age + 5" rule, a 6-year-old should consume 11 grams fiber/day

SOURCE: *Pediatrics*, 1995; 96:1023-1028

## Using the food guides

In both the US and Canada, health authorities have devised charts that recommend a range of servings from each of the four food groups. Whether it's The Food Pyramid (in the US) or Canada's Food Guide to Healthy Eating, the message is very much the same: Enjoy a variety of healthy foods every day, and keep high-sugar and other non-nutritious foods to a minimum.

The four food groups are described briefly below, followed by the charts themselves.

BREADS AND CEREALS are an essential source of carbohydrates, vitamins and minerals, and provide fiber as well.

FRUITS AND VEGETABLES provide another variety of carbohydrates, vitamins (particularly vitamin C) and minerals, as well as fiber.

MEAT AND ALTERNATIVES are an important source of proteins, fats, vitamins and minerals (particularly iron).

MILK AND DAIRY PRODUCTS provide a balance of proteins, carbohydrates and fats, and are an important source of calcium and vitamin D.

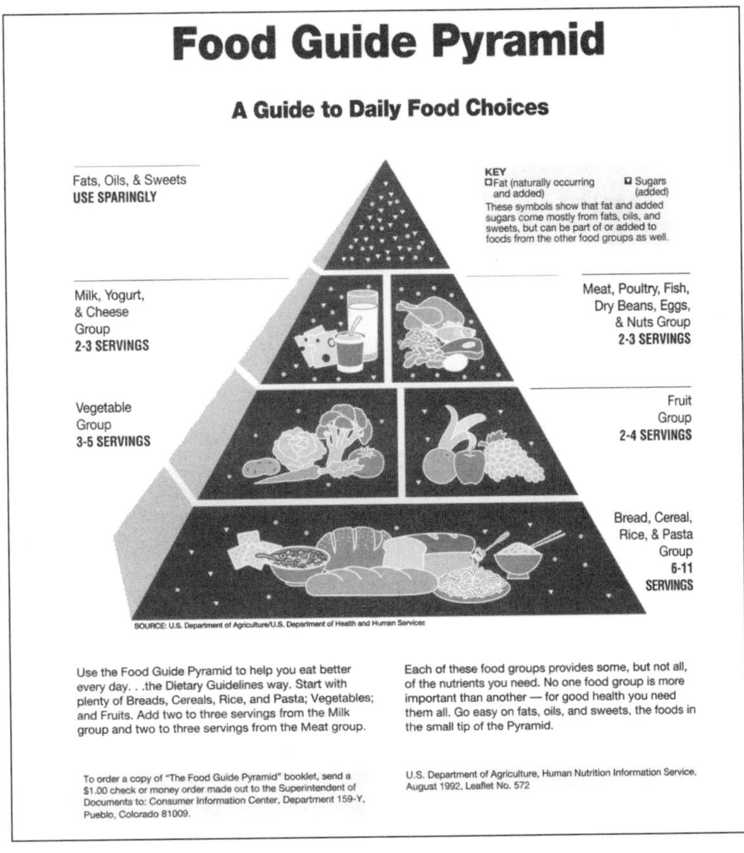

Health Canada Santé Canada

CANADA'S
Food Guide
TO HEALTHY EATING
FOR PEOPLE FOUR YEARS AND OVER
Enjoy a variety of foods from each group every day.
Choose lower-fat foods more often.
YOGOURT 2.2%
0.1%
SKIM MILK CHEESE
EVAP MILK
POWDER
2%
SKIM
TOFU

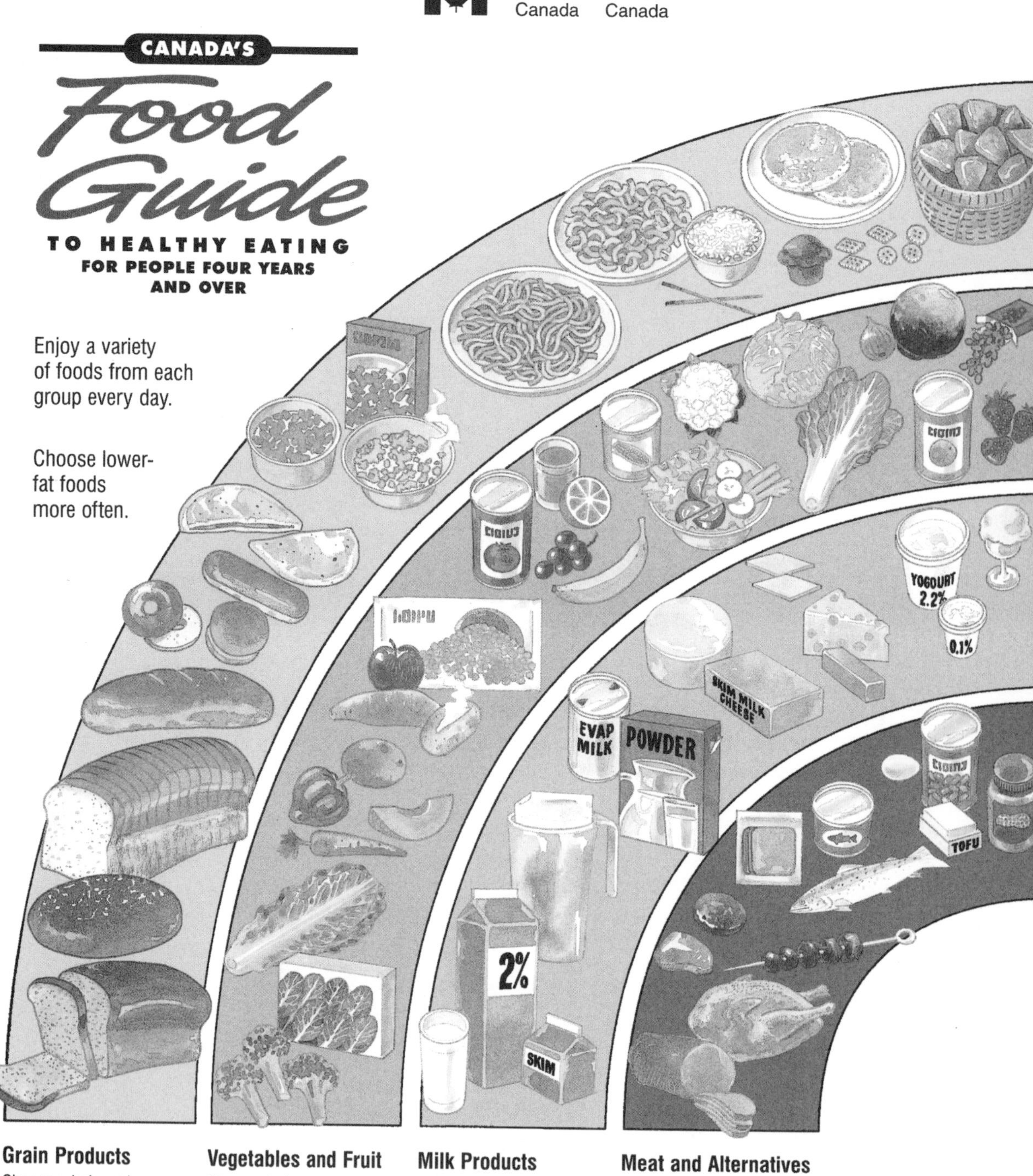

**Grain Products**
Choose whole grain and enriched products more often.

**Vegetables and Fruit**
Choose dark green and orange vegetables and orange fruit more often.

**Milk Products**
Choose lower-fat milk products more often.

**Meat and Alternatives**
Choose leaner meats, poultry and fish, as well as dried peas, beans and lentils more often.

Canada

**Grain Products**
**5 – 12**
**SERVINGS PER DAY**

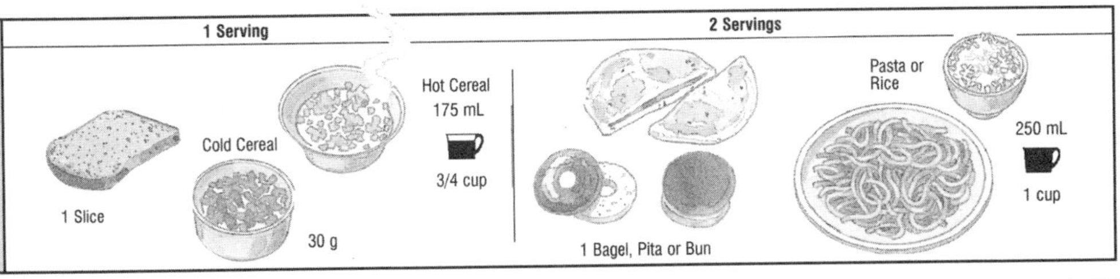

**1 Serving**

1 Slice

Cold Cereal 30 g

Hot Cereal 175 mL 3/4 cup

**2 Servings**

1 Bagel, Pita or Bun

Pasta or Rice 250 mL 1 cup

**Vegetables and Fruit**
**5 – 10**
**SERVINGS PER DAY**

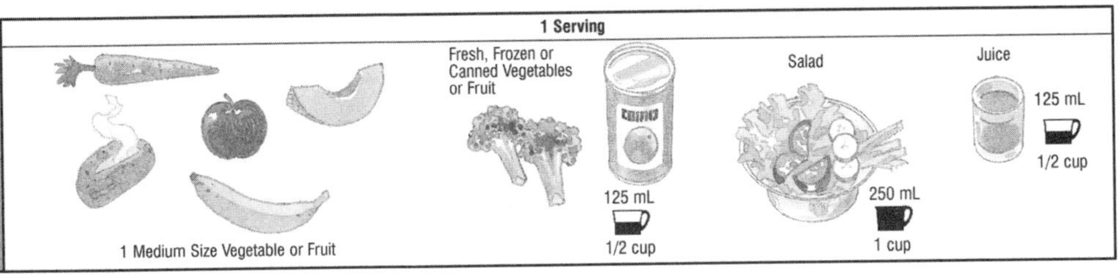

**1 Serving**

1 Medium Size Vegetable or Fruit

Fresh, Frozen or Canned Vegetables or Fruit 125 mL 1/2 cup

Salad 250 mL 1 cup

Juice 125 mL 1/2 cup

**Milk Products**
**SERVINGS PER DAY**
**Children 4–9 years: 2–3**
**Youth 10–16 years: 3–4**
**Adults: 2–4**
**Pregnant and Breast-feeding Women 3–4**

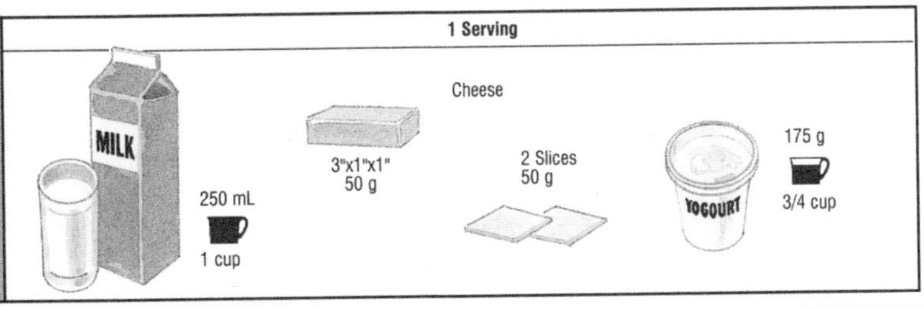

**1 Serving**

MILK 250 mL 1 cup

Cheese 3"x1"x1" 50 g

2 Slices 50 g

YOGOURT 175 g 3/4 cup

**Meat and Alternatives**
**2 – 3**
**SERVINGS PER DAY**

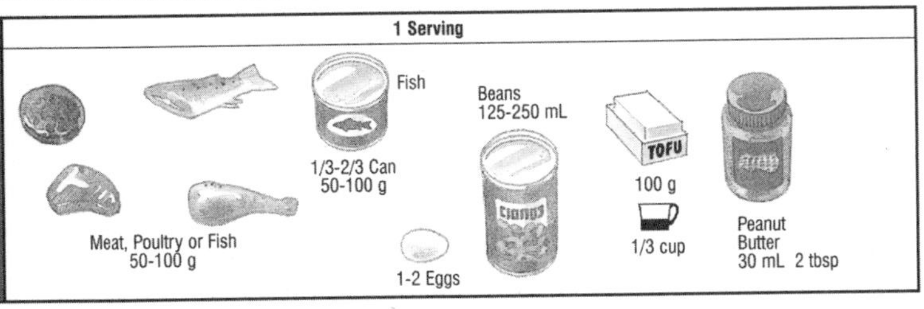

**1 Serving**

Meat, Poultry or Fish 50-100 g

Fish 1/3-2/3 Can 50-100 g

1-2 Eggs

Beans 125-250 mL

TOFU 100 g 1/3 cup

Peanut Butter 30 mL 2 tbsp

## Other Foods

Taste and enjoyment can also come from other foods and beverages that are not part of the 4 food groups. Some of these foods are higher in fat or Calories, so use these foods in moderation.

## Different People Need Different Amounts of Food

The amount of food you need every day from the 4 food groups and other foods depends on your age, body size, activity level, whether you are male or female and if you are pregnant or breast-feeding. That's why the Food Guide gives a lower and higher number of servings for each food group. For example, young children can choose the lower number of servings, while male teenagers can go to the higher number. Most other people can choose servings somewhere in between.

Consult *Canada's Physical Activity Guide to Healthy Active Living* to help you build physical activity into your daily life.

*Enjoy eating well, being active and feeling good about yourself. That's* VITALITÉ®


Cat. No. H39-252/1992E ISBN 0-662-19648-1

## Understanding food labels

When you buy commercially prepared food, how do you find out what's in it? Chances are you'll look at the nutritional information printed on the label or package. This information is something that most of us take for granted today, although it wasn't many years ago that food manufacturers were only required to list ingredients. Now we're provided with data such as the number of calories per serving, as well as the amount of carbohydrates, protein, and fat

Historically, nutrition labeling in the US has been more comprehensive than in Canada, providing a standard format of presentation for nutrients per unit of serving size, as well as a "calculated daily value" which indicates what percentage of the recommended daily amount of a given nutrient (iron, for example) is contained per serving. (Note that the percent daily value is based on *adult* requirements, not on children's needs.)

In 2001, however, Health Canada, along with the Canadian Food Inspection Agency, proposed a new system of labeling that is similar in many respects to that used in the US. The labels provide nutrient information in a standardized format, and will allow certain health-related claims where warranted (and backed by research). For example, a product containing a good source of calcium (along with vitamin D) may be allowed to display the health claim that calcium is good for bones and may help prevent osteoporosis. Other approved nutrition claims include "a low-sodium diet reduces the risk of high blood pressure"; "a diet that includes plenty of fruits and vegetables reduces the risk of some types of cancer"; and "diets low in saturated and trans fats reduce the risk of heart disease." Manufacturers of food products will not be able to make claims about their products unless they are proven to be true.

The proposed new regulations, are designed to ensure that a standard nutrition label appears on all suitable food products, with a few exceptions (such as fresh fruits and vegetables, poultry or fish).

### Look for the CDV

For the recipes in this book, we have provided the "% children's daily value" (%CDV) for calcium and iron per serving. This is based on a child's daily needs, using as a reference a 6-year-old child.

### Orders of magnitude

When reading the list of ingredients in a product, remember that they are listed in decreasing order of quantity used in the product. This is a good way to judge which cereals, for example, have a higher proportion of sugar relative to other (more healthful) ingredients.

CHAPTER 4

# Important

## *Vitamins and minerals*

*In terms of quantity consumed, vitamins and minerals represent only a tiny fraction of what we eat. Yet they are absolutely essential to our health. In this chapter we take an in-depth look at the most critical of these substances – calcium, iron, vitamin C, and zinc – and how they relate to children's nutrition. A survey of other vitamins and minerals is supplied in a convenient chart on page 56.*

### Calcium for bones and teeth

While calcium is an essential mineral for people of all ages, it is especially crucial for growing children. Between the ages of 2 and 6 years, a child's bones and teeth grow rapidly, and their normal development is ultimately dependent on an adequate supply of dietary calcium. (In fact, it is in the bones and teeth that about 99% of the body's calcium is located.)

The essential role of calcium in a young child's diet has been stated by the American Academy of Pediatrics, as follows: "Of most importance in this age group is the development of eating patterns that will be associated with adequate calcium intake later in life." A high calcium intake during childhood may not prevent osteoporosis in later years – at least, if not sustained during adolescence. However, it will reinforce the importance of eating a balanced diet, including foods rich in calcium, to help maintain bone development and strength throughout adulthood.

### How much calcium is enough?

The Dietary Reference Intake (DRI) for calcium is 500 mg/day for children from 1 to 3 years and 800 mg/day for children from 4 to 8 years. This is the equivalent of 2 to 3 servings of

### Why you need vitamin D

While calcium is essential for the normal development of bones and teeth, it cannot be used properly without vitamin D. Sources of this vitamin include milk (for preschoolers, 2 cups [500 mL] provides a sufficient amount), as well as exposure to sunshine. Vitamin D works by helping to increase the deposit of calcium and phosphorous in teeth and bones. (Phosphorous is another mineral that works with calcium, and is found in meat, poultry, milk and milk products, fish, and eggs.)

milk or milk products daily. (Note that the DRI is a relatively new standard that replaces the RDA and RNI measures formerly used, respectively, in the US and Canada.)

In the nutrient analyses that accompany the recipes in this book, you will notice that we provide a "percent children's daily value" (% CDV) for calcium. This figure uses the DRI of 800 mg/day (the amount of calcium required for a 4- to 8-year-old) as a reference. So if the CDV for a recipe is 20%, it means that a serving provides 20% (or 160 mg) of the calcium needed by a child.

## Finding calcium you can use

As shown in the table on page 47, the best dietary sources of calcium include milk and milk products, salmon and sardines, bok choy, almonds and molasses. Moderate sources (not listed in the table) include broccoli, oranges, beans and legumes. A food's calcium content is only part of the story, however; the critical factor is how much of that calcium your body is able to absorb.

Certain factors can increase or decrease the absorption of calcium:

- Lactose. A sugar found in milk, lactose enhances the absorption of calcium.
- Fiber. The fiber content of foods may decrease calcium absorption. Fiber increases the bulk of food in the intestines, which speeds its travel through the digestive tract, and reduces the time during which calcium can be absorbed. As noted in the previous chapter, however, fiber is not something that should be cut from a child's diet. It is better to compensate for fiber's effects by increasing the amount of dietary calcium.
- Phytates and Oxalates. **Phytates** are minerals found in some plant foods, and **oxalates** are found in vegetables and some berries. Both compounds can reduce calcium absorption.

## BONE-FRIENDLY FOODS

**Foods that provide at least 300 mg calcium per serving**

| **MILK AND MILK PRODUCTS** | **SERVING SIZE** |
|---|---|
| Milk: skim, 1%, 2%, whole, lactose-reduced, buttermilk, chocolate | 1 cup (250 mL) |
| Milk, evaporated | 1/2 cup (125 mL) |
| Milk, powdered | 6 tbsp (90 mL) |
| Ice milk | 1 cup (250 mL) |
| Yogurt, plain or flavored | 3/4 cup (175 mL) |
| Yogurt, frozen | 1 cup (250 mL) |
| Cheese, firm (e.g. brick, Cheddar, Colby, etc.) | 1.5 oz (45g) |
| Grated Parmesan cheese | 4 tbsp (60 mL) |
| Ricotta cheese, regular/light varieties | 1/2 cup (125 mL) |
| Puddings made with milk (e.g. rice, instant, baked custard) | 1 cup (250 mL) |
| **NON-DAIRY BEVERAGES** | **SERVING SIZE** |
| Soy beverage, calcium-fortified | 1 cup (250 mL ) |
| Rice beverage, calcium-fortified | 1 cup (250 mL) |
| Orange juice, calcium-fortified | 1 cup (250 mL) |
| **CANNED FISH** | **SERVING SIZE** |
| Salmon (with bones) | Half 7.5 oz (213 g) can |
| Sardines (with bones) | 7 medium |
| **SOY-BASED FOODS** | **SERVING SIZE** |
| Tofu, firm or extra firm, set in calcium* | 1/2 cup (125 mL) |
| Tofu, silken or regular, set in calcium | 1 cup (250 mL) |
| Soybeans, cooked | 2 cups (500 mL) |
| Soybeans, roasted | 1 cup (250 mL) |
| * Where calcium is the ingredient listed immediately after "soy milk" or "soybeans and water" | |
| **VEGETABLES** | **SERVING SIZE** |
| Bok choy, pak-choi, cooked | 1 cup (250 mL) |
| Turnip greens, cooked | 1 cup (250 mL) |
| Kale, mustard greens, turnip greens, cooked | 1 1/2 cups (375 mL) |
| Seaweed, dry (hijiki, arame, wakame) | 1 oz (25 g) |
| **OTHER** | **SERVING SIZE** |
| Almonds | 3/4 cup (175 mL) |
| Blackstrap molasses | 2 tbsp (25 mL) |

SOURCES: *Sunnybrook & Women's College Health Science Centre Multidisciplinary Osteoporosis Program / Bowes & Church's* Food Values of Portions Commonly Consumed, 6th Edition, *1994 /* Bone Vivant! *Jan Main, 1997 / Osteoporosis Society of Canada:* Building Better Bones: A Guide to Active Living.

- **Protein.** A high-protein diet can increase urinary losses of calcium. However, foods that are high in protein also contain phosphorous which can offset the calcium loss.

### Non-dairy sources of calcium

If your child is unable to drink milk – because of allergy or lactose intolerance, for example – it will be necessary to find alternate sources of calcium. These may include some of the high-calcium foods of non-dairy origin, such as fortified soy or rice drinks, which are listed in the table on page 47.

When substituting cow's milk with an alternate product for a child, however, parents must exercise caution in choosing the appropriate beverage. Many soy or rice drinks, even when fortified with added calcium, do not contain adequate amounts of other nutrients, such as protein or vitamin D, or they may not provide sufficient calories. Since children typically derive a lot of their nourishment from milk, such deficiencies can have a serious effect on nutrition. So if you are unsure about the ingredients and nutritional composition of a milk substitute, check with a dietitian or family doctor before giving it to your child.

If non-dairy food sources are inadequate for your child's calcium needs, you may be advised to provide a calcium supplement. These are available in many different forms, and your doctor will choose the one that is best for your child. Calcium carbonate, for example, is one of the most widely used supplements (it is also used in antacid tablets), with an absorption rate of 39%. Other alternatives, with their respective absorption rates, are shown on page 49.

#### How kids absorb calcium

When children eat foods that contain calcium, about 75% of the mineral is actually absorbed. (Adults do not absorb calcium as well.) This figure varies with the amount of calcium being consumed at any given time. If the amount is relatively high, less is absorbed; where smaller amounts are consumed, then more is absorbed. This regulating mechanism helps to maintain an adequate calcium supply.

### Calcium-added O.J.

As awareness of its nutritional importance has grown, calcium is now being added to an increasing number of products. Of these, calcium-fortified orange juice is one of the most popular, and you may be wondering whether it is worth buying for your child. First, keep in mind that it is not a substitute for milk, which contains vitamin D and other important nutrients not found in fortified orange juice. However, between 30 and 35% of the calcium added to this type of juice can be absorbed (which is similar to cow's milk), so it is a good choice if calcium intake needs to be increased.

| Calcium compound | Absorption |
|---|---|
| Carbonate | 39% |
| Acetate | 32% |
| Lactate | 32% |
| Gluconate | 27% |
| Citrate | 30% |

## Preventing iron deficiency

Iron is essential for the normal growth and development of a child. Yet in North America this nutrient is often deficient in a child's diet – thereby increasing the risk of iron-deficiency anemia.

Iron is found in hemoglobin, a component of the blood which carries oxygen to different parts of the body. Since this oxygen is used to form energy, children with iron-deficiency anemia may appear to be pale, more tired, and have a decreased tolerance for exercise. Iron deficiency can also affect a child's behavior, appetite and ability to learn. In fact, according to one well-publicized study, iron deficiency in infants affected their learning ability well into childhood.

How serious is this problem? Serious enough: It is estimated that 9% of young children (1 to 2 years) are deficient in iron (although not anemic), while about 3% actually have iron-deficiency anemia (where the hemoglobin levels in the blood fall below the normal range).

One reason for the disturbingly high incidence of iron deficiency may be that the diet of young preschoolers is unbalanced, with an excessive intake of juice or milk, which can displace the intake of other foods that contain iron. Not surprisingly, the American Pediatric Society suggests limiting juice to a maximum of 6 oz (175 mL) per day in order to encourage children to eat a greater variety of foods.

## Iron intakes

**Which food sources contain the most iron**

| Food | Serving size | Iron (mg) |
|---|---|---|
| Cream of wheat, iron-enriched, cooked | 3/4 cup (175 mL) | 11.3 |
| Infant cereal | 8 tbsp (120 mL) | 8.0 |
| Infant formula, fortified with iron | 8 oz (250 mL) | 5.0 |
| Spinach, cooked | 1/2 cup (125 mL) | 3.2 |
| Liver, beef, pan-fried | 1.75 oz. (45 g) | 3.0 |
| Potato, baked, skin on | 6.5 oz (190 g) | 2.6 |
| Beef, lean, broiled | 3.5 oz (100 g) | 2.8 |
| Raisins | 2/3 cup (150 mL) | 2.2 |
| Beans, navy, canned | 1/2 cup (125 mL) | 2.4 |
| Avocado | 1 medium | 2.0 |
| Prune juice | 1/2 cup (125 mL) | 1.5 |
| Chicken, light/dark, no skin | 3.5 oz (100 g) | 1.2 |
| Strained infant meat | 4 tbsp (60 mL) | 0.9 |
| Halibut | 3 oz (75 g) | 0.8 |
| Whole wheat bread | 1 slice | 0.8 |
| White bread | 1 slice | 0.7 |
| Broccoli, cooked | 1/2 cup (125 mL) | 0.7 |
| Apricots, raw | 3 medium | 0.6 |
| Rice, wild, cooked | 1/2 cup (125 mL) | 0.5 |

SOURCE: *Food Smart Professional Edition 2.0, Sasquatch Corp. © 1994-1996*

### How much iron does your child need?

The Dietary Reference Intake (DRI) for iron is 7 mg/day for children from 1 to 3 years and 10 mg/day for children from 4 to 8 years. In the nutrient analyses that accompany the recipes in this book, you will notice that we provide a "percent children's daily value" (% CDV) for iron. This figure uses the DRI of 10 mg/day (the amount recommended for a 4- to 8-year-old) as a reference. So if the % CDV for a recipe is 20%, it means that a serving provides 20% (or 2 mg) of the iron needed by a child.

### How much iron are you getting?

If you study the table on page 50, it seems quite clear that some foods contain more iron than others. But the amount of iron in a food is often less important than the *type* iron.

There are two types of dietary iron: HEME iron, which is most easily absorbed by the body; and NON-HEME iron, which is less easily absorbed.

Heme iron is found in meat, fish and poultry. Especially high in this type of iron are organ meats, such as liver, as well as red meat. Non-heme iron is found in plant foods such as nuts, vegetables and grains, in dairy products such as milk and cheese, and in eggs.

> **Iron regulation**
>
> As with calcium, the body adjusts its absorption rate for iron according to how much the body needs. So if your child's iron supply is low, the rate of iron absorption increases.

Because non-heme iron is not as well absorbed as heme iron, it is important to know which type is contained in your child's diet. For example, a vegetarian child's diet contains only non-heme iron, so he or she will need more of it (provided by foods such as tofu) to get the amount of iron required. (Other sources include iron-fortified foods such as textured proteins, vegetarian "meat" slices and patties.) To enhance the absorption of non-heme iron, it is also a good idea to accompany meals with a small amount of orange juice or with a serving of fruit high in vitamin C (which helps iron absorption). Eating sources of heme iron, such as red meat, also increase the absorption of non-heme iron.

### Treating iron-deficiency anemia

If your child is diagnosed with iron-deficiency anemia, your pediatrician or family doctor will prescribe an iron supplement. These supplements may darken the color of a child's stool.

Of course, it's much better to avoid this condition in the first place. So encourage your child to eat iron-rich foods – and limit excess milk and juice intake – to maintain iron stores at healthy levels.

## Vitamin C

Since fruit juices are a popular addition to many children's diets today, it makes sense to look at the role of vitamin C. Many parents consider fruit juice to be important for their children precisely because it contains this nutrient – and children need lots of vitamin C, right? But how much vitamin C do children actually need, and how much vitamin C is too much? What does vitamin C actually do for us?

### *Vitamin C in history*

Descriptions of scurvy – a severe form of vitamin C deficiency that results in dry, cracked skin, aching bones and joints, and bleeding gums – were recorded as early as 1500 BC. Throughout history, it caused many deaths among soldiers and sailors (whose rations consisted largely of preserved meats and bread), often proving more lethal than swords and guns. It was not until the 1600s that the link between scurvy and diet was recognized. Today, with the widespread availability of fruit and vegetables, scurvy is extremely rare.

### How vitamin C works

Humans need to obtain vitamin C from the foods they eat. This distinguishes us from most other mammals, which are able to manufacture their own vitamin C from sugar (glucose) in their diet. Vitamin C has many functions in the body, including:

Dietary antioxidant. Vitamin C helps to reduce the damage done to the body's cells by "oxidizing free radicals." As a dietary antioxidant, it converts these free radicals into harmless substances that the body can eliminate. It has been suggested that vitamin C (and other antioxidants) can help prevent cancer or cardiovascular disease, but this has yet to be confirmed definitively by research.

Collagen formation. Vitamin C plays an important role in the formation of collagen – a type of protein found in connective tissue, bones, teeth, and skin. This why a vitamin C deficiency can result in conditions such as scurvy (see sidebar) or wounds not healing properly, or bones becoming weakened and eventually distorted.

Improves absorption of other nutrients. Vitamin C helps the body absorb non-heme iron (the iron found in plants). It also helps the body absorb calcium. Vitamin C also helps convert folic acid into its active form, so that it can do its job in the body.

## Where to get your vitamin C

*per 1/2-cup (125 mL) serving unless otherwise indicated*

| Food | Vitamin C (mg) |
|---|---|
| Orange juice, fresh | 62 |
| Broccoli, cooked | 58 |
| Cantaloupe | 34 |
| Cauliflower, cooked | 34 |
| Orange, half | 34 |
| Honeydew melon | 21 |
| Spinach, cooked | 9 |
| Frozen peas, cooked | 8 |
| Prune juice | 5* |
| Apple, half | 4 |
| Carrots, cooked | 3 |
| Apple juice | 1* |
| Grape juice | 0.12* |

* 18 to 50 mg per 1/2 cup (125 mL) if fortified

SOURCE: *Food Smart Professional Edition 2.0, Sasquatch Corp. © 1994-1996*

### Does vitamin C cure the common cold?

In 1970 the Nobel-prize winning scientist Linus Pauling stirred up considerable debate with his book *Vitamin C and the Common Cold*, in which he suggested that vitamin C could offer protection against the common cold and relief from its symptoms. Since then, much research has been done on whether or not this theory holds true. Most of the current literature does not support the idea that vitamin C reduces the incidence of colds, although it may help people to recover faster and suffer less severe symptoms.

### How much vitamin C does your child need?

The Dietary Reference Intake (DRI) for vitamin C is 15 mg/day for children from 1 to 3 years and 25 mg/day for children from 4 to 8 years. While this may seem like very little – particularly to adults who are accustomed to taking megadoses of this vitamin (see "Can you have too much vitamin C?" on page 54) – it is all that's required to prevent vitamin C deficiency.

Children can get all the vitamin C they need from plant foods, especially citrus fruits and their juices, broccoli, spinach and melon. The vitamin C content of food can be enhanced by eating fruits when they are ripe, by refrigerating fruits and vegetables, and by not overcooking foods.

#### Can you have too much vitamin C?

The maximum amount of vitamin C recommended for 1- to 3-year-olds is 400 mg/day and 650 mg/day for children 4 to 8 years old. Beyond these levels, studies suggest there is the potential for negative effects from excess vitamin C. It is estimated that between 20 and 25% of the US population takes vitamin C supplements, in doses that range from 100 mg to 10 g (or 10,000 mg!) daily. Regardless of whether you think such large doses contribute to adult health, it is generally unwise to give supplements of vitamin C (or any other vitamin) to children. Most children do not need any more vitamin C than they get from eating half a fresh orange every day.

## Zinc

Because of its role in growth and development, zinc is a particularly important mineral for children. The good news is that the body requires very small amounts of zinc. And since zinc is found in a wide variety of food sources, cases of severe zinc deficiency are extremely rare in North America.

Zinc is involved with the function of every cell in the body, particularly in cell division and multiplication (hence its importance for growing children). It also plays a role in our ability to fight infection, which is especially important for the sick or elderly. It helps to maintain a healthy appetite, and is involved with the sense of taste. Zinc is also required for adequate night vision.

#### How much zinc does your child need?

The Dietary Reference Intake (DRI) for zinc is 3 mg/day for children from 1 to 3 years and 5 mg/day for children from 4 to 8 years. The body is very good at controlling its own zinc level – adjusting its absorption rate according to the amount of zinc present in the diet. This being said, when a child's diet is too low in zinc, there may still be some risk of deficiency.

While severe clinical zinc deficiency is rare in North American children, studies have shown that the zinc intakes among these children often fall below recommended levels, and that they may be at risk for mild zinc deficiency. This can affect growth, immune function, as well cognitive development.

The best food sources for zinc include beef, chicken, milk and eggs. (The protein in these foods helps to improve zinc absorption.) Moderate amounts of zinc are also contained in some vegetables and cereals, although these foods contain high amounts of fiber and phytates, which inhibit zinc absorption.

## WHERE TO FIND ZINC

| Food | Serving size | Zinc (mg) |
|---|---|---|
| Oysters | 1 medium | 12.7 |
| Lean ground beef, cooked | 3 1/2 oz (100 g) | 6.3 |
| Chicken breast, cooked | 3 1/2 oz (100 g) | 1.0 |
| 2% milk | 1 cup (250 mL) | 0.9 |
| Oatmeal, cooked | 1/2 cup (125 mL) | 0.6 |
| Egg, boiled | 1 large | 0.6 |
| Halibut, cooked | 3 oz (90 g) | 0.5 |
| Whole wheat bread | 1 slice | 0.4 |
| Broccoli, cooked | 1/2 cup (125 mL) | 0.3 |
| Apple | 1 medium | 0.06 |

SOURCE: *Food Smart Professional Edition 2.0, Sasquatch Corp. © 1994-1996*

## VITAMINS AND MINERALS • *What they do, where to find them*

| Vitamin/mineral | Type | Assists in | Sources |
|---|---|---|---|
| Vitamin A (from beta-carotene) | Fat-soluble | Vision, growth, bone development, healthy skin, may reduce risk | Liver, eggs, whole milk, dark green leafy vegetables, yellow and orange vegetables and fruit |
| Vitamin B1 (thiamin) | Water-soluble | Enzyme activity, metabolism of nutrients | Oatmeal, enriched breads and grains, rice, dairy products, fish, pork, liver, nuts, legumes |
| Vitamin B2 (riboflavin) | Water-soluble | Growth, metabolism of nutrients | Dairy products, eggs, organ meats, enriched breads and grains, green leafy vegetables |
| Vitamin B3 (niacin) | Water-soluble | Tissue repair, metabolism of nutrients | Organ meats, peanuts, brewer's yeast, enriched breads and grains, meats, poultry, fish and nuts |
| Vitamin B6 (pyridoxine) | Water-soluble | Metabolism of nutrients (primary role) | Brewer's yeast, wheat, germ, pork, liver, whole grain cereals, potatoes, milk, fruits and vegetables |
| Folic Acid (part of B vitamin group) | Water-soluble | Growth, enzyme activity, prevents neural tube defects | Liver, lima and kidney beans, dark leafy vegetables, beef, potatoes, whole wheat bread |
| Vitamin B12 | Water-soluble | Metabolism of nutrients, prevents anemia | Liver, kidneys, meat, fish, dairy products, eggs |
| Biotin (part of B vitamin group) | Water-soluble | Enzyme activity; deficiency can lead to a type of dermatitis | Liver, milk, meat, egg yolk, vegetables, fruit, peanuts, brewer's yeast |
| Vitamin C | Water-soluble | Many cellular functions, promotes healthy teeth, skin and tissue repair | Citrus fruits such as oranges and grapefruits leafy vegetables, tomatoes, strawberries |
| Vitamin D | Fat-soluble | Essential for normal growth, development, bones and teeth | Liver, butter, fortified milk, fatty fish (fish liver oils), exposure to sunlight |
| Vitamin E | Fat-soluble | Antioxidant function protects cells; assists neurological function, prevents anemia | Vegetable and fish oils, nuts, seeds, egg yolk, whole grains |
| Vitamin K | Fat-soluble | Blood clotting | Green leafy vegetables, liver, wheat bran, tomatoes, cheese, egg yolk |
| Zinc | Mineral | Growth and development, immune system | Meat, poultry, eggs, dairy products |

SOURCES: *Advanced Nutrition and Human Metabolism.* J. L. Groff, S. S. Gropper, and S. M. Hunt, ed. St Paul: West Publishing Co. 1995. *Food, Nutrition and Diet Theory, 6 ed.* M. V. Krause and L. K. Mahan. Philadelphia: W. B. Saunders 1979

CHAPTER 5

# Vegetarian Diets

*Increasingly today, many people are adopting a vegetarian lifestyle. Such dietary decisions are typically made by adults, but often affect children within the same family. And since children have special nutritional needs, it is important to make sure that they follow a well-balanced vegetarian diet.*

## What is a vegetarian?

Vegetarians are generally defined as people who consume mainly plant foods, including vegetables, fruits, legumes, grains, seeds and nuts. However, there are actually many types of vegetarians in North America, and their diets can differ greatly.

SEMI- OR PARTIAL VEGETARIANS generally avoid red meat, but may continue to eat some poultry and fish while primarily consuming vegetarian fare.

PESCO-VEGETARIANS avoid red meat and poultry but continue to consume fish and/or seafood.

LACTO-OVO VEGETARIANS avoid all animal flesh, including meat, poultry and fish. However, they still include dairy (lacto) and egg (ovo) products as part of their diet. It has been estimated that 90 to 95% of all vegetarians in North America consume dairy and/or eggs.

VEGANS avoid all foods of animal origin, including meat, poultry, fish, eggs, dairy, gelatin and honey. Many vegans also extend this prohibition beyond what they eat, eliminating from their lifestyles other animal-based products such as leather, wool and tallow candles.

MACROBIOTIC VEGETARIANS often follow highly restrictive diets that can involve the elimination of entire food groups. These types of diets are not recommended for children.

It is important to remember that even within these subgroups of vegetarianism, there can be many variations in diet.

## Vegetarianism and health

What's behind the growing popularity of vegetarianism? While a number of people become vegetarians for reasons of principle (ethical, environmental, economic or religious), for many others it's simply a matter of believing that a vegetarian diet is healthier. And there's some justification for this belief: Although vegetarianism is not for everyone, it can provide a number potential health benefits, including a lower incidence of several chronic diseases.

**It's a way of life**

In addition to dietary considerations, of course, vegetarians tend to be healthier because they often make positive lifestyle choices, including weight maintenance, regular exercise, abstinence from smoking, alcohol and drugs.

HEART DISEASE. Vegetarian diets tend to be "heart healthy." They are typically lower in total and saturated fat, as well as dietary cholesterol. They are also generally higher in fiber and polyunsaturated fat, which helps to lower LDL (popularly known as "bad cholesterol") levels in the blood. Vegetarians are statistically less likely to have high blood pressure or to die from coronary artery disease.

CERTAIN TYPES OF CANCER. Vegetarians have lower rates of certain types of cancer. The precise reason for this is unknown, although one suggestion is that vegetarians consume more antioxidants, such as vitamins C and E. Other possible factors include lower fat consumption and increased fiber intake.

Vegetarians are also less likely to suffer from obesity and non-insulin dependent diabetes.

## Vegetarian diets for children

Given all its apparent benefits, why don't we all adopt a vegetarian lifestyle? And if a vegetarian diet is good for adults, is it also healthy for children?

A vegetarian diet is not for everyone. Vegetarian diets can be healthy, but must be carefully planned so that they provide all the proper nutrients. This is especially important for children. If this done, vegetarian (and even vegan) children can be well nourished and develop normally. So let's examine some of the specific nutritional considerations required.

## Energy

Because many plant foods are not concentrated sources of calories, vegetarian diets have the potential to be low in energy. It is important that vegetarian children, especially vegan children, receive adequate energy for growth and health. This is less of a challenge in the case of lacto-ovo vegetarian children, since milk and eggs are concentrated sources of energy. Vegan children, on the other hand, need to boost their energy intake by including high-calorie plant foods – such as avocado, nuts and nut butters – as a part of their daily eating regimen.

## Protein

As noted in Chapter 3 (see page 36), proteins consist of amino acids. There are 20 different amino acids, and they can be found in a variety of the foods we eat. The body can make many of these (called *non-essential* amino acids) on its own, so we don't need to obtain them from our diet. But there are 9 amino acids that our bodies cannot make, and we must get them from the foods we eat. These are called *essential* amino acids.

Amino acids perform many different jobs in our bodies and it is important to ensure that we consume an adequate amount of all 9 essential amino acids daily. For meat eaters this is not a concern, since meats contain all 9 essential amino acids and are therefore described as *complete* proteins. On the other hand, because plant proteins are missing one or more essential amino acids, they are called *incomplete* proteins. Consequently, vegetarians need to eat plant proteins in combination, consuming a variety of foods which, together, make the proteins complete.

This is not difficult. We do it inadvertently every day, by consuming plant foods in pairs – like toast and peanut butter or split-pea soup with a roll. For planning purposes, the process is essentially this: If Food A is missing only Essential Amino Acid X, and Food B is missing only Essential Amino Acid Y, then together they are not missing Essential Amino Acids X or Y, and therefore make a complete protein.

### Where's the protein?

**Sources of protein for vegetarians**

| Food type | Examples |
|---|---|
| Grains | Wheat, oats, rice, quinoa |
| Legumes | Peas, lentils, peanuts, beans |
| Nuts and seeds | Walnuts, sesame seeds, almonds, nut butters |

NOTE: Few vegetables contain significant amounts of protein but do provide essential amino acids needed to help complement the amino acids in other plant-based proteins.
For vegetarians who consume them, milk and eggs are good sources of protein.

## Fiber

Fiber is found only in plant foods and has many benefits for children and adults alike. It helps to maintain regular bowel movements, lower cholesterol and may help in the prevention of certain types of cancers. (See page 38 for more information.) For vegetarian children, however, there is a risk that they may be getting too much of a good thing. Because high-fiber diets have the potential to be deficient in the energy (calories) needed to ensure proper growth, and are high in "bulk" (which can make you feel full more quickly), it is important to balance a child's diet with foods that are concentrated sources of calories and fat, such as nuts, cheese and eggs.

## Iron

Vegetarian children need to ensure they receive sufficient iron, since this mineral plays an important role in the function of blood cells. As noted in Chapter 4 (see page 51), there are two types of dietary iron. Heme iron is found in meats and is generally well absorbed by the body. Non-heme iron, which is not as readily absorbed, is found in plant foods. For children consuming a plant-based diet, then, it is important to ensure that they obtain enough iron.

Plant sources of iron include tofu, prunes, legumes and dark, leafy green vegetables. Infant cereal is also a terrific source of iron that can be added to pancakes, cereals and other foods. Enhancers of iron absorption can affect the percentage of non-heme iron that the body receives. Vitamin C, for example, helps with iron absorption. Try offering a small glass of orange juice with meals.

## Vitamin $B_{12}$

Like iron, vitamin $B_{12}$ is essential to the proper functioning of red blood cells. It also helps in nerve conduction by maintaining the protective sheath that surrounds nerve fibers. Since it can only be found in animal products, vegans need to be particularly concerned about this vitamin. Lacto-ovo vegetarians should receive adequate vitamin $B_{12}$ from milk and eggs. Vegans, on the other hand, need to take a supplement or consume reliable food sources of vitamin $B_{12}$, such as fortified commercial breakfast cereals, soy beverages or nutritional yeasts. Alternatively, children's multivitamins generally contain enough vitamin $B_{12}$ to avoid deficiency.

### *Vegan moms and vitamin $B_{12}$*

Children of vegan mothers are particularly at risk of vitamin $B_{12}$ deficiency, since there is a reduced amount of this vitamin that crosses the placenta during pregnancy, as well as decreased amounts present in breast milk.

## Calcium

Getting enough dietary calcium is especially important for children to maximize bone mass during growth and to minimize the bone loss that occurs later in life. Calcium is generally not a concern for lacto-vegetarians who consume adequate amounts of milk and milk products. For others, however, it can be a problem. While many plant foods contain calcium, it is often difficult for the body to absorb because the plant also contains phytates and oxalates, which inhibit the absorption process. And of those plant foods that do contain bioavailable calcium – such as kale, broccoli, bok choy and soybeans – the calcium content is so low that foods must be consumed in very large amounts to meet a child's dietary requirements of between 500 and 800 mg/day. (See page 47 for information on the calcium content of selected foods.) For children who do not consume dairy products, it may be necessary to add calcium-fortified foods or supplements to their diet.

## Vitamin D

Like calcium, vitamin D also plays a role in bone health, and is an important vitamin for all growing children. The most common food source of vitamin D is milk, so lacto-vegetarian children who drink an adequate amount of milk need not worry about getting enough vitamin D. However, children who do not drink fortified cow's milk or an acceptable fortified alternative – or who do not receive 10 to 15 minutes daily exposure to sunlight (which the allows the body to manufacture its own vitamin D) – may require a vitamin D supplement.

## Zinc

Because zinc is important for growth and development (see page 54), it is important to ensure that vegetarian children (and non-vegetarians too, of course) receive adequate amounts of this mineral. This is rarely a problem for vegetarians, since zinc can be obtained from foods such as grains, legumes and nuts.

## TERRIFIC TOFU

One of the best plant-based sources of protein is tofu. Manufactured from soybeans (which is why it's sometimes called "soybean curd"), tofu is a soft, cheese-like food that, when fortified (as it usually is), can also be a source of calcium. Tofu is quite bland on its own, but has an amazing ability to soak up the flavors of whatever food it is cooked with.

There are 3 main types of tofu available:

**Firm** or **Extra-firm.** Dense and solid, this type of tofu is great in stir-fries, soups or on the grill. It will maintain its shape as it cooks. This type of tofu also contains the most protein and fat (see below).

**Soft.** Less solid than the firm variety, this type of tofu is often used in Asian-style soups.

**Silken.** With its creamy, custard-like consistency, silken tofu works well in puréed or blended dishes, and is often used in tofu desserts or soups.

## HOW THEY COMPARE

**Nutrients per 4-oz (100 g) serving for different types of tofu**

| | FIRM TOFU | SOFT TOFU | SILKEN TOFU |
|---|---|---|---|
| Calories | 120 | 86 | 72 |
| Protein (g) | 13 | 9 | 10 |
| Carbohydrate (g) | 3 | 2 | 3 |
| Fat (g) | 6 | 5 | 2 |
| Calcium (mg) | 120 | 130 | 40 |

SOURCE: *Composition of Foods: Legumes and Legume Products.* United States Department of Agriculture Human Nutrition Information Service, Agriculture Handbook 0-16. Revised December 1986.

## 7 STEPS TO HEALTHY VEGETARIAN EATING

1. Be sure to include a variety of foods from all four "vegetarian food groups" at each meal. These groups include grains, vegetables and fruits, beans and bean alternatives, as well as milk and milk alternatives (if consumed). This will ensure that your child receives a balance of energy and nutrients every day.
2. Preschoolers should receive 16 to 20 oz (500 to 625 mL) daily of whole cow's milk or a nutritionally acceptable replacement. School-aged children should receive 16 oz (500 mL) daily. Milk is a valuable source of energy, calcium, vitamin D and riboflavin. For vegan children ages 2 to 5 years, a fortified soy infant **formula** will provide all the vitamins and minerals necessary to prevent deficiency.
3. Include protein-rich foods with every meal. Lacto-ovo vegetarian children can obtain high-quality protein from milk and eggs. High-quality vegan sources of protein include fortified soy infant formula or milk, tofu, quinoa, or legume and grain combinations. Non-dairy beverages such as rice milk or potato milk are very low in protein and should not be used for vegetarian children until they are 6 years old and are consuming a wide variety of other foods.
4. Balance high-fiber foods with those that are concentrated sources of energy and fat, such as cheese or yogurt (for those who consume dairy products) or, for vegan children over the age of 4, nuts and nut butters. A vegan diet can be very high in fiber and bulk, making it difficult for children to meet their daily caloric requirements.
5. Provide plant foods each day that are good sources of iron and zinc.
6. Include 5 or more servings of vegetables and fruits each day. These foods are great sources of vitamins and minerals, including vitamin A, vitamin C and folic acid. Try to eat at least one serving of fruit or vegetables at each meal.
7. Include a reliable source of vitamin $B_{12}$ in the diet. Lacto-ovo vegetarian children can meet their daily vitamin $B_{12}$ requirements from about 1 1/2 glasses of milk or from 1 glass of milk and 1 egg. Since this vitamin is not found in plant foods, vegan children must obtain it from fortified foods such as soy infant formula, or by taking a vitamin $B_{12}$ supplement.

*Adapted from *Being Vegetarian*. V. Melina, B. Davis and V. Harrison. Toronto: Macmillan Canada, 1994.

CHAPTER 6

# Avoiding Food contamination

*There are hundreds of microorganisms presents in our everyday lives. Many of these are harmless to humans, while others, such as the bacteria that ferment cheese and yogurt, are actually beneficial. But some of these "bugs" are harmful and, when they get into our food, are capable of causing serious illness. As a parent, you need to be aware of what these microorganisms are, and how to prevent them from making your child sick.*

## The bugs in our food

The microorganisms that cause illness are known as *pathogens*. These are mostly bacteria, which are responsible for more than 90% of all food-poisoning cases.

Food-borne bacteria can cause illness in two ways:

INFECTION. This is caused by bacterial growth in the food itself. Generally, cooking foods thoroughly to an internal temperature of at least 155° F (68° C) can prevent infections.

INTOXICATION. Here it is not the bacteria that cause harm, but rather the toxins produced by the bacteria. In most cases, these toxins are unaffected by heat, and cannot be destroyed by cooking.

Bacterial contamination occurs primarily in cases where products or ingredients are eaten raw, or where food is improperly handled or stored.

Which bacteria cause food poisoning? There are many different varieties, but here are some of the worst offenders.

STAPHYLOCOCCUS AUREUS. Although this common bacteria is found in the nose, throat, hair or skin of about 50% of

### Signs of sickness

Symptoms of food poisoning can include stomach cramps, diarrhea, vomiting, sweating or chills. They usually commence within 12 to 18 hours of eating the contaminated food.

healthy people, it is also responsible for about 1 in 4 cases of all food-borne illness in North America. Staph aureus contamination is found in foods such as meat, fish, poultry, dairy products and salads.

ESCHERICHIA COLI (E. COLI). This bacteria can be found in the intestinal tract of both animals and humans. It is occasionally found in raw meats or poultry, but can be eliminated by thorough cooking. Other potential sources of E. coli include unpasteurized milk and cheese, as well as contaminated water (see sidebar: "Hamburger Disease").

SALMONELLA ENTERITIDIS. Most commonly found in raw or partially cooked eggs, as well as raw or undercooked chicken. Salmonella poisoning often results when foods containing uncooked egg ingredients (such as Caesar salad dressing or the meringue topping on a pie) have not been properly refrigerated.

LISTERIA MONOCYTOGENES. Unusual for its ability to survive in the cold (in fact, it thrives at normal refrigerator temperatures), this bacteria can be found in cooked meats or seafood, prepared salads, soft cheeses, as well as unpasteurized milk and milk products. Listeria is also very resistant to heat, requiring a minimum of 2 minutes at 160° F (70° C) to significantly reduce its numbers.

TRICHINELLA SPIRALIS. This bacteria comes from a parasitic worm that infects pigs. Now rare, trichinella infection (or trichinosis) from pork consumption was once a major health problem in the US. Today fewer than 100 cases are reported each year.

CLOSTRIDIUM BOTULINUM. Found most often in canned goods, usually where the can has been damaged slightly, allowing the bacteria to enter. In this oxygen-free, low-acid environment, the bacteria grows, producing a dangerous neurotoxin which can only be destroyed by exposure to temperatures of 180° F (85° C) or greater for at least 10 minutes. To avoid C. botulinum, do not purchase goods in dented cans. The bacteria has occasionally been found in unpasteurized honey, which is why this sweetener should not be given to infants less than 1 year of age.

### Hamburger disease

Named for the undercooked ground beef that is often its source, "hamburger disease" is caused by a particularly nasty strain of E. coli, called *verotoxigenic E. coli*, or VTEC. In addition to hamburger, it is also found in unpasteurized milk or contaminated water, as well as other foods such as cheese, yogurt or cold cuts. This bacteria produces a toxin that breaks down the lining of the intestines and, in severe cases, can damage the kidneys. Symptoms include severe stomach ache and bloody diarrhea. In severely affected children, a specific kind of kidney failure can develop, called hemolytic uremic syndrome (HUS). Hamburger disease can be prevented by observing standard rules of safe food preparation (see at right) and by never eating undercooked meat or unpasteurized milks and cheeses.

## Clean and safe

The following are some suggestions to help minimize the risk of food-borne illnesses in your home:

- Always wash your hands before preparing or serving foods.
- Avoid breathing, coughing or sneezing on foods, especially if you have a cold.
- Keep your preparation area and utensils clean.
- Keep highchair trays clean. Wash down with hot soapy water after each meal. Once a week, be sure to clean with a diluted solution of bleach and water.
- Always keep raw foods and cooked foods separate. Use separate cutting boards or clean the boards thoroughly between uses.
- Never place cooked foods on a plate that held raw food unless that plate has been thoroughly washed.
- Store uncooked meats, poultry or fish on the lowest refrigerator rack to avoid juices spilling onto other fresh foods.
- Wash fruits and vegetables thoroughly under running water.
- Thaw frozen foods overnight in the refrigerator or use a microwave. Foods thawed on the counter are at risk of microbial contamination.
- Cook meats thoroughly to kill bacteria.
- Always keep hot foods hot (over 165° F [72° C]) and cold foods cold (less than 40° F [4° C])
- Do not eat food from any can that is swollen or dented.
- Always check the expiration date on foods. Do not consume foods beyond the expiration date.
- Don't eat raw eggs or fish.
- Do not eat moldy or spoiled foods.

## Packing a safe lunch

Many school-aged children take a lunch to school in the morning, where it remains for several hours, usually at room temperature, before being eaten. To minimize the risk of bacterial contamination and/or growth, there are a number of steps you can take when packing the lunch.

## MEALS FOR MICROBES

**Foods that carry a high risk of contamination**

| FOOD TYPE | EXAMPLE(S) | CONTAMINANT |
|---|---|---|
| Raw or undercooked eggs | Caesar salad dressing, soft-cooked eggs, meringue pies, some puddings and custards, mousse, sauces made with raw eggs | Salmonella enteritidis |
| Raw dairy products | unpasteurized milk; some soft cheeses, such as Brie and camembert | Listeria monocytogenes<br>E. coli<br>Salmonella<br>Campylobacter |
| Raw or rare meat | hamburger | E. coli<br>Salmonella |
| Raw fish | sushi, tuna | Parasites |

NOTE: For an expanded list of high-risk foods, see information at *www.foodsafety.gov*

### *If in doubt, throw it out*

A refrigerator slows down the rate of bacterial growth, but doesn't stop it. So don't keep foods in the fridge too long. Fresh poultry should be stored for no longer than 2 days, and other fresh meats no longer than 3 to 5 days. Cooked leftovers can be kept for up to 4 days. If you're unsure how long food has been in the refrigerator, it's better to throw it out than risk illness.

- PUT SOMETHING COLD IN THE BAG. A frozen juice box or small water container will act like a freezer pack to help prevent against food-borne illness. (By lunchtime, the drink will have thawed, but still be cold and refreshing.)
- FREEZE THOSE SANDWICHES. This works better with coarse-textured breads that won't get soggy when they thaw. Veggies or mayonnaise will need to be packed separately.
- INSULATE YOUR FOOD. An insulated lunch bag with a freezer pack inside will keep foods cold. This is especially helpful when packing highly perishable foods such as cold cuts, poultry, fish or egg sandwiches. Use an insulated container (thermos) to keep liquids hot or cold.
- FIND SOMEPLACE COOL. Keep your lunch in the coolest part of the room – or at least away from warm places, such as hot air vents or sunny window sills. If the school has a refrigerator available, use it.
- KEEP IT CLEAN. Wash the inside of lunch boxes/bags with warm soapy water every night. Once a week, clean with a diluted solution of bleach and water. While you're at it, remind your kids to wash their hands before eating.

CHAPTER 7

# Conventional vs Organic foods

*Many parents are concerned about the environment – particularly about the use of pesticides and other chemicals in the production of our food. While regulatory agencies in both the US and Canada have declared the levels of these substances in food to be safe for human consumption, some parents still worry that chemicals may be having (as yet unknown) effects upon their children. In fact, the presence of these agents in food is often blamed for the overall increase in child allergies and asthma.*

*For all of these reasons, organic foods – which are produced without pesticides, antibiotics or growth hormones – have become increasingly popular. Are they safer than conventional foods? What kinds of chemicals are actually in conventional foods, anyway? These are some of the questions we'll examine in this chapter.*

## What's in the food we eat now?

Modern agricultural practices have helped farmers to make huge gains in the quantity and quality of food they are able to produce, which has made that food much cheaper and more widely available to a larger number of people. But questions of safety still persist.

### Pesticides

Agricultural pesticides (including herbicides and other chemicals) control many different types of pests, including insects, rodents, weeds, and microbial pests such as bacteria, fungi and viruses. Pesticides can be chemical, biological, natural or synthetic. The widespread use of insecticides began in the 1950s with the introduction of DDT (dichlorodiphenyltrichloroethane).

While often effective in eradicating specific problems, pesticides can have larger effects that are not intended. And, as most people now realize, we need to consider the entire ecological system in which the pests live. Because all pesticides are made to kill some organism, no single agent is considered to be "completely" safe. Indeed, safety is always a relative term, in which minimal risks are weighed against major benefits. For this reason, the effects of pesticides (which are widely speculated about in the media) have alarmed many consumers, even though most of the scientific community consider the risks from pesticide use to be minimal.

**North American cows remain sane**

In recent years, beef production in Britain and other European countries has suffered from outbreaks of "mad cow disease", or bovine spongiform encephalopathy (BSE), which causes a slow deterioration of the nervous system. It is not considered a threat in North America, despite some alarming reports in the media. Both Canada and the US have inspections for the symptoms of BSE which have been in place for years. Animal feeds in the US do not contain sources of the harmful agent. For more information on this disease, search for "BSE" on government websites in both the US and Canada.

### Antibiotics

Antibiotics are chemicals that inhibit the growth of harmful microorganisms. Originally used in medicine to fight infection in humans, they are now used in agriculture – typically in relatively small doses added to feed to promote or enhance growth in animals. In the US, over 100 antibiotics have been approved for use in animal feed. It is estimated that two-thirds to three-quarters of all domestic animals raised for food in the United States have been treated with antibiotics at some time.

There is much public concern about the safety of antibiotics and the effects of possible antibiotic residue in the foods we eat. One major concern is that the use of antibiotics in animals may cause certain microorganisms to develop a resistance that could make them difficult to control in humans, or that antibiotic residues could trigger human allergic reactions. To minimize this risk, Food and Drug Administration (FDA) regulations specify maximum allowable doses, minimum times before slaughter that administration of antibiotics must be stopped, as well as limits on antibiotic residues permitted in animal products.

### Hormones

Hormones are used increasingly today in animal breeding to produce larger, leaner animals. In the United States, the FDA restricts the amount of hormones that can be given to livestock – specifically, no more than 1% of the amount normally produced by the animal. Since animals absorb only a fraction of an orally administered hormone, the possibility that consumers ingest significantly increased amounts of these hormones is negligible.

### Tainted tuna?

Tuna is one of the most widely consumed fish in the world. So when media reports started to appear about elevated levels of mercury in tuna, they received serious attention. Mercury is often released into marine ecosystems through industrial waste, where it accumulates in fish. At high enough levels it can cause damage to the body's nervous system; however, the effects of trace amounts of mercury are unclear.

In Canada, canned tuna is tested to ensure that mercury levels are below an acceptable minimum (5 parts per million). But tuna harvested for sale as fresh or frozen fish are not. Because tuna is a predatory fish (that is, it eats other smaller fish), it is more likely to accumulate mercury than other species. Because this type of tuna is not routinely tested, consumers may want to limit their intake of fresh or frozen tuna to no more than one meal per week. Young children and women of childbearing years should limit their intake to no more than one meal per month. Since most North Americans do not consume fresh and frozen tuna every week, this does not pose a concern for most consumers. It is important to remember that fish (including tuna) is an excellent source of protein, low in saturated fat, and high in polyunsaturated fat.

### PCBs in food

Polychlorinated biphenyls (PCBs) are dangerous compounds that, in sufficient quantities, damage the immune system, rendering it less capable of fighting infection. While they are no longer allowed to be used in products (such as insulation), they are still found in our environment, where they persist in places such as soil and water. PCBs typically enter our food supply through dairy products, meat and other processed foods.

Young children and infants are especially vulnerable to PCBs. Breast milk can be a major source of PCBs in infants if their mothers have consumed a lot of fatty fish (such as salmon) that have been harvested from contaminated waters. It is prudent for pregnant women (as well as infants and young children) to limit their consumption of fatty fish harvested from fresh waters where contamination is either known or suspected.

## Environmental contaminants

While not used deliberately (in the same way that pesticides are, for example), environmental contaminants can enter the food supply by various means, including exposure to air, water or soil that contains industrial wastes and other environmental pollutants. Many of these chemicals are not biodegradable, so once they enter the food chain they can accumulate in parts of the body (human or animal), including the liver, brain or fats. Examples of environmental contaminates include increased levels of mercury in tuna or swordfish (see sidebar), contaminated water from lead pipes, or increased cadmium levels in soil.

## Are organic foods worth the cost?

As noted earlier, conventional agricultural techniques have helped to make farming more efficient. So you might expect that organic farming – which does not use pesticides, antibiotics or hormones – would be less efficient, with higher costs for each unit of production. And you would be right: the increased costs of producing organic foods make them more expensive – up to 40 % higher in some cases.

Are these foods worth their cost? Many studies have been conducted on the levels of chemicals and pesticides found in conventionally produced foods, and these have been determined to be safe for human consumption. Food production is also strictly regulated by government. So you may not be any "safer" buying organic foods – particularly since these foods are not completely isolated from the environment, and may still contain traces of pollutants beyond the farmer's control. In addition, organic foods have generally not been shown to offer any nutritional benefits over conventional foods.

Still, when it comes to feeding their children, many parents take a certain comfort from organic foods. They should realize, however, that they are paying a high price for foods that have no nutritional advantages over their non-organic counterparts.

### *Scrub that food*

To remove chemicals that may be deposited on the surface, wash all fruits and vegetables thoroughly under running water.

## Food science

Technology is continuously advancing to make it possible to produce more and more food for the world's population. For example, genetic manipulation has created crops that are resistant to pests, thereby reducing the need for chemical pesticides. This is desirable, of course, but often leads consumers to trade one worry for another – in this case, about the possible hazards of changing plant genetics.

### Novel foods

### *Is it certified?*

In order to qualify as organic food, the originating farm or processing facility must meet the requirements of (and be inspected by) a government-recognized certification body.

Also known as genetically engineered foods, novel foods are typically those where a gene from one food has been inserted into the genetic make-up of another food. In some cases, this is to make the food more resistant to damage from pests or disease; in others, it is to increase its nutritional profile. These foods are always tested thoroughly before they reach the consumer. For example, genes from Brazil nuts were used to enhance the protein content of soybean meal (feed for animals) a few years ago. However, it was discovered that the genetically modified soy contained a nut protein that caused allergy, so the product was never brought to market.

Novel or genetically modified foods have not been shown to be any less safe than traditional foods. Governments in North America regulate the types of foods that are allowed to appear on grocery shelves. For example, it is the responsibility of the FDA and Health Canada to ensure that, in their respective countries, products derived through biotechnology are assessed for their potential impact on human health. (For information on probiotics, see page 94.)

### Irradiation

How do you keep food fresh and safe for human consumption? One technique is irradiation – where food is subjected to gamma rays from radioactive cobalt-60 or cesium-137. This process kills most bacteria, insects and mold that are normally responsible for causing both decay and many food-borne illnesses.

### *Wired on sugar and food additives?*

A study of children age 3 to 10 years has revealed that, contrary to what many people believe, neither sucrose (sugar) nor aspartame make any significant contribution to hyperactivity. One-half of these children were described by parents to be sensitive to sugar. Another study looked at the effects of artificial food colors on behavior. Parents who had previously attributed behavioral changes to the consumption of food colors were generally not able to detect behavioral changes after food colors were given during the study. In yet another study, intolerance to additives (food colorings or preservatives) was confirmed in only 16% of suspected children. What is the message? The majority of children believed to have intolerances to sugar, color or additives are likely not affected – although a minority do have reactions, which may include rashes, respiratory problems or behavioral changes.

Irradiation does not cause the food to be radioactive and does not form harmful compounds in the food. In fact, the FDA and Health Canada both consider it to be a safe, effective and economical way of preserving food. But the general public has not responded well to the idea of eating anything that has been in contact with radioactive materials, and food retailers have had trouble promoting irradiated foods in the US, where irradiated foods must be identified as such. In Canada, there are currently no means of identifying foods that have been treated with radiation.

## Sweet nothings

Many artificial sweeteners have been approved by the FDA and Health Canada for use in our food supply. Sweeteners are found in a variety of food products, including baked goods, puddings, frozen desserts, yogurts, soft drinks and chewing gum. They are also available in the form of tabletop sweeteners as alternatives to sugar.

Most health authorities do not recommend artificial sweeteners for children under the age of 2 years. This is because they do not provide calories in the diet, and very young children should never have their caloric intake compromised. In addition, the safety of artificial sweeteners has not been determined for children under the age of 2.

It is safe for healthy children over the age of 2 years to consume artificial sweeteners; however, it is important to remember that children of all ages need sufficient calories to grow and develop normally. Children generally do not need to eat lower-calorie foods containing artificial sweeteners, although there is no harm in a child consuming a yogurt or the occasional diet soda containing sweetener. The key is the amount of sweetener eaten daily. The FDA and Health Canada set "Acceptable Daily Intakes" (or ADIs) for all sweeteners, and normal consumption of the occasional sweetened product should never reach these limits.

There are a number of sweeteners on the market, each of which has different characteristics.

ASPARTAME (sold as Nutrasweet® or Equal®) is a non-nutritive sweetener that is composed of 2 amino acids (the building blocks of protein): phenylalanine and aspartic acid. Many foods naturally contain these 2 amino acids. Aspartame is 200 times sweeter than sugar. It is safe to eat by virtually all individuals expect those who have a rare disorder called phenylketonuria or PKU, and need to control their phenylalanine intake. The acceptable daily intake for aspartame in the US is 50 mg per kilogram of body weight per day (40 mg/kg/day in Canada). This means a 15 kg or 33 lb child can safely consume up to 750 mg (600 mg) of aspartame daily or the equivalent of 10 (8) cans of diet soda every day.

SACCHARIN (sold as Sweet n Low®) was one of the first artificial sweeteners available. It is 300 times sweeter than table sugar, but has a slightly bitter aftertaste. Saccharin has received much media attention over the years because of its alleged connection with cancer; however, research has not been able to determine a direct association.

CYCLAMATE (sold as Sugar Twin®) is 30 times sweeter than table sugar. Cyclamate has no aftertaste and can be used in both hot and cold foods. In Canada, cyclamate is available only as a tabletop sweetener.

SUCRALOSE (sold as Splenda®) is a calorie-free sweetener created from ordinary sugar. It looks and tastes just like sugar, but the body is not able to break it down and use it as energy. Sucralose is 400 to 800 times sweeter than sugar, and is available in a wide variety of products, including hot and cold drinks, as well as other commercial foods.

ACESULFAME POTASSIUM or ACE-K (sold as Senett®) is about 200 times sweeter than sugar. People who are on restricted potassium diets or who have sulfa allergies should talk to their doctor before using Ace-K.

SUGAR ALCOHOLS (sold as Xylitol or Dentec®) are different from other artificial sweeteners in that they contribute calories to the diet. However, they are endorsed for use in chewing gum by the Canadian and American Dental Associations because they help prevent cavities. Sugar alcohols are also used in products such as hard candies, jams, and cough lozenges.

It is important to remember that although artificial sweeteners are safe for use in foods and beverages, there is no need for healthy children to consume them. Artificial sweeteners, if enjoyed, should be used as a part of a healthy, well-balanced diet.

CHAPTER 8

# Food allergy and intolerance

*One of the most worrying aspects of feeding a child is the possibility of a food allergy (which involves an immune response) or a food intolerance (which does not). Reactions to food can be serious, and it is important for parents to be knowledgeable about this subject – particularly where there is a family history of allergy or intolerance.*

## Immune responses to food

Food allergy or "hypersensitivity" is defined as an immune system response to a food protein that the body identifies as foreign. It has been estimated that approximately 3 to 6% of children have an allergy to at least one food.

One predictor of whether or not a child may develop an allergy is a strong family history of allergy. If a parent or sibling has a food allergy, the child's risk of developing an allergy to food is increased.

It is important to note that allergies in general are inherited, although specific allergies are not. For example, if one parent has allergies, then the child may have a 50 to 75% chance of also having an allergic problem, even though the specific allergy or allergies may be different from those of the parent.

Breastfeeding may also protect against certain allergies.

Signs and symptoms of allergy generally fall into the following categories:

- Skin: rash, hives, eczema
- Digestive: nausea, vomiting, stomach cramps, diarrhea

- RESPIRATORY: runny nose, nasal congestion, difficulty breathing, wheezing
- CARDIOVASCULAR: increased heart rate

## How to diagnose a food allergy

There are many different ways to diagnose food allergy. Let's review some of the most common methods.

SKIN TEST. This type of test (also known as a "prick test") is widely used to diagnose food allergy. A small amount of an allergen is introduced by pricking the skin with a small needle. The skin is then monitored for a reaction.

ELIMINATION DIET. With this technique, highly allergenic foods are eliminated from the diet for several weeks. The eliminated foods are then slowly reintroduced in an attempt to identify which foods are causing symptoms. This diet should be done under medical supervision and should not last more than 2 weeks, after which it can lead to nutritional deficiencies.

ORAL FOOD CHALLENGE. In this test, a small amount of the suspected food is given under controlled conditions. The patient is then monitored for a reaction.

There are other techniques for diagnosing allergy. If you suspect your child may have a food allergy, speak with your physician or pediatrician. Remember that you should always seek professional assistance in cases of suspected allergy. Don't attempt to eliminate multiple foods from your child's diet unless advised to do so by a physician. An unbalanced diet due to eliminating foods can cause poor weight gain and/or vitamin or mineral deficiencies.

### Extreme reactions

Anaphylaxis is an immediate, life-threatening response involving several organ systems. Symptoms can include hives, swelling of any part of the body (such as the mouth and face), itching, difficulty breathing, nausea and diarrhea. Severe cases can lead to anaphylactic shock or even death. Anaphylactic symptoms usually occur within minutes of food ingestion, although they may take as long as 1 or 2 hours. Because of these dangers, parents of a child with anaphylactic reactions should take strict measures to avoid the offending foods, and carry with them (or have older children carry themselves) an injection containing epinephrine (such as Epipen®) at all times. (Epinephrine is a drug that will help to keep the airways open if an allergen has been ingested.) A prescription can be obtained through your physician, pediatrician or allergist. If the injection is used, it is still important to go to the nearest hospital after the pen has been injected.

## Types of allergies

There are many types of food allergies prevalent in children. Here we provide some general information about the more common types.

## Milk allergy

It has been estimated that between 2 to 3% of infants have an allergy to cow's milk protein. The good news is that up to 85% of children who are diagnosed with this allergy as infants will grow out of it by the time they are 3 years old. However, if a child develops a sensitivity to cow's milk protein after the age of 3, he or she will probably be sensitive for life. Milk allergy is much more common in children than adults.

**Allergy or intolerance?**

It is important to differentiate the difference between a cow's milk protein allergy, which is an immune response to the protein in milk, and lactose intolerance, which is an inability to digest the sugar in milk (lactose). Lactose intolerance does not involve an immune response. For more information on lactose intolerance see page 88.

Common symptoms of cow's milk allergy include: skin rash or hives (the most frequently reported symptom); gastrointestinal disturbances, including abdominal pain or bloating, gas, diarrhea and nausea; and blood loss in stool (occasionally reported in infants, this can lead to iron deficiency anemia). Respiratory symptoms may include coughing or wheezing.

There are more than 30 proteins in milk and most children with a milk allergy will react to more than one of these proteins. Since many milk proteins are not broken down when heated, a child will be as allergic to cold milk as to cooked milk or cooked products containing milk.

Once a child has been diagnosed with a milk allergy, it is important to avoid all milk and foods containing milk or milk products. This includes:

- All liquid and evaporated milks
- Yogurt, buttermilk
- Cream
- All cheeses, including hard cheeses, soft cheeses, cottage cheese and cream cheese

- Ice cream and ice milks
- Foods containing milk solids, such as butter and many margarines

### Milk alternatives

Milk and milk products are an important source of energy, protein, calcium and vitamin D in non-vegetarian infants and toddlers. Therefore, if these foods need to be eliminated from the diet due to cow's milk allergy, it is important to replace them with acceptable alternatives in order to ensure adequate growth. Energy and protein can be found in many other foods, including meats, poultry, fish, grains, vegetables and fruit. And provided we have adequate exposure to sunlight, our bodies can produce sufficient vitamin D. It is more challenging, however, to find another source of dietary calcium.

## Find the milk protein

**When you have young children with milk allergy, it is essential to read all food labels carefully for milk or words indicating milk protein ingredients. Some of these are not obvious, as the following list demonstrates.**

| | | | |
|---|---|---|---|
| milk | cheese | cream | casein |
| condensed milk | cottage cheese | cream cheese | sodium caseinate |
| evaporated milk | sour cream | quark® | potassium caseinate |
| milk powder | yogurt | ice cream | whey |
| butter | buttermilk | sherbet | lactoglobulin |
| milk solids | curd | feta/ricotta | lactose |

SOURCE: Vickerstaff-Joneja, J. *Managing Food Allergy and Intolerance: A Practical Guide.* 1995

**Fortified milk alternatives** contain calcium and vitamin D. Acceptable choices include:

- *Soy formula or soy milk.* This may not be appropriate for all children with cow's milk allergy, since some children may also be intolerant of soy protein. Check with your doctor to see which is the best choice for your child. Remember, too, that while all infant soy formulas on the North American market are fortified, all soy milks are not. Check the label to make sure that a soy milk has been fortified with calcium and vitamin D, and that it is a good source of energy (since some varieties are low in fat).
- *Protein hydrolysate formulas* (such as Nutramigen® or Neocate®) are appropriate for infants with cow's milk and soy protein allergy.
- *Some rice beverages.* Rice Dream® is a rice beverage appropriate for children who are over the age of 2 years and have a cow's milk and/or soy protein allergy. Again, it is important to ensure that a rice beverage has been fortified with calcium and vitamin D. Rice beverages are also low in calories and protein, so it is important to ensure that the child's diet contains adequate energy and protein from alternate sources.

***Unacceptable*** choices include:

- *Goat's milk.* Between 70 and 80% of children with cow's milk protein allergy will also be allergic to goat's milk.
- *Nut milks (such as almond milk).* Many children with cow's milk allergy may also be allergic to nuts. In addition, many nut milks are not fortified.
- *Fruit juices.* Nutritionally speaking, fruit juices are no substitute for milk. For young children, 6 oz (175 mL) is the maximum recommended daily juice intake.

**Green leafy vegetables.** Broccoli, spinach and kale provide some calcium, although it is not easily absorbed by the body, so they will probably not provide adequate dietary calcium on their own.

CANNED FISH WITH THE BONES INCLUDED. Canned salmon with bones may be a good source of calcium for milk-allergic children. To reduce choking risk, make sure that the bones are well mashed before serving.

TOFU. Since this product is made from soy, it is clearly not suitable for a child with soy allergy. Otherwise, tofu is a good source of calcium, although the silken variety is less so.

NUTS AND LEGUMES. These may contain some calcium.

It may be difficult to obtain enough calcium in the diet if your child is not consuming a fortified alternative beverage. For these milk-allergic children, a calcium supplement may be recommended. Speak with your physician for more information.

## Soy protein allergy

True soy protein allergy is rare and occurs in only about 4 to 7% of the population. The symptoms of soy protein allergy are similar to those of an allergy to cow's milk

### HIDDEN SOY

**Because soy and soy products are found in so many commercially prepared foods today, it can be very difficult to follow a soy-free diet. With adequate education and information, however, it is possible to maintain a well-balanced diet that is free of soy proteins. Read food labels carefully for ingredients that indicate the presence of soy protein; many are not obvious.**

| | | | |
|---|---|---|---|
| emulsifiers* | lecithin* | miso | shoyu |
| Sobee | soy | soy albumin | soy beans |
| soy flour | soy lecithin | soy milk | soy nuts |
| soy oil | soy protein | soy protein isolate | soya |
| soy sauce | soy sprouts | soy-based infant formulas | stabilizers* |
| tempeh | tofu | unspecified sprouts* | vegetable broth* |
| vegetable gum* | vegetable oil* | vegetable paste* | vegetable protein* |
| | vegetable shortening* | vegetable starch* | |
| | textured vegetable protein (TVP)* | hydrolyzed vegetable protein (HVP)* | hydrolyzed plant protein (HPP)* |

**These items may or may not contain soy; the source is seldom listed on a food label.*

SOURCE: Vickerstaff-Joneja, J. *Managing Food Allergy and Intolerance: A Practical Guide.* 1995

protein. In infants and young children these may include: abdominal pain; loose stools or diarrhea; vomiting; respiratory symptoms, such as cough or wheeze; and eczema or hives.

Many unlabeled products – including bulk foods, unwrapped breads and baked goods – contain soy, especially when flour is an ingredient. If your child has been advised to follow a soy-free diet because of a soy allergy, it is important to also avoid these foods.

Although pure soy oil should not cause an allergic reaction (technically, it contains no protein), there is a risk that it could have been contaminated with soy protein during the manufacturing process. To be safe, it makes sense to avoid soy oil in cases of soy allergy.

For children over the age of 2 years on a milk-free, soy-free diet, it is essential to find an acceptable milk alternative. We recommend a rice beverage fortified with calcium and vitamin D as the best alternative when cow's milk or fortified soy milk cannot be used.

## Egg allergy

Eggs are a terrific source of many nutrients, including energy, protein, fat, and vitamins such as riboflavin and vitamin $B_{12}$. However, there are many different types of protein in eggs – found primarily in the whites – to which some children may be allergic. Cooking can break down some of these proteins, in which case a child who is allergic to raw eggs may tolerate eggs when they are cooked. Keep in mind, however, that some egg proteins are not broken down during the cooking process, and can still cause an allergic reaction.

### *What's in that vaccine?*

Some vaccines for common illnesses contain traces of egg protein. If your child has an egg allergy, be sure to check with your doctor that a vaccine does not contain egg.

### Cooking without eggs

While an egg allergy can make it unsafe to eat commercially prepared foods (since so many egg ingredients are not clearly identified on food labels), it need not be a problem if you prepare the food yourself. For example, there are many recipes that call for eggs, but can be made egg-free by using egg substitutes. This allows children with egg allergies to enjoy foods (baked goods, say) that might otherwise be too risky for them to eat.

For egg-free baking and cooking, try some of the following substitutions for eggs in recipes.

WHERE EGG IS USED AS A LEAVENING AGENT. For each egg required, use

1 tbsp (15 mL) egg-free baking powder + 2 tbsp (25 mL) liquid

OR

2 tbsp (25 mL) flour + 1/2 tbsp (7 mL) egg-free baking powder + 2 tbsp (25 mL) liquid

You can make your own egg-free baking powder (see page 85) or buy an egg-free commercial variety (such as Magic brand). Use whatever liquid is appropriate for the recipe (water, vinegar, fruit juice, broth, etc.).

## EGG HUNTING

**Avoiding eggs on their own is fairly simple. But eggs or egg proteins may be hidden in many prepared foods, including baked goods, salad dressings and sauces. The following is a list of words that indicate the presence of egg protein in food.**

| | | | |
|---|---|---|---|
| albumin | mayonnaise | egg | egg powder |
| baking powder | egg powder | ovalbumin | ovoglobulin |
| egg white | egg protein | ovomucin | ovomucoid |
| egg yolk | frozen egg | ovovitellin | pasteurized egg |
| globulin | simplesse® | livetin | vitellin |

SOURCE: Vickerstaff-Joneja, J. *Managing Food Allergy and Intolerance: A Practical Guide*. 1995

For recipes that call for only 1 egg and a relatively large amount of baking powder (for example, 2 tsp [10 mL] baking powder or 1 1/2 tsp [7 mL] baking soda), try replacing the egg with 1 tbsp (15 mL) vinegar.

WHERE EGG IS USED AS A BINDER. For each egg required:

In a saucepan combine 1/3 cup (75 mL) water and 3 to 4 tsp (15 to 20 mL) brown flaxseeds. Bring to a boil; reduce heat and simmer for 5 to 7 minutes or until a slightly thickened gel begins to form. Strain through a sieve, discarding seeds. Use gel for egg in recipe.

OR use

1/3 cup (75 mL) water + 1 tbsp (15 mL) arrowroot powder + 2 tsp (10 mL) guar gum

OR use

2 oz (50 g) tofu

WHERE EGG IS USED AS A LIQUID. For each egg required use:

1/3 cup (75 mL) apple juice

OR

4 tbsp (60 mL) puréed apricot

OR

1 tbsp (15 mL) vinegar

TO MAKE EGG-FREE BAKING POWDER. Combine 1 part baking soda + 2 parts cream of tartar + 1 part cornstarch. Mix well and store in airtight container.

SOURCE: Vickerstaff-Joneja, J. Managing Food Allergy and Intolerance: A Practical Guide. 1995

### Egg-free eggs

Check out your local health food store for some of the "egg replacer" products that are now available. These products do not contain egg protein, which allows children with egg allergies to enjoy "eggs" for breakfast. Be sure you don't confuse these specialized egg-replacers with the low-cholesterol egg products commonly sold in grocery stores; they may be healthier, but they are *not* egg free.

## Peanut allergy

Of all food allergies, peanut allergy is one of the most dangerous, and a leading cause of anaphylactic reactions. Peanut allergy is a food allergy that affects 1 to 2% of the population. Unlike milk and egg allergies, it is one that most children do not outgrow.

Symptoms of peanut allergy may not necessarily be as serious as anaphylaxis, but can include: skin rash, eczema and hives; respiratory symptoms, such as wheezing; nausea or vomiting; and itching. Where the risk of anaphylactic reactions does exist, children with peanut allergies (or their parents and/or daycare providers) should carry an Epipen® – and should know how to inject it – in case of emergencies.

Children with peanut allergy are not necessarily allergic to all nuts, and may be able to eat other tree nuts – such as pecans, walnuts, and cashews – without effect. However, if your child has a peanut allergy, it is safer to avoid all nuts. Even when nuts are identified as being something other than peanuts (or, in the case of nut mixtures, as not containing peanuts), trace amounts may still exist. Also, be sure to read labels carefully for foods that "may contain" peanuts.

Avoid pure peanut oil which, although theoretically free of peanut protein, may also contain trace amounts. This type of oil is often used in Thai and Chinese cooking, so you may wish to avoid restaurants that serve this food. In fact, whenever dining out with an allergic child, it makes sense to call ahead and ask about any ingredients that may cause a reaction.

## Allergies and pregnancy

Can eating peanuts during pregnancy cause the unborn child to be allergic? While some have theorized that eating peanuts or other highly allergenic foods during pregnancy may cause allergies in infants and children, it is now thought to be unlikely. This is true even in cases where mothers have a strong family history of allergy.

Avoiding many foods during pregnancy can cause nutritional deficiencies, which is more likely to be dangerous to the fetus than any risk of developing an allergy. If the mother herself has an allergy, of course, she should continue to avoid the same allergenic foods that she did before becoming pregnant.

For mothers who are not necessarily allergic themselves, but have a strong family history of allergy and are very concerned about their babies developing food allergies, we suggest the following:

- Consume a well-balanced diet and do not eliminate foods during pregnancy (other than the foods to which the mother herself is allergic)
- Breastfeed exclusively for the first 4 to 6 months of life
- Avoid the consumption of peanuts or other nuts while breastfeeding, since the protein from these foods may cross into the breastmilk.
- Delay the introduction of solids or infant formula until at least 4 to 6 months

It is important to note that delaying the introduction of certain foods has not been shown to reduce food allergies. Such delays provide no guarantee that a child will not go on to develop a food allergy. Skin testing, and a food challenge under controlled conditions by an allergist, may be advised for those children who have a strong family history of allergy.

## Dealing with multiple food allergies

It is not common for children to be allergic to a number of foods. The majority are allergic to one food only, although some may be allergic to 2, 3 or 4 foods. Allergies to 5 or more foods are highly unusual and are more likely to be the result of incorrect diagnoses. The most common food reactions in infancy are those to milk and dairy products, eggs, soy, peanuts, nuts, wheat, fish and shellfish.

While it is important to eliminate all allergens from the child's diet, it is also necessary to ensure that proper alternatives are provided to meet the child's nutritional needs for growth. The elimination of many foods without cause can be dangerous. Allergy to a specific food should be confirmed before eliminating it from a child's diet, and should only be done under a physician's supervision. Occasionally, supplements may be required and dietary counseling may be beneficial for some families.

## Food intolerances

While there are different types of food intolerance (which is distinguished from food allergy by its not involving an immune response), one of the most common among children is lactose intolerance.

### Lactose intolerance

Unlike a milk allergy (where the immune system reacts to cow's milk protein), lactose intolerance is caused by a deficiency of lactase. This enzyme (located in the small intestine) is responsible for breaking down the sugar lactose, which is found in milk and milk products.

When lactose is not broken down, it builds up in the digestive system, causing excess water to be drawn into the intestines, which can cause diarrhea. Other symptoms include abdominal pain and discomfort. Bloating and gas are caused by the fermentation of lactose bacteria in the digestive tract.

Lactose intolerance in infancy is extremely rare (since lactose is present in breast milk). However, many people lose the ability to produce lactase later in life. This is most common among people of Asian, African-American and Mediterranean descent, up to 80% of whom lose the ability to digest lactose starting at around age 5 (compared to only 20% of people with Northern European ancestry).

The good news for anyone suffering from lactose intolerance is that there are many products available to make your life easier. By taking lactase supplements at mealtime (usually in pill form), you can enjoy dairy and other foods containing lactose without discomfort. Lactose-free milks are also available for those who are lactose intolerant.

CHAPTER 9

# Disturbances in bowel function

*Any parent will tell you that the bowel habits of their child has caused concern at some point in their lives. Indeed, the main point of discussion during routine visits to the family doctor or pediatrician is often focused on whether a child's bowel movements are too infrequent or too frequent. The information presented here may help parents to understand more (and worry less) about this subject.*

## Establishing patterns

During infancy, there is great variation in the frequency, color and consistency of bowel movements. This continues from the first few weeks of life to later months, when a wider variety of foods is introduced. By the age of 2, bowel patterns usually become established, with more regular and predictable consistency and number of movements per day. After this age, normal stools are soft and usually occur 1 or 2 times per day, although frequency may be less in some children. With the commencement of toilet training, however, and with other new routines – for example, when starting daycare – a change in bowel habits may be observed.

### How digestion works

When food is chewed and swallowed, it is mixed with juices in the stomach and ground down to very small particles. This mixture is then released into the small intestine, where digestion and absorption take place. Once it reaches the large intestine, or colon, the mixture moves much more slowly, and much of the water is "pulled" out.
Fiber in the diet, which allows the "undigested" material to reach the colon, results in a softer mass of stool by increasing its water content.

### Family ties

In addition to its other causes, the tendency to become constipated may also have a genetic component. As a result, parents who have had problems with bowel movements may find that their children have the same difficulty.

## Coping with constipation

Constipation occurs when there is reduced water content in the stool. When children are constipated, their stools, which are normally soft, become harder, usually larger in volume, and less frequent. It is estimated that this prompts some 3% of all visits to the general practitioner, and 15 to 25 % of pediatric gastroenterology consultations. Constipation may start out with only one or two episodes of withholding stools due to painful stooling. But if left untreated, the condition may become chronic and can last for years. Chronic constipation is believed to be one of the main causes of repeated abdominal pain in children.

## Causes of childhood constipation

Only a very small percentage of children become constipated as a result of disease or other "medical" factors. Rather, the causes are much more likely to be dietary or behavioral. Your family doctor will be able to evaluate the cause and sort out the best treatment for your child.

The most common causes of childhood constipation are dietary, behavioral (deliberately withholding stool), toilet training, and change in daily routine. When children begin to be toilet trained, they may "hold in" their stool so that they do not have to try to use the toilet, or sometimes they are "just too busy" to make the trip to the bathroom. When held in, the stool stays in the colon (the last part of large intestine) for a longer period, with the result that more water is drawn out of the stool and reabsorbed into the colon, thus making the stool drier and harder to pass. (Sometimes children who are constipated will have soiling in their underwear, which occurs when loose stool passes around the hard stool mass. Children are unable to withhold or control this loose stool.) The size of the stool becomes larger and this also makes it more difficult to pass. This is naturally distressing for the child, who may have already experienced a hard stool that was pushed out with great effort, resulting in both pain and, occasionally, a small amount of blood (from a small tear in the bowel wall). Constipation can result in abdominal pain and create a decrease in appetite which, in extreme cases, may result in weight loss.

## Methods of treatment

Experts agree that a number of factors can help relieve or reduce constipation and suggest a variety of treatments.

First, make sure the child's diet includes adequate amounts of fiber and fluid. If the child is not eating the recommended number of fresh vegetables and fruits, these should be increased (see page 40 for more information on sources of fiber). Encourage consumption of whole grain cereals and breads, along with plenty of water. If the child prefers a cereal that is low in fiber, mix it together with a higher-fiber variety.

Second, set a regular bowel routine to help improve training and decrease the straining. This involves setting a specific time each day to sit quietly on the toilet. If you wish, set up a system of rewards, such as a sticker chart to recognize successes, as well as other positive reinforcements.

Some fruit juices, such as prune and apple, contain higher-than-average amounts of sorbitol, a sugar that remains in the small intestine and moves to the large intestine (or colon), where it is broken down into smaller particles, which pull water back into the stool. This has the effect of softening the stool, making it easier to pass. It may be worthwhile to try giving a child juices that contain sorbitol in order to relieve constipation.

If constipation persists for a long period, your family doctor may recommend intervention with some form of laxative. Mineral oil is sometimes used for children older than 2 to 3 years. Lactulose and sorbitol are also considered to be safe and effective treatments. Always consult your family doctor before beginning any laxative treatment. Prolonged use of laxatives should be avoided, if possible, and then only under the supervision of your doctor.

If the stool is impacted (and the child is unable to pass it voluntarily), then an oral or rectal medication may be given, including an enema. Any non-dietary treatments should be given under the supervision of the family doctor. Prolonged use of any treatment should be evaluated on a regular basis by medical personnel. Once the stool is passed, encourage a regular bowel routine, as well as the regular consumption of adequate fluids and fiber.

If these therapies fail, or if it is suspected that the constipation is caused by factors other than behavioral or functional, or if management becomes complex, then the case should be referred to a specialist.

## Dealing with diarrhea

Childhood diarrhea is defined as a change in bowel pattern which can result in more frequent or looser, watery stools. Every year, about 16% of all children require a visit to the family doctor because of diarrhea – making it the most common of all reasons for seeing the doctor. Guidelines have been developed by a number of medical groups, including the American Academy of Pediatrics, on the appropriate treatment for diarrhea.

### *Rehydration solutions*

When children become dehydrated, they lose electrolytes (for example, sodium, potassium and chloride). To restore these compounds, a doctor may recommend using an electrolyte solution, which can be found in pharmacies and in many grocery stores.

## Causes and treatment of childhood diarrhea

The most frequent cause of acute (or sudden) diarrhea is viral infection. In these cases, stools may be more mucousy and have a distinctly different odor than usual. Viral illness causing diarrhea may also be accompanied by vomiting. Since dehydration is typically the result (a particularly dangerous condition for infants, because of their small size), the focus of treatment is on rehydration with fluids such as an appropriate electrolyte solution (see sidebar, page 92). Your family doctor will tell you the volume required for your child, as well as the period over which they should be given (usually 24 hours).

After rehydration, a normal diet – including milk and servings of all food groups – can and should be resumed, even with continued diarrhea. (Be sure to remain watchful for signs of dehydration; your doctor can tell you what to look for.) A child should not be offered only juices, for example, or plain cereals until the diarrhea subsides. This may only prolong their diarrhea and result in weight loss. Note that if vomiting is severe, a return to normal diet may have to be delayed until symptoms subside.

Sometimes diarrhea is caused by a carbohydrate or lactose intolerance (which itself may be the temporary result of viral illness). Lactose is a sugar found in milk which is normally broken down by an enzyme, called lactase, found in the wall of the intestine. When the supply of lactase is inadequate, the undigested lactose has the effect of "pulling" water through the intestine, causing watery and more frequent stools. In these cases, it may be advisable to give a child lactose-free milk. Your family doctor can advise you, if necessary, on the type of milk to choose.

Chronic diarrhea is less common, and may be caused by excessive juice intake. As an alternative to juice, children should be offered water between meals to quench their thirst. Daily juice consumption of more than 6 oz (175 mL) can result in a decreased appetite for foods that make up a varied diet; and this lack of variety can itself be a cause of diarrhea.

There are other causes of chronic diarrhea that may be medical. Your family doctor will investigate further if necessary.

### Are probiotics helpful?

Probiotics are "safe bacteria" that are used to treat certain conditions, such as gastrointestinal ailments. These bacteria are normally found in the human intestine. The theory behind the use of probiotics is that they can improve the immune response of the gut and protect it against the invasion of harmful bacteria or viruses. In other words, they may promote healing. Research results have not been conclusive. More studies will be required to determine how probiotics work, and to confirm whether they are beneficial.

CHAPTER 10

# Choking Hazards

*Between the ages of 2 and 6, children become much more adept at the art of self-feeding. They are better able to chew and swallow a wider range of foods with different textures, so the risk of choking is much less than when they were younger. Still, the risk is not entirely eliminated (in fact, it remains for people of all ages), and children can still choke on foods that are too hard, or not chewed well enough. In this chapter, we'll look at how you can minimize choking risks.*

## Still learning

As toddlers continue to learn new feeding skills, it is important to remember that they are still learning and are at high risk of choking from foods – or other small non-food items that may be around the house. Small children are more susceptible to choking than older children and adults. This is because their airways are smaller, and their teeth may have yet to emerge completely, with the result that infants and toddlers can swallow food before it is fully chewed.

## Safe feeding

Within the 2- to 6-year-old age group, the highest risk of choking is between the ages of 2 and 4 years. During this time, it is especially important that children be watched while eating. They should always be seated when eating a meal or snack, as this can prevent the sudden inhalation of

## Hard to swallow

**Foods you shouldn't give to children under 4 years old**

popcorn

cough drops

sunflower seeds

whole carrots

hard candies

whole raisins

fish with bones

chewing gum

peanuts/nuts

snacks with toothpicks /skewers

a food piece that is not yet chewed. (It's also easier to keep an eye on them if they are seated in one place.)

While we have listed many of the higher-risk foods to avoid (see sidebar, at left), use your common sense to determine which items are safe. Many can present a danger, including foods such as hard carrots (when bitten in large pieces), as well as whole grapes or hot dog round slices which, although soft, can block a young child's airway if swallowed without chewing.

## Choking-prevention strategies

How can you minimize a child's risk of choking? Here are some important tips.

- Avoid giving foods considered unsafe to children who are less than 4 years of age. (See sidebar.) Or modify unsafe foods – by slicing hotdogs lengthwise, for example, or by grating carrots, quartering grapes and chopping sticky foods such as dates.
- Give children foods and beverages only if they are sitting upright. Do not provide liquid in a bottle while they are lying down; they may choke on the fluid.
- Children should not be force-fed.
- For young children who do not yet have their incisors or primary molars, be sure to cut food into small pieces.
- A child should always be sitting while eating. Do not let toddlers walk (and especially run) around while eating.
- Always watch your toddler while eating. The risk of choking can be minimized if parents and caregivers are aware of their toddlers' chewing and swallowing abilities, and are able to react quickly at the first signs of choking.
- Choose toys that are appropriate for your child's age. Keep him or her away from older children's toys, which may be unsafe.
- Most importantly, be prepared to help children in the event that they do choke. Learn how to perform the Heimlich maneuver – and other first-aid techniques. If you don't know how to provide this assistance, contact your local community center or the Red Cross to organize a training session.

CHAPTER 11

# Childhood Obesity

*For the first few years of life, weight gain is both healthy and desirable for children. But after the age of 3, a child who is significantly heavier than his or her peers may be heading for a weight problem. Throughout this book, we have stressed that children should never be put on a "diet" which restricts food intake in order to promote weight loss. And we continue to stress this. What we would add, however, is that weight problems can and should be avoided by teaching your child the importance of healthy living (which includes eating and exercise) from an early age.*

## Kids are getting fatter

Childhood obesity is the most common nutritional problem among children in North America today. It has been estimated that, of all school-aged children, about 14% are now obese, while another 11% are overweight and at risk of becoming obese. While the incidence of obesity among younger children (in the age range for this book) is not as high, the trend also points upward.

In 1998, the World Health Organization declared obesity a "global epidemic" for both adults and children. Obese children have an increased risk of developing childhood hyperinsulinemia (which may be a risk factor for the development of non-insulin dependent diabetes mellitus), as well as high blood pressure and dyslipidemia (abnormal blood cholesterol levels).

With each year after the age of 3, the probability that an obese child will become an obese adult continues to increase. It is generally estimated that overweight children are twice as likely to be obese as adults when compared with children who are not overweight. This risk increases when one or more of the child's parents are also overweight.

The health risks of obesity in adulthood are well known. Obesity has been associated with high blood pressure, high cholesterol, non-insulin dependent diabetes mellitus, some cancers (including colon, breast and pancreatic), skin disorders, orthopedic conditions and other psychosocial illnesses, including depression.

## Prevention is the key

Once a child (or adult) becomes obese, experience has shown that treatment programs often prove ineffective for long-term weight management. Therefore, prevention is the key.

The early childhood years are the best time to prevent obesity, since this is when lifestyle behaviors are being established. Poor dietary and activity habits have not yet been formed, and parents continue to have an influence over the lifestyle of their children. The question is: How do we prevent obesity in children without causing them to become obsessed (as so many adults are) with their weight? Here we recommend the following four fundamental strategies: encourage healthy eating habits; maintain physical activity; establish a positive outlook towards food and eating; and encourage a positive body image.

## Healthy eating habits

The hectic lifestyle experienced by today's families makes it challenging to develop healthy eating habits – for adults and children. Families dine out more than they did in previous generations, and may make less nutritious choices. When families dine in, they may often choose prepackaged meals or convenience foods because some parents have less time to cook and have busy schedules that continue once they get home from work.

All these things do not escape the notice of young children who, unlike infants (typically fed on their own schedules), are now joining the family for meals. Therefore, it is important for parents to set a good example and choose healthy foods and meals for the entire family.

Parents' eating habits and beliefs mold children's food preferences and eating patterns. If parents follow healthy eating patterns, their children will likely follow. If parents have poor eating habits, then that is what children will accept as the norm. Children also pay attention to the foods that come home from the grocery store, so it is important that moms and dads make healthy choices when they go to the market.

Severe restrictions should not be placed on the consumption of high-energy and/or high-fat foods for young children. Turning any kind of food into a "forbidden fruit" may simply focus the child's attention on that food and make it more desirable. Nutrient-dense, high-energy or higher-fat foods play an important role in a growing child's diet. Nutritious food choices should not be eliminated or severely restricted in a young child's diet simply because of their fat content.

### *Born to eat junk food?*

While it has been said that young children have an innate preference for high-sugar or high-fat foods, there is no evidence to suggest this. Children can learn to like healthy, nutritious foods just as easily as sweets or other junk foods.

### Putting Fat into Perspective

Thanks to widespread media reports, it is now almost accepted wisdom that a high-fat diet is bad for your health and causes obesity. The fact is that no single nutrient causes obesity, although consuming an excess number of total calories (in relation to activity) certainly will. Nutrition experts suggest that healthy individuals should derive no more than 30% of the calories in the diet from fat and no more than 10% of calories from saturated fat. But these figures are intended for older children and adults. Infants tend to have a higher-fat diet, in which approximately 50% of calories come from fat. Many health authorities now recommend a slow, gradual transition from the high-fat diet of infancy to the lower-fat diet of an adult. This transition should take place from the age of 2 years until a child has reached his or her full height potential at the end of adolescence. During this transition period, energy intake should be adequate to support normal growth and development.

As you help to develop healthy eating habits in your children, remember that there are no "good" or "bad" foods. It is the overall diet that is important. Kids need a variety of nutrient-rich foods throughout the day. These foods should include grains, cereals, fruit and vegetables, lower- and full-fat milk products (or other calcium-rich foods), as well as protein-rich foods such as beans, lean meats, poultry, or fish.

## Physical activity

Young children tend to be naturally active, and enjoy playing and running about. As they get older and start preschool or grade school, it is important that they continue to be active. Yet with technological advances and societal changes, today's children have become generally less active, spending more time participating in sedentary activities such as watching television or playing computer games. In fact, it has been estimated that young children in North America today expend about 25% fewer calories than current recommendations for caloric intake. And when more energy is consumed than expended, it is stored as fat.

Apart from television and computer games, there are other societal factors that contribute to the decline in children's activity levels. Today's parents are generally more safety-conscious (or risk averse) than those of previous generations. As a result, children who were once free to play outdoors at every opportunity now have their activity restricted to supervised recreational activities and playgrounds – which may or may not be available for much of the time. Some school-aged children may come home after school to an empty house until mom or dad comes home from work. These "latch key" children are often forbidden to play outside by parents because of safety concerns.

### Activity for life

Encouraging physical activity does not mean embarking on an ambitious fitness program. Instead, it should be seen as a program of maintenance – taking familiar activities (such as walking) and making them part of your (and your child's) life. Maintaining an active lifestyle is always easier than trying to make big changes to lifestyle habits.

### A FAMILY THAT PLAYS TOGETHER...

Spontaneous physical activity should be a part of daily life for children. These lifestyle activities are easier to sustain than regimented exercise programs. Children are more likely to continue with an activity if they are allowed to choose an activity in which they are interested, rather than having one chosen for them. Forcing children to exercise can decrease chances of success.

Parents should participate in activities with their children. This provides a wonderful opportunity for parents to spend time with their children and increases the physical activity of the entire family. Activities may include things such as family walks or bike rides. Research has shown that parents who are inactive tend to have children who are inactive. Likewise, parents who enjoy an active lifestyle tend to have children who also enjoy being active.

Other strategies for maintaining physical activity may include encouraging children to reduce time spent in sedentary pursuits. Limits should be set on the amount of television watched and computer games played. Research has shown that setting these limits can be just as (or more) effective as trying to get kids to go outside and exercise.

## Overcoming the power of television

**Body and soul**

Too much television can have a negative effect on body image, nutrition and dieting behaviors of young children and adolescents.

It has been estimated that the average North American child watches approximately 3 hours of television per day. When combined with computer games and other physically undemanding activities involving other media (watching movies, for example), this figure may be in excess of 6 hours per day. The exposure of American children and adolescents to television is estimated to exceed the time they spend in the classroom: By the time they graduate, children will have spent an average of 12,000 hours in the classroom and 15,000 hours in front of a television set.

Studies have shown a significant link between television watching and the prevalence of obesity. The time spent watching television or other media can displace other activities that are more enriching for the mind and body, including reading, exercise and playing with friends.

Television can also cause an increase in between-meal snacking. Children may snack on less nutritious foods while watching television and may not be aware of how much they are actually eating.

Commercials also affect a child's eating patterns by encouraging the consumption of foods advertised on television. Television advertising has been shown to influencing a parent's grocery-store purchases, often because children make requests for specific foods. Even brief exposures to televised food commercials have been shown to have an influence on the food preferences of young children. Commercials typically aired during children's programming are often for calorically dense foods such as sugared breakfast cereals, chocolate bars, cakes, cookies and soda pop. One recent Australian study found that 63% of food advertisements during children's programming were for high-fat and/or high-sugar foods.

While there are some worthwhile, educational benefits of watching television – including the promotion of many positive social behaviors such as sharing, manners and cooperation – there are also many negative health effects, apart from increasing the prevalence of obesity. These include the depiction (not always unfavorably) of violent or aggressive behavior, substance use and abuse, sexual activity, as well as decreased school performance. A recent US study found that 32% of children between the ages of 2 and 7 years old have a television in their bedroom. In such cases, it is not surprising that parents are often not aware of what their children are watching, or that they do not limit the amount of television their children watch. Many young children are not able to distinguish between what they see on television and what is real, and children's programs can be some of the most violent on television.

Both the American and Canadian Pediatric Societies have published suggestions for parents regarding the television that their children watch. These suggestions for parents include:

- Limiting television viewing to a maximum of 1 to 2 hours per day
- Emphasizing alternative activities, including reading, athletics, hobbies and creative play
- Participating in the selection of programs to be viewed
- Watching TV with children and discussing it with them
- Being a good media role model for children
- Removing television sets from children's and adolescent's bedrooms
- Avoiding using the television as an "electronic babysitter"

## Positive outlook towards food and eating

How you as a parent help to shape your child's attitudes towards eating and towards his or her body image could be the most important factor in preventing obesity and other eating disturbances.

### The proper role of food

Food should not be used as a tool for reward, bribery or punishment. Parents will often use tactics to get kids to eat, to calm temper tantrums or to promote good behavior. Examples include "Eat all your vegetables and then you may go and watch television" or "If you stop fighting with your sister, you may have a cookie." These feeding techniques can result in children who have a poor ability to regulate their caloric intake, and may contribute to overeating behavior and obesity.

Children's food preferences are influenced when foods are related to performing non-food related tasks. For example, the child who is offered a cookie to stop fighting with his sister learns that a cookie must be a really good thing if he is rewarded with it. Likewise, children often learn to dislike certain foods that they are required to eat in order to obtain non-food related rewards. For example, the child who is made to eat her vegetables before she can watch television learns that a vegetable must be a terrible thing to eat, if she must be bribed to do so. (This also reinforces the perceived value of television watching.)

### Food is not a controlled substance

Parents should not try to control their child's food intake. Those who attempt to control their child's eating patterns are more likely to have children who are less capable of self-regulating their caloric intake. In other words, their children are less aware of using hunger to determine their eating habits – specifically, that they should eat when they are hungry and stop eating when they are full. Controlling a child's eating patterns includes forcing children to eat when they are told to, and to "eat what's on your plate."

Parents should provide healthy food choices, but must allow their children to assume control of their own intake. This can be difficult, since it is often tempting to place severe restrictions on a child's access to palatable foods that may be high in fat or sugar. While this may seem to be an easy, straightforward way of decreasing the intake of these foods, it only focuses more attention on these "forbidden" foods, and can increase a child's desire to obtain and eat them. Ultimately, the strategy is self-defeating.

### Mothers and daughters

Between moms and dads, it is mothers who appear to play a particularly important role in determining whether or not their daughters will develop diet and other eating problems. This is especially true in the case of mothers who attempt to control their own weight or have a history of dieting. Some studies have suggested that daughters of "dieting mothers" have a comparable focus on dieting themselves. Parents must remember that their own dieting behavior influences their daughter's ideas and beliefs about dieting.

## Promoting a positive body image

Parents who are concerned about their own body image or their child's weight need to be especially careful. It has been suggested that young girls, even as early as 5 years old, are more likely to develop a more negative self-perception of their weight when their parents are concerned about their own body image or their daughter's weight. One study found that parental concern about their child's weight – and the restriction of specific foods as a result – was associated with negative self-evaluations by young children.

Concerned parents often criticize their children (either directly or indirectly) or exert strict control over the types or quantities of foods to which their children have access. While their intent is well-meaning – that is, to encourage a behavior change, foster healthy eating habits or prevent an increase in weight gain – these attempts at control only send a message to children that their weight status is undesirable and that they are not capable of controlling their own eating habits. These messages, especially when the child is visibly overweight, can cause a child to have a poor body image and sense of self.

Research has shown that by 6 years of age, children have learned societal messages that say being overweight is undesirable. This can be especially detrimental to children who are already overweight, since these children are at an increased risk of having psychosocial problems that may persist into adulthood. Children need to be encouraged to have a positive body image and to be reassured about the range of healthy and acceptable body weights and shapes. Children also need to feel valued for their abilities and talents – not just their appearance – if they are to foster a positive self-image.

CHAPTER 12

# Daycare and nutrition

*When a child starts going to daycare (or some other facility outside the home) and, eventually, to school, the important role of feeding the child is no longer exclusively that of the parent. Instead, it becomes shared with outside providers, who will also have an influence on your child's attitudes towards food and nutrition. In this chapter, we'll look at some of the issues involved, and how you can ensure that your child eats healthy meals away from home.*

## Eating away from home

Working parents are a fact of modern life. It is a reality for approximately 30 to 40% of American households. And finding the right kind of care for your child can be a most stressful time. Once the daycare setting is selected, many parents assume that the nutritional needs of their children will be met by experienced individuals who have a good knowledge about nutrition. Although this may be true in many instances, research indicates that it is not always so.

It is up to the parent to become familiar with the menus and other specific choices of foods offered to their child. This is important because, as parents in one study indicated, a childcare setting is equal to, if not more important than, home for establishing specific food likes and dislikes.

Typically, where children are enrolled in a full-time program of 8 hours a day, a daycare facility provides about 50 to 60% of a child's daily energy needs. In other words, a majority of nutrients are consumed away from the watchful eye of the parent.

### Shared failings

As one study has revealed, daycare facilities are not always exclusively to blame for failing to provide adequate nutrition for a child. In this study, which set out to evaluate the intake of children both at home and at the daycare, it was discovered that in either setting, the intake of vegetables was inadequate. There was an overconsumption of foods containing fat, oils and sweets while the children were at home, and there was inadequate intake of breads and cereals while at the daycare. For parents who want to ensure that their child is properly nourished, home is the place to start.

It is essential to appreciate the importance of providing children with a varied diet, and that foods given at the daycare and at home must complement each other. If one food group is not taken well in one setting, then it should be encouraged in the other. Of course, it is possible to offer a variety of foods from all food groups if the nutrition program at the daycare and at home are balanced and well planned. (In fact, nutrition standards for daycare programs have been published by the American Dietetic Association.)

Here are some things you can do to ensure that you are familiar with what your child consumes.

- Check the menu each week. For the first few weeks, look at the menu and review the food choices offered, both at mealtimes and for snacks. If you have any questions about why certain foods are not offered, ask the director of the daycare. Find out how the menu selection was evaluated, and who was involved in the decision making.
- Monitor your child's intake. If you are concerned about your child's intake, ask the daycare to keep a record of what he or she eats each day – at least for the first few weeks of care.
- Ask about fruits and vegetables. Ensure that there are plenty of fresh fruits and vegetables offered, and that they are age-appropriate (for chewing and swallowing).
- What are they drinking? Make sure that the daycare provides water as the main beverage of choice and that juice is limited. Where fruit beverages are served, make sure that they are fruit juices – not fruits drinks, which are not as nutritious and typically contain more added sugar.
- Check out the snack menu. Evaluate the type and quality of the snacks provided. Are they nutritious?
- Offer a complementary menu at home. Daycare facilities obviously can't tailor their menus to the needs of each child's family, so take the initiative and complement the foods offered at the daycare with the meals that you provide at home. If pasta was served at the daycare, try to provide something different for supper.

- What is your child learning about nutrition? Find out if the daycare offers any type of education about nutrition and health. If so, what is being taught?

## School meal programs

Research indicates that students who eat breakfast and are well nourished do better academically. They have longer attention spans and have been shown to have fewer academic and behavior problems than children who are hungry.

A recent Minnesota state study demonstrated that children who ate breakfast had higher scores in math and reading. Other studies have shown that children who are not hungry demonstrate less irritability, anxiety and aggression. Such children are also less likely to be late or absent from school.

### *Critical nutrients*

While all nutrients are important to a child's health, one study of children's intakes at daycare has suggested that the nutrients of greatest concern were iron, zinc and energy. See pages 50 and 55 for information on foods that contain adequate amounts of iron and zinc.

In Canada, although there are no federally funded school breakfast or lunch programs, many schools do have cafeteria-style facilities which offer food choices at economical prices. It is up to parents and the school system to ensure that children are educated about making healthy food choices for themselves.

In the US, there are federally funded Breakfast and Lunch Programs, which are administered by Food and Nutrition Services of the United States Department of Agriculture (USDA). The mandate of these programs is to provide nutritionally balanced meals and snacks at low cost (or no cost) to children in public schools, not-for-profit private schools, and residential childcare facilities. Both programs must meet the recommendations of the Dietary Guidelines for Americans, which state that no more of 30% of the day's calories come from fat, and no more than 10% of the day's calories come from saturated fat.

The School Breakfast Program started in 1966 as a pilot project and has been a permanent program since 1975. It is currently available in more than 72,000 schools and institutions across the US. As mandated by the program, the breakfast must provide at least one-quarter of the recommended dietary allowances (RDAs) for energy, protein, calcium, iron, as well as vitamins A and C. In the year 2000, the school breakfast program provided a morning meal each day to an average of 7.55 million American children. In 2001, congress appropriated US$1.5 billion for the school breakfast program.

The National School Lunch Program (NSLP) provides lunches and snacks to even more children than the school breakfast program. In 2000, the NSLP provided nutritionally balanced lunches and snacks to more than 27 million children each day. The lunches must provide at least one-third of the RDA for energy, protein, iron, calcium as well as vitamins A and C. Although these school lunches must meet federal nutrition requirements, the school boards or institutions themselves are able to make their own decisions about specific foods to serve.

CHAPTER 13

# Dental Care *for kids*

*By the time children reach the age of 2 years, most of their teeth have come in, except for the second molars. Teeth do not begin to fall out until children are about 6 years of age, usually starting with the teeth that were first to come in. During this period, dental hygiene is important, even though many of the child's teeth are not permanent.*

## Keeping teeth clean

Dental hygiene involves brushing teeth at least twice a day – in the morning and evening – as well as after eating any foods that are sweet and sticky. Encourage your child to drink water after meals and snacks. This is a good habit to develop, since it helps to clean out the mouth and rinses teeth of leftover food. If the mouth is not cleansed properly, bacteria in the mouth digest the carbohydrate from foods – which can come from many sources, including milk, juice or sweets – and create an acid that leads to tooth decay.

Frequent sipping of juice can cause cavities by providing a constant supply of carbohydrate or sugar to newly developing teeth. As recommended by the American Pediatric Society, limit juice to a maximum of 6 oz (175 mL) per day and offer water as the child's primary beverage.

## Nursing bottle syndrome

When an infant or child falls asleep with a bottle – typically containing milk or juice – in his or her mouth, it can lead to something called "nursing bottle syndrome." This is believed to occur in 3 to 6% of children under 4 years of age. The syndrome involves deterioration of the front teeth because of prolonged exposure to carbohydrates in the mouth, causing bacterial action that results in tooth decay.

While it's true that a bottle is helpful in soothing a child, it should contain water. Early exposure of an infant or child to water will encourage him or her to accept it as a replacement for milk at bedtime. Studies reveal that a child who wakes up crying more frequently at night is at higher risk of nursing bottle syndrome, because soothing techniques used by parents may include giving milk or juice in a bottle. Some parents are not aware of the syndrome, or believe it is only milk that can cause tooth decay.

### Water? What's that?

Excessive juice consumption may seem like a relatively new phenomenon (about the same age as the juice box) but, as early as 1957, a study reported that 29% of children between the ages of 6 months and 5 years had never had a drink of plain water! Since then the situation has not improved: A recent study in the UK of 2- to 7-year-olds showed that, over a 48-hour period, 50 to 70% never drank plain water, but consumed milk, juice, sweetened drinks and other beverages. The message to parents: Encourage your child to drink water!

## Teaching children to brush

Children between the ages of 2 and 6 can learn to brush their own teeth, and brushing skills will improve with age. Only a small amount of toothpaste, less than the size of a pea, is needed. Once the child has finished brushing, parents should follow with a quick brush to ensure that cleaning is thorough. (Be sure to encourage your child to spit out the toothpaste.)

Toothpaste should provide all the necessary fluoride protection when combined with municipal water supplies that contain fluoride concentrations of at least 0.6 ppm (parts per million). If the drinking water contains less than this concentration, fluoride supplements are necessary. If you are unsure about the fluoridation of your drinking water, check with your family doctor or dentist, or your local water company.

### Finding fluoride

Your local water supply is just one source of fluoride. You can also find it in a number of commercial beverages and foods.

Too much fluoride can lead to a condition known as fluorosis. In severe cases, this can cause a brownish discoloration of the teeth – although it is not considered a health risk. Infants are more susceptible to fluorosis than older children. To regulate fluoride consumption, encourage children to limit the use of toothpaste to a pea size, not to swallow any, to spit out excess toothpaste, and to rinse well with water after each brushing. Another option is to choose a children's toothpaste without fluoride.

CHAPTER 14

# Food to Go

*Traveling with a young child presents many challenges – not the least of which is ensuring that their nutritional needs are being met throughout the duration of the trip. The possible effects of food and water from unfamiliar sources may also cause problems. Still, you shouldn't let these things keep you at home. Here are some practical tips on how to feed your child when traveling.*

WATER. Depending on your destination, you may have to purchase bottled water. Always check the water safety of any country you are visiting – and remember that the quality of water is not guaranteed just because it's in a bottle. Be sure to purchase bottled water from a reliable source. Even if the drinking water is considered to be safe, you may want to purchase bottled water to be sure it is safe for you and your children. Your travel agent should be able to provide you with information on the water in the area being visited. Keep in mind that water quality can vary even between different parts of the US and Canada.

FRESH FRUITS AND VEGETABLES. Fresh produce is usually available in most countries, although specific varieties will obviously vary according to the country, climate and season. This is a good opportunity to try different fruits and vegetables with your child. If you are unsure about the quality of the drinking water in the area, take the same caution with produce; peel the fruit or vegetables before serving. Also, just because you are eating in a restaurant, this does not mean that the vegetables used in a salad (for example) have been rinsed with "safe water." When in a foreign country where food contamination is a risk, be careful of the food choices you make when eating out.

DRINKING TO RELIEVE THE PRESSURE. When the plane in which they are traveling is landing or descending, some young children may experience earaches as the pressure in the cabin is adjusted. Try to offer a beverage during this part of the travel, so that your child is swallowing constantly, which may help to prevent the pressure changes from causing any problems. Older children can be offered gum to keep them chewing and swallowing.

**Food for car trips.** Ensure that you always have some snacks to offer, since mealtimes may not be as regular as they are at home. Try bringing containers of your child's favorite cereal mix or plain cookies for the trip. Offer plenty of fluids, especially if travelling in hot weather. (You may forget to drink adequate fluids yourself, and not be aware of your child's fluid needs.) For younger children, provide fluids in a spill-proof cup. When traveling by car, the best foods to bring are those that are easy to eat and not too messy – such as soft cheese, cookies and fruit pieces. To minimize the risk of choking, make sure that someone is observing your child while he or she is snacking. Children are more likely to choke when traveling by car, which can hit unexpected bumps in the road, or come to a stop suddenly. If possible, stop the car before consuming snacks. It is always handy to keep wet wipes in the car.

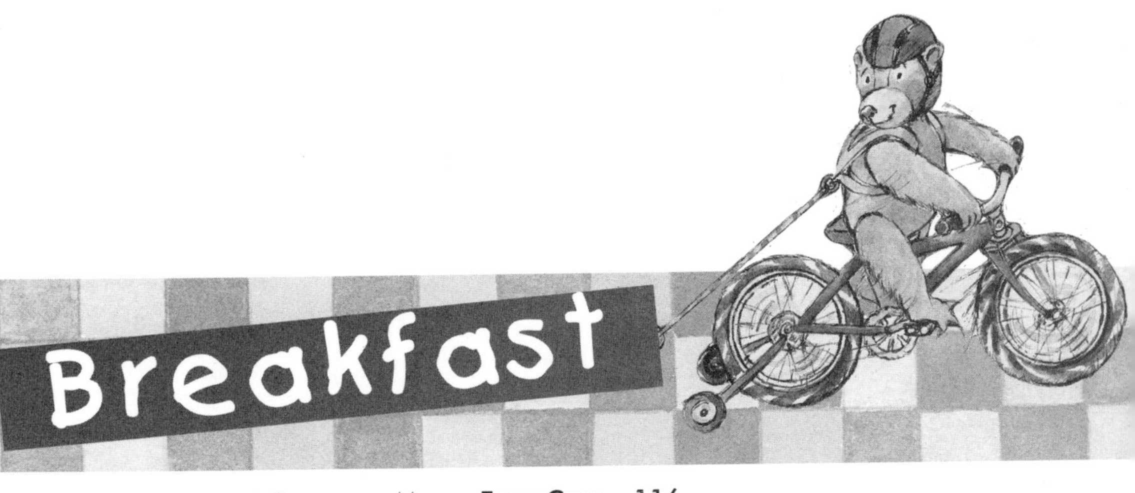


# Breakfast

# Grape and Melon Fruit Cups

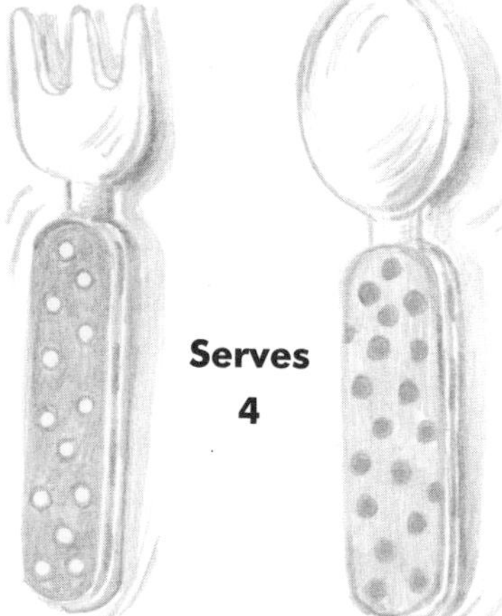

**Serves 4**

*Fruit dishes don't get much simpler (or more delicious) than this.*

| | | |
|---|---|---|
| 1 cup | seedless grapes (see Safety Tip, at left) | 250 mL |
| Half | cantaloupe, seeded, peeled and cut into bite-size pieces | Half |
| 2/3 cup | water | 150 mL |
| 1 to 2 tbsp | granulated sugar | 15 to 25 mL |
| 1 tsp | ground ginger | 5 mL |

1. Arrange fruit into 4 small serving cups.
2. In a small saucepan over high heat, combine water and sugar; cook, stirring, until sugar dissolves and light syrup forms. Stir in ginger. Remove syrup from heat and allow to cool before pouring over fruit.

### Safety Tip

To minimize the risk of choking for children under the age of 4, you may wish to cut whole grapes in half.

### Kitchen Tip

Try this dish with any combination of fruit your children enjoy, such as pears and mandarin oranges.

If you wish, omit the syrup in Step 2.

| Nutritional Analysis | Energy | Protein | Carbohydrate | Fat | Calcium | Iron |
|---|---|---|---|---|---|---|
| per serving | 75 kcal | 0.9 g | 18.7 g | 0.5 g | 2 % CDV | 3 % CDV |

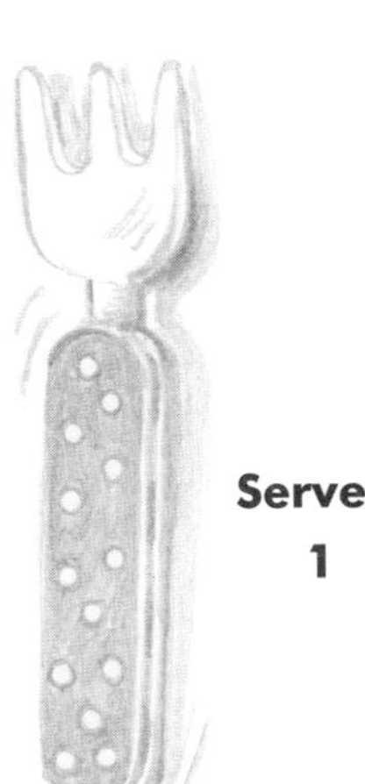

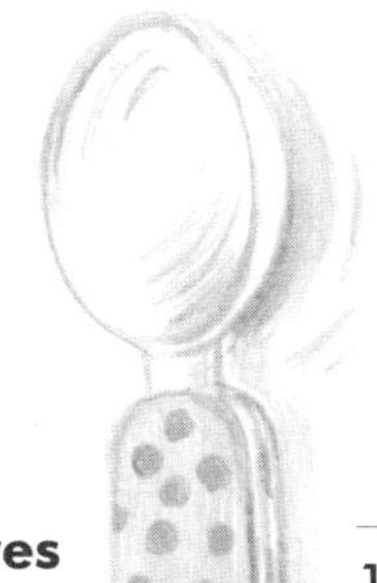

# Creamy Breakfast Fruit Mix

**Serves 1**

*Try this easy and delicious dish using one or more of your child's favorite fruits. Add toast squares and you've got a healthy breakfast.*

| | | |
|---|---|---|
| 1/4 cup | cottage cheese | 50 mL |
| 2 tbsp | sour cream (see Tip, at left) | 25 mL |
| 1/4 cup | chopped fresh fruit (such as orange, pineapple, banana, apple, strawberry, kiwifruit, peach or pear) | 50 mL |
| Pinch | brown sugar | Pinch |
| Pinch | ground cinnamon | Pinch |

1. In a small bowl, stir together cottage cheese, sour cream and fruit. Sprinkle with brown sugar and cinnamon.

### Kitchen Tip

Instead of sour cream, try using plain or fruit-flavored yogurt.

### Food Safety Tip

To avoid spoilage, be sure to store perishable foods in the refrigerator (set no higher than 40° F [4° C]) or in the freezer.

| Nutritional Analysis | Energy | Protein | Carbohydrate | Fat | Calcium | Iron |
|---|---|---|---|---|---|---|
| per serving | 305 kcal | 10.1 g | 59.2 g | 5.8 g | 16 % CDV | 16 % CDV |

# Homemade Fruit Yogurt

**Makes 2 cups (500 mL)**

*Delicious served by itself, this yogurt is also wonderful served over cottage cheese, or with pancakes or waffles. Youngsters love it as a dip for fresh fruit.*

| | | |
|---|---|---|
| 1 cup | raspberries or sliced strawberries or sliced peaches | 250 mL |
| 1 tbsp | granulated sugar | 15 mL |
| 1 tbsp | frozen orange juice concentrate | 15 mL |
| 1 cup | plain yogurt | 250 mL |
| | Fresh fruit, such as mandarin orange sections, whole strawberries, banana chunks, apple or pear slices | |

1. In a food processor or blender, purée fruit with sugar and orange juice until smooth. Transfer mixture to a microwave-safe container.
2. Microwave, covered, on High for 2 minutes or until warm and sugar is dissolved. Cool before whisking in yogurt. Serve as a topping or sauce or as a dip with a variety of fruit.

| Nutritional Analysis | Energy | Protein | Carbohydrate | Fat | Calcium | Iron |
|---|---|---|---|---|---|---|
| per 1/2-cup (125 mL) serving | 72 kcal | 3.7 g | 12.2 g | 1.2 g | 16 % CDV | 2 % CDV |

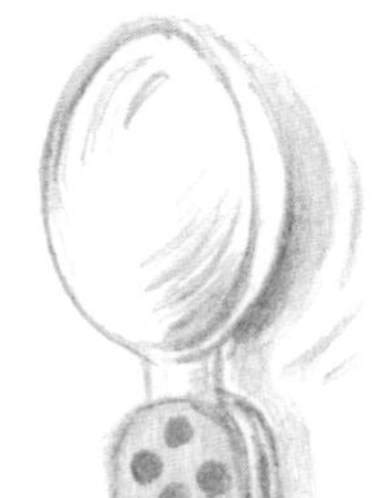

# Spiced Bananas

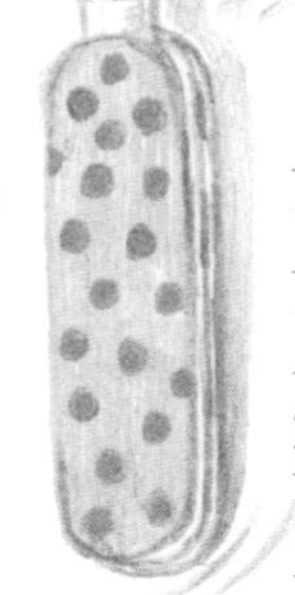

**Serves 4**

*Here's a zesty variation on bananas that will start your child's day (and yours) with a bang. Serve alone, with a slice of toast on the side, or as an accompaniment to pancakes or toaster waffles.*

| | | |
|---|---|---|
| 1/4 cup | orange juice | 50 mL |
| 1 tsp | grated orange zest | 5 mL |
| 2 tbsp | cream cheese | 25 mL |
| Pinch | ground cinnamon | Pinch |
| Pinch | ground ginger | Pinch |
| 1/4 cup | liquid honey | 50 mL |
| 4 | medium bananas, cut into slices | 4 |

1. In a bowl with an electric mixer, combine orange juice and zest, cream cheese, cinnamon and ginger; beat until smooth. Transfer mixture to a large nonstick skillet. Add honey and cook, stirring, over medium heat until mixture is warm and thoroughly blended.
2. Add bananas to skillet; cook, turning slices frequently, until bananas are softened and warm. Serve banana slices topped with some sauce.

| NUTRITIONAL ANALYSIS | Energy | Protein | Carbohydrate | Fat | Calcium | Iron |
|---|---|---|---|---|---|---|
| per serving | 188 kcal | 1.8 g | 43.5 g | 2.7 g | 2 % CDV | 6 % CDV |

# Breakfast Fruit Smoothie

**Makes 2 cups (500 mL)**

*This fast and delicious beverage is a breakfast favorite at our house. It also makes a great snack.*

| | | |
|---|---|---|
| 1 cup | 2% milk | 250 mL |
| 1/2 cup | fresh or frozen strawberries or raspberries | 125 mL |
| 1 tbsp | liquid honey | 15 mL |
| 1/2 cup | vanilla-flavored yogurt | 125 mL |
| 1 tbsp | wheat germ | 15 mL |

1. In a blender process milk and fruit until very smooth. (If there are too many seeds, strain through a sieve, discard seeds and return mixture to blender.) Add honey, yogurt and wheat germ; process until smooth. Pour into glasses and serve.

| Nutritional Analysis | Energy | Protein | Carbohydrate | Fat | Calcium | Iron |
|---|---|---|---|---|---|---|
| per 1/2-cup (125 mL) serving | 85 kcal | 4.5 g | 12.8 g | 2.0 g | 18 % CDV | 4 % CDV |

# Strawberry-Banana Smoothie

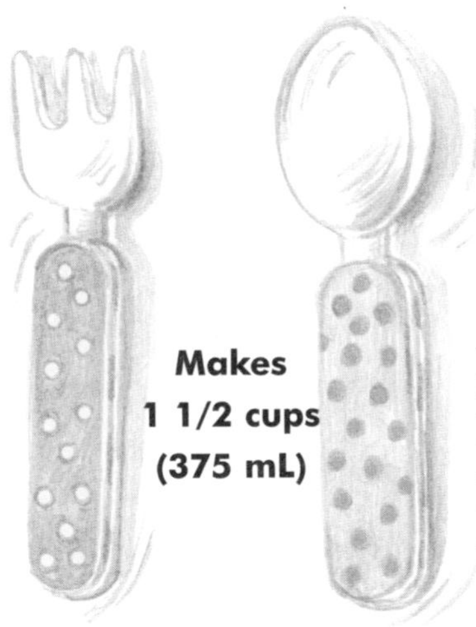

**Makes 1 1/2 cups (375 mL)**

*Smoothies are what you get from blending just about any fruit or fruits with a dairy product such as milk or yogurt. This combination is one of our favorites.*

| | | |
|---|---|---|
| 3/4 cup | sliced strawberries | 175 mL |
| 1 | small banana, sliced | 1 |
| 1/2 cup | plain yogurt | 125 mL |
| 1/4 cup | orange juice | 50 mL |
| 2 tbsp | granulated sugar | 25 mL |
| 1/2 tsp | vanilla extract | 2 mL |

1. In a blender process strawberries, banana, yogurt and orange juice until very smooth. Add sugar and vanilla; process until blended. Pour into glasses and serve.

| NUTRITIONAL ANALYSIS | Energy | Protein | Carbohydrate | Fat | Calcium | Iron |
|---|---|---|---|---|---|---|
| per 1/2-cup (125 mL) serving | 103 kcal | 2.9 g | 21.9 g | 1.0 g | 11 % CDV | 3 % CDV |

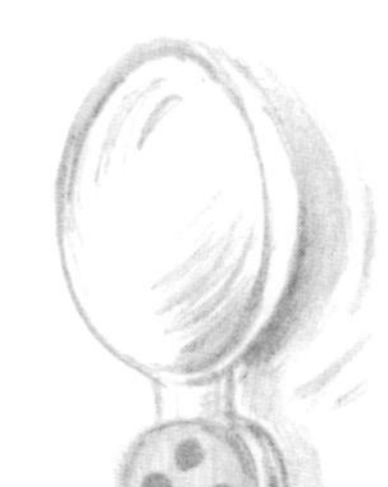

# Homemade Pancake Mix

**Makes about 3 cups (750 mL)**

| | | |
|---|---|---|
| 1 cup | rolled oats | 250 mL |
| 1 1/2 cups | whole wheat flour | 375 mL |
| 1/2 cup | skim milk powder | 125 mL |
| 2 tbsp | wheat germ | 25 mL |
| 2 tbsp | brown sugar | 25 mL |
| 4 tsp | baking powder | 20 mL |
| 1/2 tsp | baking soda | 2 mL |
| 1/2 tsp | salt | 2 mL |

*Preparing your own pancake mix is easy – and rewarding since, unlike commercial mixes, you know exactly what's in it.*

1. In a food processor, process oats until finely ground. Add flour, milk powder, wheat germ, brown sugar, baking powder, baking soda and salt. Process until thoroughly mixed and transfer to an airtight container. Store mix in refrigerator for up to 2 weeks or freeze for up to 3 months.

**KITCHEN TIP**

Serve pancakes with maple syrup or our Tangy Fruit Sauce (see recipe, page 268).

## COOKING PANCAKES FROM A MIX

**Makes 6 large or 10 medium pancakes**

1. In a bowl whisk together 1 egg, 1 tbsp (15 mL) vegetable oil, 1/2 cup (125 mL) milk and 1/4 tsp (1 mL) vanilla extract. Stir in 3/4 cup (175 mL) Homemade Pancake Mix. Let mixture stand for 2 minutes.
2. In a nonstick skillet over medium heat, heat another 1 tbsp (15 mL) vegetable oil until hot. Using a 1/4-cup (50 mL) measure, pour batter into hot skillet; cook for 3 minutes or until bubbles break on surface and underside is golden brown. Turn pancakes with a spatula and cook just until bottom is slightly browned. Repeat with remaining batter.

| NUTRITIONAL ANALYSIS | Energy | Protein | Carbohydrate | Fat | Calcium | Iron |
|---|---|---|---|---|---|---|
| per medium pancake | 130 kcal | 6.2 g | 24.9 g | 1.1 g | 14 % CDV | 19 % CDV |

# Dad's Pancakes

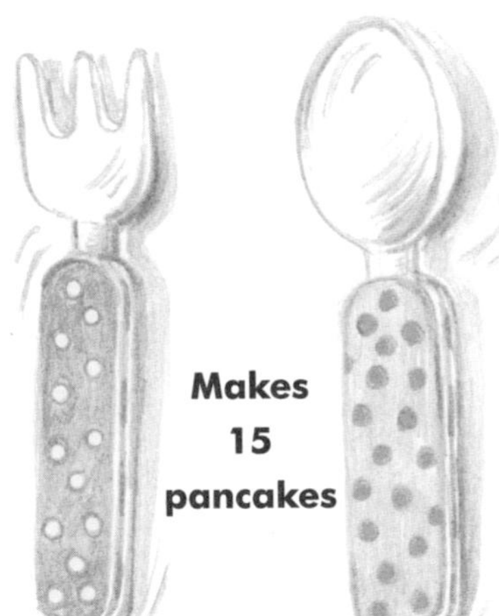

**Makes 15 pancakes**

*Daina's dad used to make these for the kids on weekends. They were considered quite a treat!*

**Kitchen Tip**

For a delicious variation, add apple slices to this recipe. Peel 1 apple and cut into thin slices; add slices to batter at the end of Step 1.

| | | |
|---|---|---|
| 1 | egg, lightly beaten | 1 |
| 1 cup | 2% milk, divided | 250 mL |
| 3/4 cup | all-purpose flour, divided | 175 mL |
| 1/2 tsp | salt | 2 mL |
| 1 tsp | granulated sugar | 5 mL |
| 2 tbsp | butter, divided | 25 mL |

1. In a large bowl, combine egg with 1/2 cup (125 mL) of the milk, 1/2 cup (125 mL) of the flour, as well as salt and sugar; stir until batter is smooth and free of lumps. Stir in remaining milk and flour; mix until smooth.
2. In a nonstick skillet over medium-high heat, melt 2 tsp (10 mL) of the butter. For each 2-inch (5 cm) pancake, pour about 2 tbsp (25 mL) batter into skillet. (Vary amount according to size of pancake desired.) Cook on one side for about 2 minutes or until pancake starts to bubble. Turn pancake over and cook for another 1 minute until browned. Repeat procedure for remaining batter, adding another 1 tsp (5 mL) butter for each batch.

| Nutritional Analysis | Energy | Protein | Carbohydrate | Fat | Calcium | Iron |
|---|---|---|---|---|---|---|
| per pancake | 53 kcal | 1.6 g | 5.4 g | 2.6 g | 3 % CDV | 3 % CDV |

# Sweet Potato Pancakes

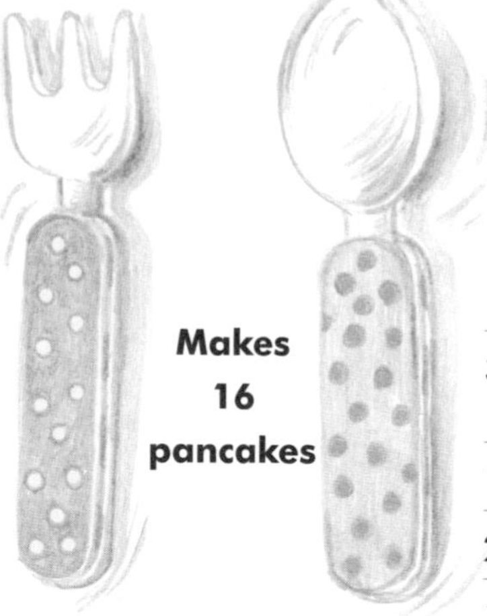

**Makes 16 pancakes**

*A nice change from traditional pancakes, these are wonderful topped with butter and maple syrup.*

| | | |
|---|---|---|
| 3/4 cup | mashed cooked sweet potato (about half large) | 175 mL |
| 1 tbsp | butter or margarine, melted | 15 mL |
| 2 | egg whites, lightly beaten | 2 |
| 1/1/2 cups | 2% milk | 375 mL |
| 1 cup | all-purpose flour | 250 mL |
| 2 tsp | baking powder | 10 mL |
| 1/2 tsp | salt | 2 mL |
| 1/4 tsp | ground cinnamon | 1 mL |

1. In a large bowl, combine sweet potato, margarine and egg whites. Stir in milk.
2. In another bowl, combine flour, baking powder, salt and cinnamon. Stir into the sweet potato mixture.
3. Heat a nonstick skillet sprayed with vegetable oil over medium-high heat. When pan is hot, pour in about 2 tbsp (25 mL) batter to make pancakes about 3 inches (7.5 cm) in diameter. Cook on one side for about 2 minutes or until pancake starts to bubble. Turn pancake over and cook for another 1 minute until browned.

### Kitchen Tip

For a slightly sweeter version of these pancakes, add 2 tsp (10 mL) granulated sugar to the batter at the end of Step 2.

These pancakes freeze very well. Simply reheat frozen pancakes in your toaster oven.

| Nutritional Analysis | Energy | Protein | Carbohydrate | Fat | Calcium | Iron |
|---|---|---|---|---|---|---|
| per pancake | 74 kcal | 2.7 g | 11.3 g | 1.9 g | 5 % CDV | 5 % CDV |

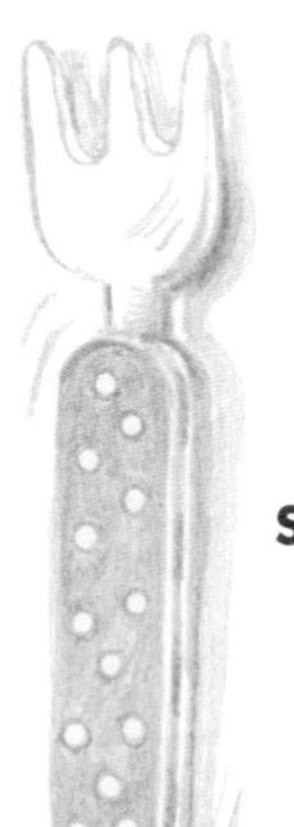

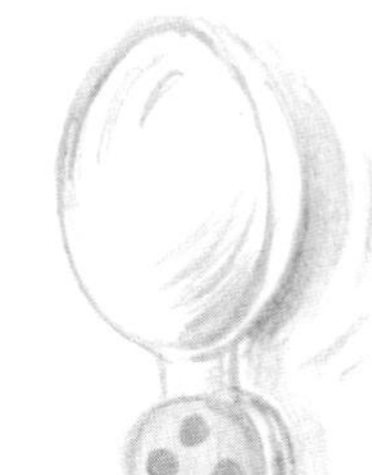

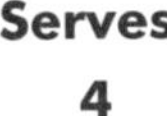

# Oven-Baked French Toast Sandwich

**Serves 4**

*Make these French toast sandwiches with jam or with the fillings suggested below. Or experiment with others to find your child's favorite. In our experience, peanut butter and banana is hard to beat!*

**VARIATIONS**

**Peanut Butter and Banana**: Replace jam with peanut butter and top with a layer of sliced bananas.

**Cheddar Cheese**: Substitute sliced medium Cheddar cheese for jam. This is much like a grilled cheese sandwich, which many kids like served with ketchup.

*11- by 7-inch (2 L) baking pan, greased*

| | | |
|---|---|---|
| 8 | slices bread, white or whole wheat | 8 |
| 1/3 cup | strawberry or raspberry jam | 75 mL |
| 3 | eggs | 3 |
| 1/3 cup | milk | 75 mL |
| 1/2 tsp | vanilla extract | 2 mL |
| | Ground cinnamon | |

1. Place 4 bread slices in prepared pan. Spread with jam. Top with remaining slices.
2. In a small bowl, whisk together eggs, milk and vanilla. Pour mixture evenly to cover each sandwich. Sprinkle lightly with cinnamon. Cover and refrigerate for 4 hours or overnight if desired.
3. Preheat oven to 350° F (180° C). Bake sandwiches, uncovered, for 35 minutes or until golden brown and set in center. Cut each sandwich into smaller pieces and serve.

| NUTRITIONAL ANALYSIS | Energy | Protein | Carbohydrate | Fat | Calcium | Iron |
|---|---|---|---|---|---|---|
| per serving | 203 kcal | 8.0 g | 25.3 g | 8.2 g | 9 % CDV | 18 % CDV |

# Eggs Fajitas

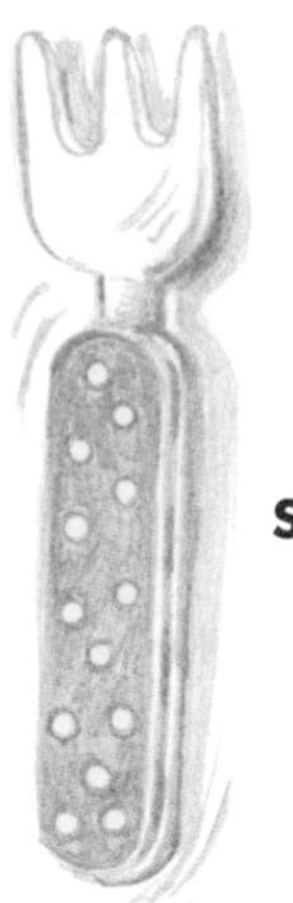
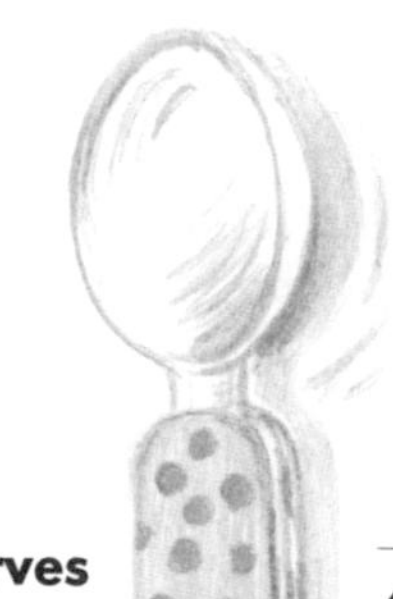

**Serves 4**

*When time is short, this makes a fast and easy breakfast. It's great for lunch too!*

| | | |
|---|---|---|
| 4 | eggs | 4 |
| 1/4 tsp | salt | 1 mL |
| Pinch | freshly ground black pepper | Pinch |
| 2 tsp | butter *or* margarine | 10 mL |
| 2 | green onions, chopped | 2 |
| 4 | 8-inch (20 cm) flour tortillas | 4 |
| 1/4 cup | mild salsa | 50 mL |

1. In a small bowl, whisk together eggs, salt and pepper. Set aside.
2. In a nonstick skillet, melt butter over medium heat. Add green onions and cook for a few minutes or until softened. Add egg mixture and cook, without stirring, until almost set. Turn over to finish cooking. Remove to cutting board. Cut egg into strips.
3. Warm tortillas in microwave oven for 45 seconds on High or until heated through. Place several egg strips in center of each tortilla; top with 1 tbsp (15 mL) salsa. Roll up tortilla to enclose egg and salsa.

| Nutritional Analysis | Energy | Protein | Carbohydrate | Fat | Calcium | Iron |
|---|---|---|---|---|---|---|
| per serving | 214 kcal | 8.9 g | 20.3 g | 10.4 g | 5 % CDV | 19 % CDV |

# Baked Vegetable Frittata

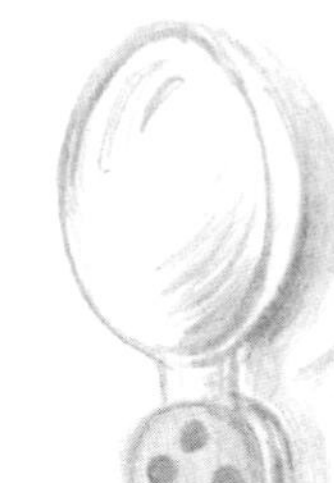

**Serves 4**

*Here's a great way to use up any leftover cooked vegetables you happen to have on hand. Just about anything works – broccoli, cauliflower, peas and corn kernels. Use your imagination!*

*Preheat oven to 350° F (180° C)*
*8-inch (2 L) square baking pan, greased*

| | | |
|---|---|---|
| 1/2 cup | chopped cooked vegetables | 125 mL |
| 1/2 cup | dried bread cubes or seasoned croutons | 125 mL |
| 4 | eggs | 4 |
| 1/4 cup | 2% milk | 50 mL |
| Pinch | salt | Pinch |
| Pinch | freshly ground black pepper | Pinch |
| 1/2 cup | grated Cheddar or mozzarella cheese | 125 mL |
| Pinch | dried basil | Pinch |

1. In a bowl combine vegetables and bread cubes. Sprinkle mixture evenly over bottom of prepared pan.
2. In a small bowl, whisk together eggs, milk, salt and pepper. Pour over vegetable mixture. Sprinkle with cheese and basil.
3. Bake in preheated oven for 20 minutes or until knife inserted in center comes out clean. Cut into 4 servings.

| NUTRITIONAL ANALYSIS | Energy | Protein | Carbohydrate | Fat | Calcium | Iron |
|---|---|---|---|---|---|---|
| per serving | 169 kcal | 11.2 g | 5.6 g | 11.2 g | 20 % CDV | 14 % CDV |

# Breakfast Cheese Melts

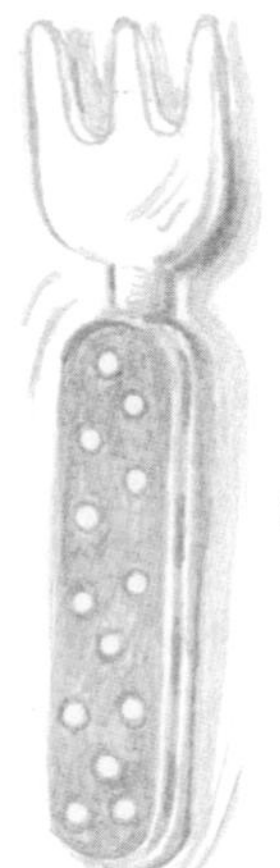

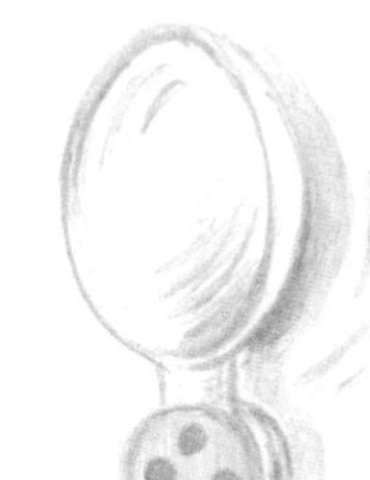

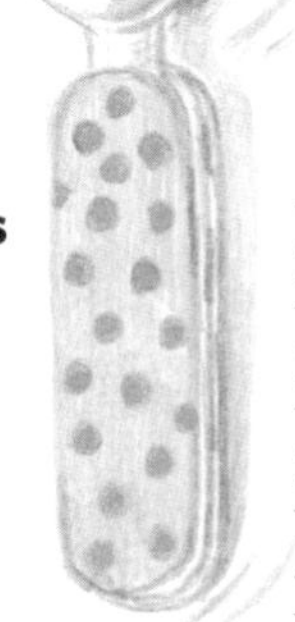

**Serves 4**

*Looking for a change from egg dishes at breakfast? Try this easy recipe next weekend.*

*Preheat broiler*

| | | |
|---|---|---|
| 2 | English muffins, halved | 2 |
| 2 | slices ham, halved | 2 |
| 2 | slices pineapple, halved | 2 |
| 4 | slices mozzarella or Swiss cheese | 4 |

1. Place muffins cut-side up on a baking sheet. Cook under broiler until golden brown.
2. Top toasted muffins with ham, pineapple and cheese. Return to broiler and cook until cheese is bubbly and melted.

| NUTRITIONAL ANALYSIS | Energy | Protein | Carbohydrate | Fat | Calcium | Iron |
|---|---|---|---|---|---|---|
| per serving | 142 kcal | 9.8 g | 12.7 g | 5.8 g | 25 % CDV | 7 % CDV |

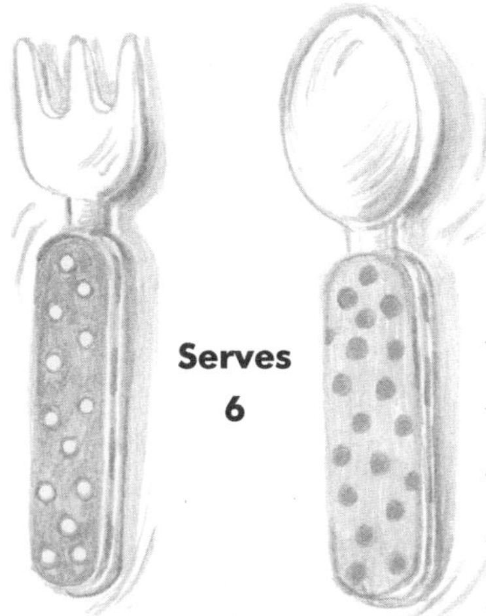

**Serves 6**

*Traditional quiche is delicious, although time-consuming to prepare. But you can make this dish in just a fraction of the time.*

# Weekend Breakfast Quiche

*Preheat oven to 375° F (190° C)*
*10-inch (25 cm) quiche pan, greased*

| | | |
|---|---|---|
| 1 cup | chopped broccoli (see Tip, at left) | 250 mL |
| 1 cup | shredded Swiss cheese | 250 mL |
| 1/2 cup | finely chopped onion | 125 mL |
| 3 | eggs | 3 |
| 1 cup | 2% milk | 250 mL |
| 1/2 cup | biscuit baking mix | 125 mL |
| 1/4 tsp | ground nutmeg | 1 mL |
| 1/4 tsp | salt | 1 mL |
| Pinch | freshly ground black pepper | Pinch |

**KITCHEN TIP**

Asparagus or corn kernels make a nice change from broccoli.

1. Sprinkle broccoli, cheese and onion in bottom of prepared pan.
2. In a bowl with an electric mixer, combine eggs, milk, baking mix and seasonings; beat at high speed for 1 minute. Pour over broccoli mixture in pan.
3. Bake in preheated oven for 45 minutes or until a knife inserted in center comes out clean. Transfer to a wire rack and allow to cool for 5 minutes before cutting into 6 wedges.

| NUTRITIONAL ANALYSIS | Energy | Protein | Carbohydrate | Fat | Calcium | Iron |
|---|---|---|---|---|---|---|
| per serving | 259 kcal | 16.7 g | 12.9 g | 15.5 g | 56 % CDV | 11 % CDV |

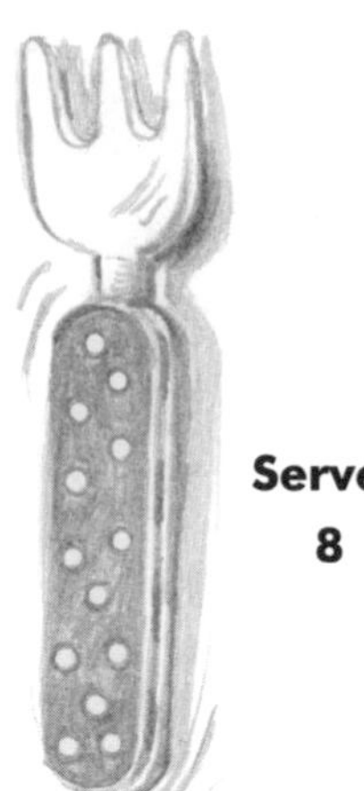

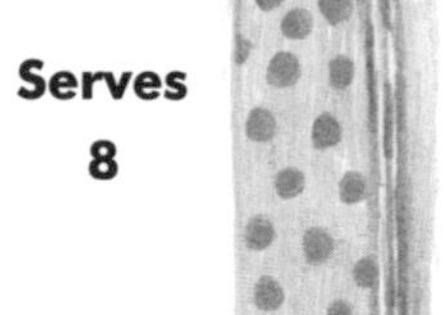

**Serves 8**

**KITCHEN TIP**

Serve this quiche with toast, bagel or English muffin.

Cooked ham or chicken make good substitutes for the bacon.

# Easy Quiche

*4-cup (1 L) microwave-safe casserole, greased*

| | | |
|---|---|---|
| 3 | eggs | 3 |
| 1 cup | 2% milk | 250 mL |
| 1/4 tsp | salt | 1 mL |
| 1/4 tsp | paprika | 1 mL |
| Pinch | ground nutmeg | Pinch |
| 2 | green onions, chopped | 2 |
| 3/4 cup | grated Swiss cheese | 175 mL |
| 1/4 cup | grated Parmesan cheese | 50 mL |
| 3 | strips bacon, chopped and cooked, fat drained | 3 |

1. In a bowl with an electric mixer, combine eggs, milk, salt, paprika and nutmeg; beat at high speed for 1 minute.
2. Place green onions, Swiss cheese, Parmesan cheese and bacon in bottom of prepared dish. Pour egg mixture over. Microwave, uncovered, on High for 5 minutes. Stir egg and microwave for another 6 minutes or until firm (not runny). Let stand for 5 minutes before serving.

| NUTRITIONAL ANALYSIS | Energy | Protein | Carbohydrate | Fat | Calcium | Iron |
|---|---|---|---|---|---|---|
| per serving | 191 kcal | 13.2 g | 3.3 g | 13.8 g | 43 % CDV | 7 % CDV |

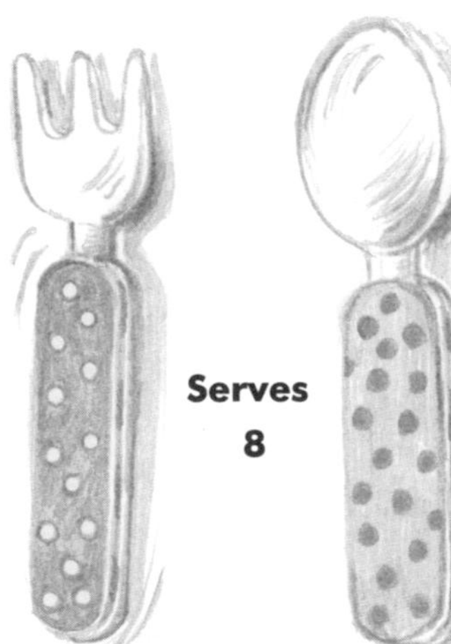

**Serves 8**

*What a great weekend treat – ham, pineapple and a cornbread batter.*

# Pineapple Ham Upside-Down Cake

*Preheat oven to 425° F (210° C)*
*9-inch (23 cm) round baking pan, greased*

| | | |
|---|---|---|
| 2 tbsp | melted butter or margarine | 25 mL |
| 1/3 cup | packed brown sugar | 75 mL |
| 1 tsp | dry mustard | 5 mL |
| 5 | slices canned pineapple, halved | 5 |
| 2 cups | minced ham | 500 mL |
| 1 cup | all-purpose flour | 250 mL |
| 1 cup | cornmeal | 250 mL |
| 1 tbsp | baking powder | 15 mL |
| 1/2 tsp | salt | 2 mL |
| 1 | egg | 1 |
| 1 cup | 2% milk | 250 mL |
| 1/4 cup | vegetable oil | 50 mL |

1. In a small bowl, combine butter, brown sugar and mustard; spread mixture to cover bottom of prepared pan. Arrange pineapple in circles on top and sprinkle evenly with ham.
2. In another bowl, stir together flour, cornmeal, baking powder and salt. Set aside.
3. In a bowl with an electric mixer, combine egg, milk and oil. Add flour-cornmeal mixture and beat at high speed until smooth. Pour batter over ham in baking pan.
4. Bake in preheated oven for 35 minutes or until a cake tester inserted in center comes out clean. Transfer to a wire rack and allow to cool for 5 minutes before cutting into 8 pieces.

| Nutritional Analysis | Energy | Protein | Carbohydrate | Fat | Calcium | Iron |
|---|---|---|---|---|---|---|
| per serving | 350 kcal | 9.8 g | 42.0 g | 15.8 g | 10 % CDV | 16 % CDV |

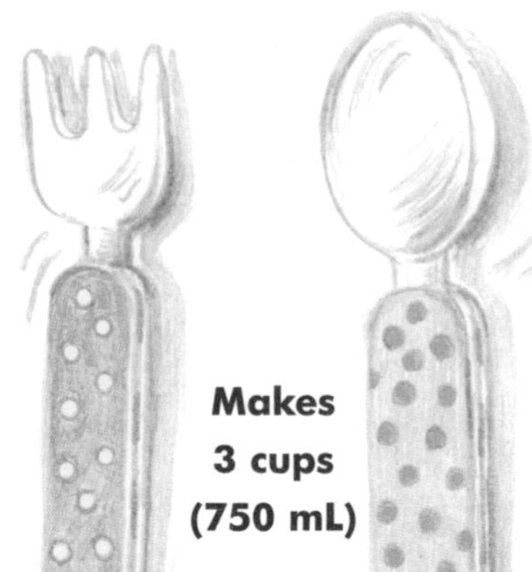

**Makes 3 cups (750 mL)**

# Homemade Microwave Granola

*4-cup (1 L) microwave-safe casserole, greased*

*Commercially prepared granola is convenient, but may contain added ingredients you don't want. Here's a homemade version that's packed with nutritious goodness. And because it's cooked in the microwave, preparation is a snap.*

| | | |
|---|---|---|
| 1 cup | large-flake rolled oats | 250 mL |
| 1/2 cup | wheat flakes (see Tip, at left) | 125 mL |
| 1/2 cup | rye flakes | 125 mL |
| 1/4 cup | unsweetened flaked coconut | 50 mL |
| 1/4 cup | natural wheat bran | 50 mL |
| Pinch | salt | Pinch |
| 1/4 cup | liquid honey | 50 mL |
| 2 tbsp | vegetable oil | 25 mL |
| 1/2 cup | chopped dried fruit, optional (see Tip, at left) | 125 mL |

1. In a microwave-safe container, combine oats, wheat and rye flakes, coconut, bran and salt.
2. In a 1-cup (250 mL) measure, whisk together honey and oil. Pour over oat mixture; toss until well mixed.
3. Microwave on High for 6 minutes, stirring well every 2 minutes, until mixture is slightly brown. Stir in fruit, if using. Allow granola to cool before storing in a tightly covered container. Keeps for up to 1 month.

### Kitchen Tip

You can find wheat and rye flakes (and other grains used in this recipe) at health food stores, as well as some supermarkets.

Use whatever fruit you like best. Good choices include dried apricots, dates, apples or raisins.

| Nutritional Analysis | Energy | Protein | Carbohydrate | Fat | Calcium | Iron |
|---|---|---|---|---|---|---|
| per 1/2-cup (125 mL) serving | 199 kcal | 3.5 g | 33.3 g | 7.2 g | 3 % CDV | 34 % CDV |

# Granola Breakfast Squares

*7- by 11-inch (2 L) baking pan, greased*

**Makes 24 squares**

*These unbaked squares are a snap to prepare in the microwave. Kids love them – and because they contain less sugar and fat than commercial granola treats, you'll love them too!*

| | | |
|---|---|---|
| 1/2 cup | corn syrup | 125 mL |
| 2 tbsp | brown sugar | 25 mL |
| 1/3 cup | peanut butter | 75 mL |
| 3 cups | Homemade Microwave Granola (see recipe, page 132) | 750 mL |
| 1/4 cup | sunflower seeds | 50 mL |
| 1/2 tsp | ground cinnamon | 2 mL |
| 1/2 tsp | ground nutmeg | 2 mL |

1. In a large microwave-safe bowl, combine syrup and sugar. Microwave on High for 2 minutes or until mixture is boiling. Stir in peanut butter until smooth.
2. Quickly stir in granola, sunflower seeds, cinnamon and nutmeg. Press firmly into prepared pan. Cut into squares when cool. Transfer to an airtight container and store in the refrigerator.

| Nutritional Analysis | Energy | Protein | Carbohydrate | Fat | Calcium | Iron |
|---|---|---|---|---|---|---|
| per square | 98 kcal | 1.9 g | 15.4 g | 3.9 g | 2 % CDV | 13 % CDV |

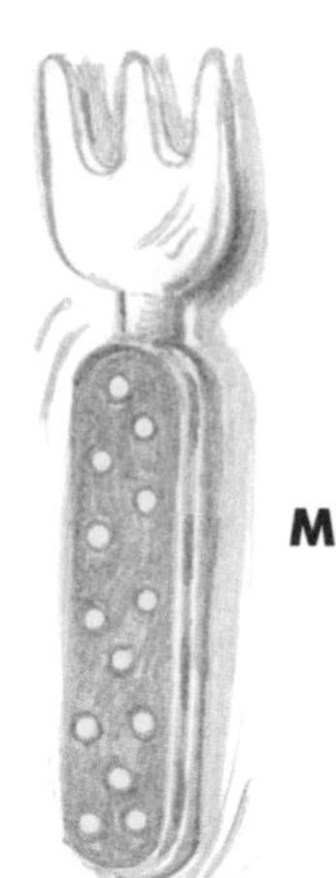
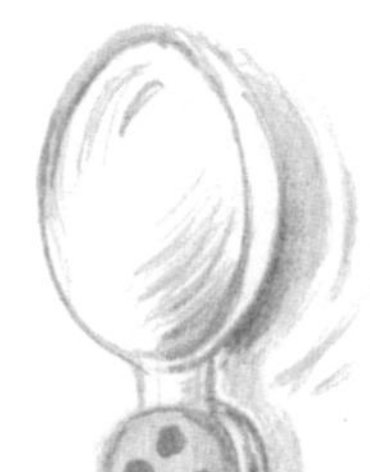

# Rolled Oat Muffins

**Makes 12**

*These great-looking muffins combine wonderful taste and texture.*

*Preheat oven to 375° F (190° C)*
*12-cup muffin tin, greased or paper-lined*

| | | |
|---|---|---|
| 1 cup | all-purpose flour | 250 mL |
| 1 cup | whole wheat flour | 250 mL |
| 1 cup | rolled oats | 250 mL |
| 1/2 cup | granulated sugar | 125 mL |
| 1 tbsp | baking powder | 15 mL |
| 1 tsp | ground cinnamon | 5 mL |
| 1/2 tsp | baking soda | 2 mL |
| 1/2 tsp | salt | 2 mL |
| 1 1/2 cups | 2% milk | 375 mL |
| 1/4 cup | vegetable oil | 50 mL |
| 1 | egg | 1 |
| 1/4 cup | molasses | 50 mL |

1. In a large bowl, combine all-purpose flour, whole wheat flour, rolled oats, sugar, baking powder, cinnamon, baking soda and salt.
2. In another bowl, combine milk, oil, egg and molasses. Add to dry ingredients; stir just until moistened.
3. Spoon batter into prepared muffin cups. Bake in preheated oven for 20 minutes or until muffins are firm to the touch.

| NUTRITIONAL ANALYSIS | Energy | Protein | Carbohydrate | Fat | Calcium | Iron |
|---|---|---|---|---|---|---|
| per muffin | 204 kcal | 5.0 g | 34.1 g | 5.7 g | 13 % CDV | 3 % CDV |

# Corn Muffins

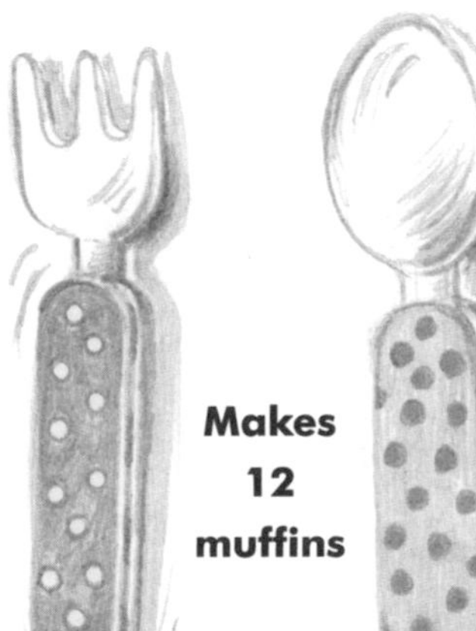

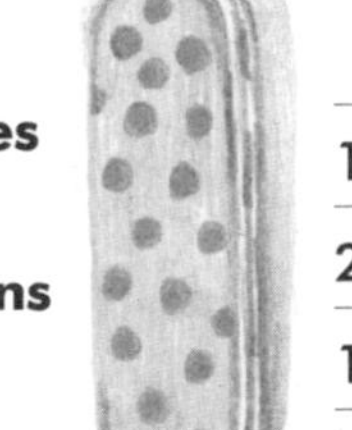

**Makes 12 muffins**

*While we've chosen to feature this recipe in our breakfast chapter, it's also perfect for accompanying hearty main meals, such as winter stews or chilies.*

**Kitchen Tip**

These muffins are best served warm from the oven. Serve with fruit jam or preserves.

*Preheat oven to 350° F (180° C)*
*12-cup muffin tin, greased or paper-lined*

| | | |
|---|---|---|
| 1 1/2 cups | all-purpose flour | 375 mL |
| 2/3 cup | granulated sugar | 175 mL |
| 1/2 cup | cornmeal | 125 mL |
| 1 tbsp | baking powder | 15 mL |
| 1/2 tsp | salt | 2 mL |
| 1 1/4 cup | 2% milk | 300 mL |
| 2 | eggs, slightly beaten | 2 |
| 1/3 cup | vegetable oil | 75 mL |
| 1/4 cup | butter or margarine, melted | 50 mL |

1. In a large bowl, combine flour, sugar, cornmeal, baking powder and salt.
2. In another bowl, whisk together milk, eggs, oil and melted butter. Add to dry ingredients; stir just until moistened.
3. Spoon batter into prepared muffin cups, filling about three-quarters full. Bake in preheated oven for 18 to 20 minutes or until muffins are firm to the touch.

| Nutritional Analysis | Energy | Protein | Carbohydrate | Fat | Calcium | Iron |
|---|---|---|---|---|---|---|
| per muffin | 236 kcal | 4.1 g | 30.3 g | 11.1 g | 6 % CDV | 9 % CDV |

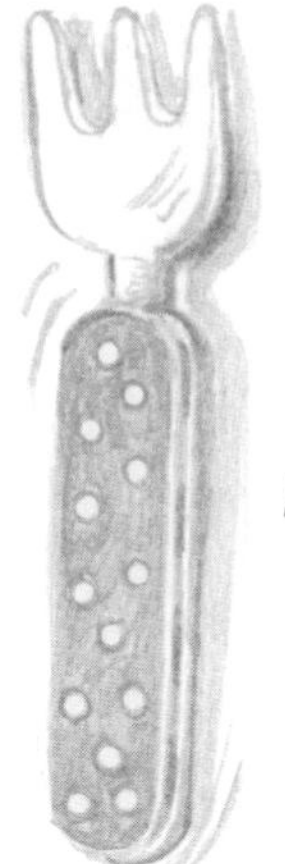
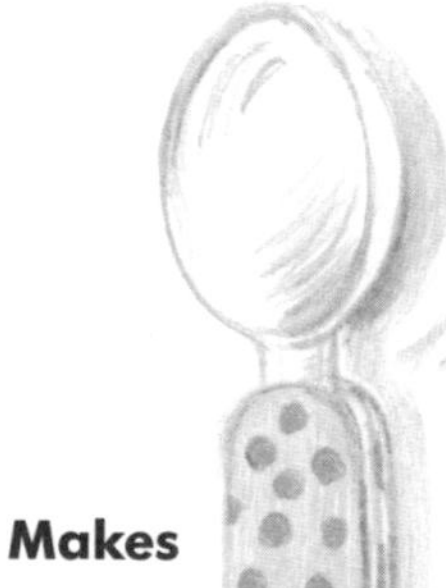

# Apple and Cheese Whole Wheat Muffins

*Preheat oven to 375° F (190° C)*
*12-cup muffin tin, greased or paper-lined*

**Makes 12**

*Wonderful and moist, these nutritious muffins have great flavor. They're sure to be a hit with the entire family.*

| | | |
|---|---|---|
| 1 1/4 cups | all-purpose flour | 300 mL |
| 1 cup | whole wheat flour | 250 mL |
| 1 cup | lightly packed brown sugar | 250 mL |
| 1 tsp | baking soda | 5 mL |
| 1/2 tsp | ground cinnamon | 2 mL |
| 1/2 tsp | ground nutmeg | 2 mL |
| 1 | egg | 1 |
| 1 cup | plain yogurt | 250 mL |
| 1/3 cup | vegetable oil | 75 mL |
| 2 cups | diced peeled apples | 500 mL |
| 1/2 cup | shredded old Cheddar cheese | 125 mL |

1. In a large bowl, combine all-purpose flour, whole wheat flour, brown sugar, baking soda, cinnamon and nutmeg.
2. In another bowl, combine egg, yogurt, oil, apple and cheese. Add to dry ingredients; stir just until moistened.
3. Spoon batter into prepared muffin cups. Bake in preheated oven for 20 minutes or until muffins are firm to the touch.

| NUTRITIONAL ANALYSIS | Energy | Protein | Carbohydrate | Fat | Calcium | Iron |
|---|---|---|---|---|---|---|
| per muffin | 250 kcal | 5.3 g | 38.2 g | 9.1 g | 11 % CDV | 16 % CDV |

# Banana Oatmeal Muffins

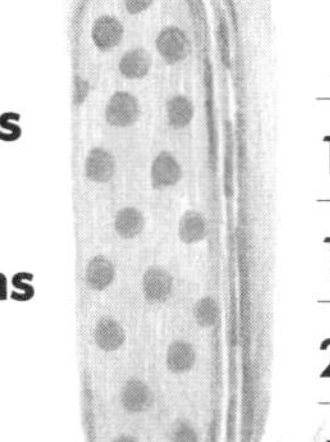

**Makes 24 muffins**

*Here's a great way to start the day. Serve with cheese and milk for a complete breakfast.*

**Kitchen Tip**

For a special treat, add 1 cup (250 mL) chocolate chips to this recipe. Stir in with bananas before baking.

*Preheat oven to 375° F (190° C)*
*Two 12-cup muffin tins, greased or paper-lined*

| | | |
|---|---|---|
| 1 cup | rolled oats | 250 mL |
| 1 cup | 2% milk | 250 mL |
| 2 cups | all-purpose flour | 500 mL |
| 1/2 cup | lightly packed brown sugar | 125 mL |
| 1/2 cup | granulated sugar | 125 mL |
| 1 tsp | baking soda | 5 mL |
| 1 tsp | salt | 5 mL |
| 1/2 tsp | ground cinnamon | 2 mL |
| 1/4 tsp | ground nutmeg | 1 mL |
| 1/2 cup | butter or margarine, softened | 125 mL |
| 2 | eggs | 2 |
| 2 tsp | vanilla extract | 10 mL |
| 2 cups | mashed bananas | 500 mL |
| 1 cup | chocolate chips (optional) | 250 mL |

1. In a bowl combine oats and milk. Set aside to soak.
2. In another bowl, combine flour, brown sugar, granulated sugar, baking soda, salt, cinnamon and nutmeg.
3. Add butter, eggs, vanilla and bananas to oatmeal mixture; stir until thoroughly combined. Add mixture to dry ingredients; stir just until moistened. If using, stir in chocolate chips.
4. Spoon batter into prepared muffin cups, filling about three-quarters full. Bake in preheated oven for 20 minutes or until muffins are firm to the touch.

| Nutritional Analysis | Energy | Protein | Carbohydrate | Fat | Calcium | Iron |
|---|---|---|---|---|---|---|
| per muffin | 154 kcal | 2.8 g | 24.2 g | 5.3 g | 3 % CDV | 9 % CDV |

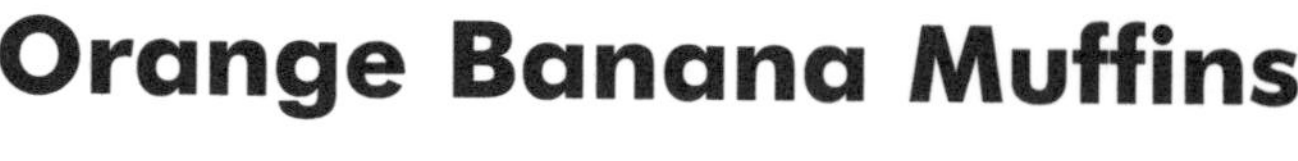

# Orange Banana Muffins

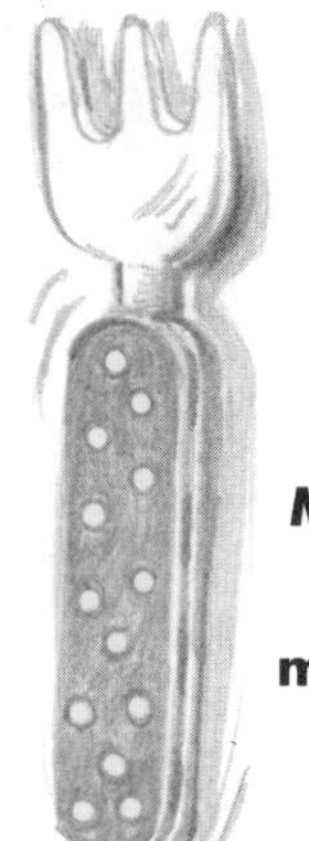

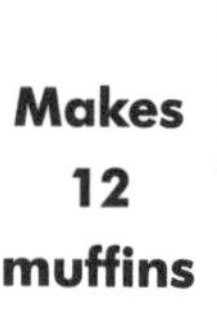

**Makes 12 muffins**

*The combination of orange juice and bananas makes these muffins incredibly moist and flavorful.*

*Preheat oven to 400° F (200° C)*
*12-cup muffin tin, greased or paper-lined*

| | | |
|---|---|---|
| 1 cup | whole wheat flour | 250 mL |
| 1 cup | all-purpose flour | 250 mL |
| 1/4 cup | cornmeal | 50 mL |
| 1 tsp | baking soda | 5 mL |
| 1 tsp | baking powder | 5 mL |
| Pinch | salt | Pinch |
| 1 cup | mashed bananas | 250 mL |
| 1/2 cup | frozen orange juice concentrate, thawed | 125 mL |
| 1/4 cup | packed brown sugar | 50 mL |
| 1/4 cup | vegetable oil | 50 mL |
| 1/4 cup | 2% milk | 50 mL |
| 1 | egg | 1 |

1. In a bowl combine whole wheat flour, all-purpose flour, cornmeal, baking soda, baking powder and salt.
2. In another bowl, stir together bananas, orange juice concentrate, brown sugar, oil, milk and egg. Add mixture to dry ingredients; stir just until mixed.
3. Spoon batter into prepared muffin cups. Bake in preheated oven for 20 to 25 minutes or until muffins are firm to the touch.

### Kitchen Tip

For added fiber, use natural bran instead of cornmeal.

| Nutritional Analysis | Energy | Protein | Carbohydrate | Fat | Calcium | Iron |
|---|---|---|---|---|---|---|
| per muffin | 179 kcal | 3.9 g | 31.1 g | 4.9 g | 3 % CDV | 11 % CDV |

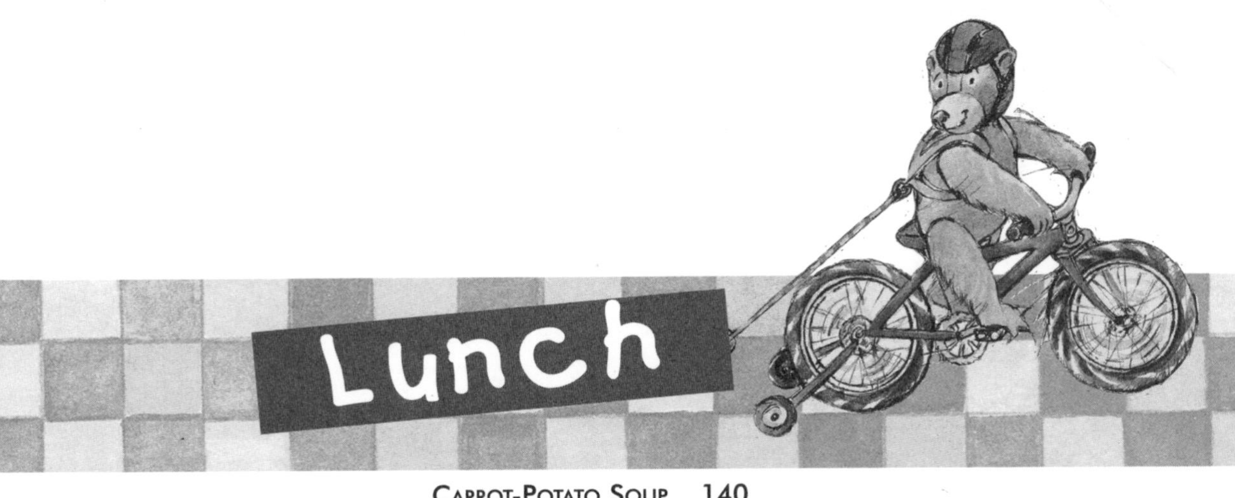


# Lunch

# Carrot-Potato Soup

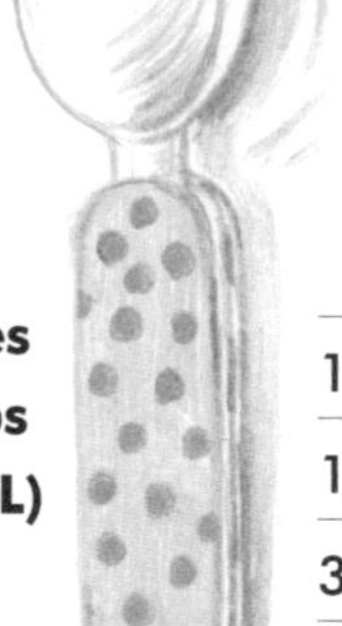

**Makes 5 cups (1.25 L)**

*The creamy texture of this soup comes from the starch in the potatoes. It's delicious – and healthy too!*

**Kitchen Tip**

If you have it (or have the time to make it), use homemade chicken stock. Otherwise, use canned chicken broth or water and chicken bouillon cubes or sachets.

Kids generally prefer their soup warm. But this recipe also makes a great summertime starter for adults when served cold.

| | | |
|---|---|---|
| 1 tbsp | olive oil | 15 mL |
| 1/3 cup | chopped onion | 75 mL |
| 3 | green onions, chopped | 3 |
| 2 cups | finely chopped carrots | 500 mL |
| 2 cups | diced potatoes | 500 mL |
| 2 tsp | grated ginger root (optional) | 10 mL |
| 3 cups | chicken stock (see Tip) | 750 mL |
| 1/4 tsp | curry powder | 1 mL |
| 1/4 tsp | ground cinnamon | 1 mL |
| 1/4 tsp | ground nutmeg | 1 mL |
| Pinch | freshly ground black pepper | Pinch |
| 1 | bay leaf | 1 |
| | Sour cream (optional) | |

1. In a large saucepan, heat oil over medium heat. Add onions and sauté for 3 minutes. Add carrots and potatoes; cook for 2 minutes.
2. Add ginger root, if using, along with stock, curry, cinnamon, nutmeg, pepper and bay leaf. Bring to a boil. Reduce heat and simmer, covered, for about 45 minutes or until vegetables are very tender. Remove and discard bay leaf. Allow soup to cool slightly.
3. Transfer soup to a blender or food processor; purée until smooth. Return mixture to saucepan and heat to serving temperature. Ladle soup into bowls and, if desired, garnish with a small dollop of sour cream.

| Nutritional Analysis | Energy | Protein | Carbohydrate | Fat | Calcium | Iron |
|---|---|---|---|---|---|---|
| per 1/2-cup (125 mL) serving | 62 kcal | 2.6 g | 9.0 g | 1.9 g | 2 % CDV | 6 % CDV |

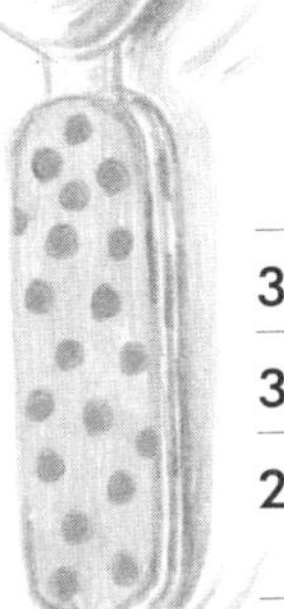

# Creamy Vegetable Soup

**Makes 4 cups (1 L)**

*Here's another wonderfully creamy soup that uses milk (not cream) and can be made with all kinds of different vegetables.*

| | | |
|---|---|---|
| 3 tbsp | butter or margarine | 45 mL |
| 3 tbsp | all-purpose flour | 45 mL |
| 2 cups | vegetable or chicken stock (see Tip, at left) | 500 mL |
| 2 cups | chopped cooked vegetables | 500 mL |
| 1 cup | 2% milk | 250 mL |

1. In a large saucepan, melt butter over medium heat. Add flour and cook, stirring, for 2 minutes or until bubbly. Gradually whisk in broth; cook until smooth and thickened.
2. Add cooked vegetables. Remove from heat and transfer soup to food processor or blender. Purée until smooth. Return to saucepan. Slowly stir in milk and heat to serving temperature.

### Kitchen Tip

Add whatever seasonings you like, depending on the vegetables used. See our Seasoning Guide, at right, for suggestions.

If using homemade stock, add salt to taste. With commercially prepared broth, however, you may find the soup is already salty enough.

This soup freezes well.

### VEGETABLE SOUP SEASONING GUIDE

| VEGETABLE | SEASONING |
|---|---|
| Asparagus | Ground nutmeg or white pepper |
| Broccoli | Lemon zest or juice |
| Carrot | Ground nutmeg, ginger, curry |
| Cauliflower | Ground nutmeg or white pepper |
| Cream-style corn | Cayenne pepper |
| Green beans | Dried tarragon or basil |
| Green peas | Dried mint or parsley; lemon zest |
| Mushroom | Ground white pepper, cayenne |
| Spinach | Lemon zest or ground nutmeg |
| Tomato | Dried thyme or basil |

| Nutritional Analysis | Energy | Protein | Carbohydrate | Fat | Calcium | Iron |
|---|---|---|---|---|---|---|
| per 1/2-cup (125 mL) serving | 90 kcal | 3.5 g | 7.2 g | 5.5 g | 8 % CDV | 7 % CDV |

# Tuscan Bean Soup

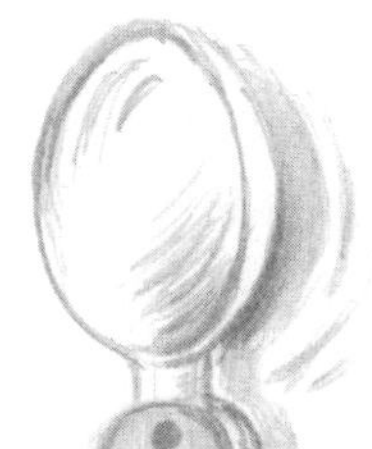

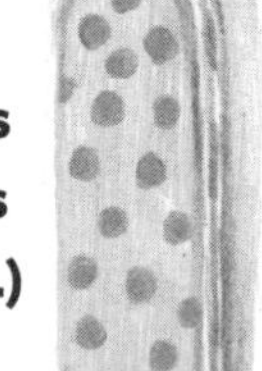

**Makes 9 cups (1.75 L)**

*Known in its native Italy as ribolitta, this thick bean soup is the ideal comfort food to fend off the winter blues.*

**Kitchen Tip**

The traditional texture of this soup is quite chunky. If your children prefer a smoother soup (as some seem to do), purée their portion and keep the remainder as is for adults.

| | | |
|---|---|---|
| 1 cup | dried cannelini or white kidney beans | 250 mL |
| 2 tbsp | olive oil | 25 mL |
| 1 | small onion, finely chopped | 1 |
| 1 | large stalk celery, finely chopped | 1 |
| 1 | sprig fresh rosemary leaves, chopped (or 1 tbsp [15 mL] dried) | 1 |
| 1 | large carrot, finely chopped | 1 |
| 2 | cloves garlic, finely chopped | 2 |
| 4 cups | chicken stock | 1 L |
| 2 tbsp | tomato paste | 25 mL |
| 2 | leeks, white part only, washed and chopped | 2 |
| 2 | zucchini, chopped | 2 |
| 1/2 cup | chopped fresh basil | 125 mL |
| | Salt and freshly ground black pepper to taste | |
| | Toasted bread slices | |
| | Grated Parmesan cheese | |

1. In a large saucepan, add sufficient cold water to cover beans. Cover and bring to a boil; reduce heat and cook for 5 minutes. Remove from heat and allow to stand for 1 hour. Drain and discard liquid. Return drained beans to saucepan and add 4 cups (1 L) cold water. Bring to a boil; reduce heat and cook for 1 hour or until beans are tender. Drain.

| Nutritional Analysis | Energy | Protein | Carbohydrate | Fat | Calcium | Iron |
|---|---|---|---|---|---|---|
| per 1/2-cup (125 mL) serving | 74 kcal | 4.3 g | 10.7 g | 1.8 g | 4 % CDV | 15 % CDV |

2. Meanwhile, in a large nonstick skillet, heat oil over medium heat. Add onion, celery, rosemary, carrot and garlic; cook for 10 minutes.
3. Add vegetable mixture to cooked drained beans. Stir in chicken stock and tomato paste; cook, uncovered, over medium heat for 10 minutes. Add leeks and zucchini; cover and cook for 15 minutes or until all vegetables are tender. Add basil and season to taste with salt and pepper.
4. Place toasted bread in each soup bowl. Ladle soup over and sprinkle with Parmesan.

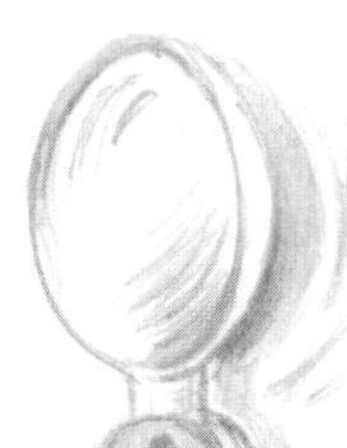

# Easy Bean Soup with Ham

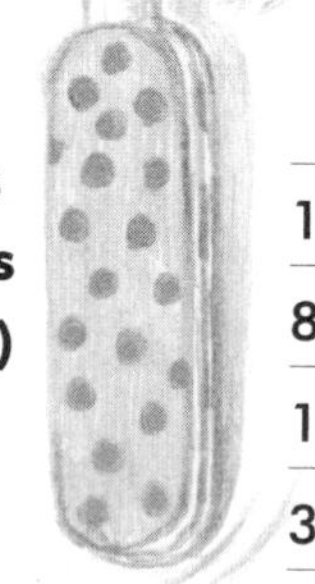

**Makes 13 cups (3.25 L)**

*Here's a simple and delicious way to use up leftover cooked ham.*

| | | |
|---|---|---|
| 1 lb | Great Northern beans | 500 g |
| 8 cups | cold water (used in Step 2) | 2 L |
| 1 | medium onion, chopped | 1 |
| 3 | carrots, chopped | 3 |
| 3 | stalks celery, diced | 3 |
| 2 cups | chopped cooked ham | 500 mL |
| 1 | bay leaf | 1 |
| | Salt and freshly ground black pepper to taste | |

1. In a large saucepan, add sufficient cold water to cover beans. Cover and bring to a boil; reduce heat and cook for 5 minutes. Remove from heat and allow to stand for 1 hour. Drain and discard liquid. Return drained beans to saucepan and add 4 cups (1 L) cold water. Bring to a boil; reduce heat and cook for 1 hour or until beans are tender. Drain.
2. In a large stockpot, stir together beans, 8 cups (2 L) cold water,, onion, carrots, celery, ham and bay leaf. Season to taste with salt and pepper. Bring to a boil; reduce heat, cover and simmer for 1 1/2 hours or until beans are soft. Remove and discard bay leaf before serving.

**Kitchen Tip**

For a more colorful soup, try adding 1/2 to 1 cup (125 to 250 mL) tomato juice.

| Nutritional Analysis | Energy | Protein | Carbohydrate | Fat | Calcium | Iron |
|---|---|---|---|---|---|---|
| per 1/2-cup (125 mL) serving | 40 kcal | 3.4 g | 4.3 g | 1.4 g | 1 % CDV | 6 % CDV |

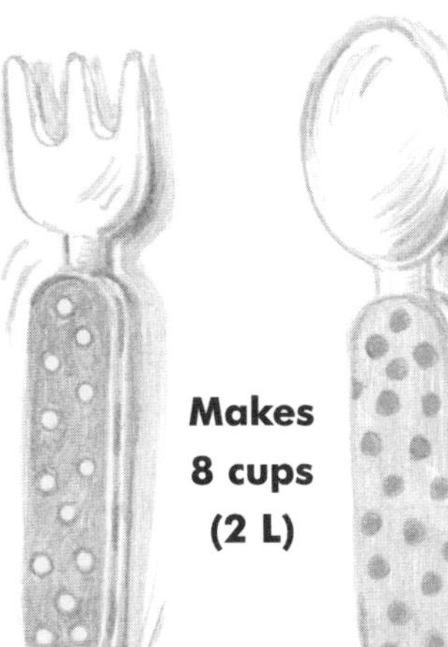

# Hungarian Chicken Soup

**Makes 8 cups (2 L)**

*Here's a good opportunity for you and your kids to try some vegetables that you may not have very often – kohlrabi and parsnips, which add a sweet flavor to this soup.*

**KITCHEN TIP**

Kohlrabi can be found at most supermarkets.

Serve this hearty soup over cooked rice or noodles.

| | | |
|---|---|---|
| 4 | bone-in chicken thighs, with skin, rinsed under cold running water | 4 |
| 5 cups | water | 1.25 L |
| 1 tsp | salt | 5 mL |
| 1/4 tsp | freshly ground black pepper | 1 mL |
| 2 | carrots, peeled and sliced | 2 |
| 2 | parsnips, peeled and sliced | 2 |
| 1 | kohlrabi, peeled and chopped | 1 |
| 3 | sprigs parsley | 3 |

1. In a large saucepan, combine chicken and water. Add salt and pepper. Bring to a boil; reduce heat and simmer, skimming off any froth from the surface, for 1 1/2 hours or until chicken falls off of the bone.
2. Remove bones from broth and add vegetables. Simmer for another 45 minutes or until the vegetables are tender. Transfer soup to a serving bowl and garnish with parsley.

| NUTRITIONAL ANALYSIS | Energy | Protein | Carbohydrate | Fat | Calcium | Iron |
|---|---|---|---|---|---|---|
| per 1/2-cup (125 mL) serving | 63 kcal | 4.4 g | 3.1 g | 3.6 g | 1 % CDV | 1 % CDV |

# Sweet Potato Soup

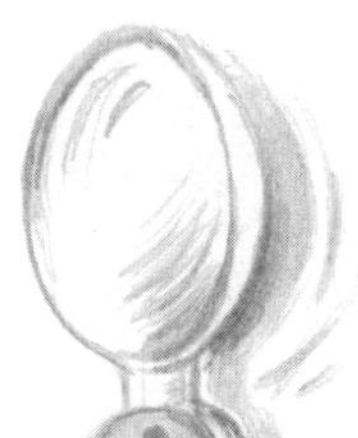

**Makes 6 cups (1.5 L)**

*Sweet and oh-so-simple, this soup is a great source of beta carotene.*

| | | |
|---|---|---|
| 1 tbsp | vegetable oil | 15 mL |
| 1 | small onion, chopped | 1 |
| 6 cups | chicken stock | 1.5 L |
| 2 | large sweet potatoes, peeled and chopped | 2 |
| 1/2 tsp | ground nutmeg | 2 mL |
| 1/4 tsp | freshly ground black pepper | 1 mL |

1. In a large saucepan, warm oil over medium-high heat. Add onions and sauté for 2 to 3 minutes or until onions are soft and translucent. Add chicken stock, sweet potatoes, nutmeg and pepper. Cover and bring to a boil; reduce heat and simmer for 25 minutes or until potatoes are tender.
2. Remove soup from heat and, in batches, purée soup in a blender or food processor until smooth. Return soup to saucepan and heat to serving temperature.

### Kitchen Tip

If using canned chicken broth, try looking for the salt-reduced or low-sodium variety.

Garnish the soup with a little plain yogurt or sour cream before serving.

| Nutritional Analysis | Energy | Protein | Carbohydrate | Fat | Calcium | Iron |
|---|---|---|---|---|---|---|
| per 1/2-cup (125 mL) serving | 173 kcal | 7.1 g | 26.5 g | 4.2 g | 5 % CDV | 12 % CDV |

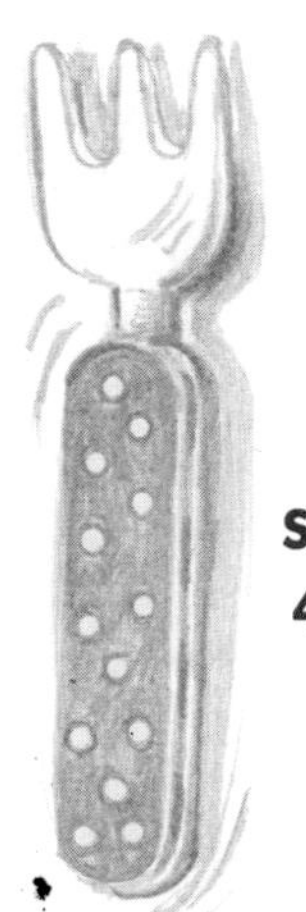

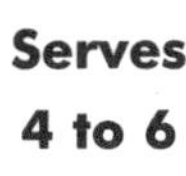

# Baked Vegetarian Cheese Chili

*Preheat oven to 325° F (160° C)*
*9-inch (23 cm) deep baking pan, greased*

**Serves 4 to 6**

*A unique and savory vegetarian dish, this chili can be served alone or with a salad and pita bread or rolls.*

| | | |
|---|---|---|
| 2 1/2 cups | shredded mozzarella cheese, divided | 625 mL |
| 3/4 cup | shredded carrots (see Tip, at left) | 175 mL |
| 6 | eggs | 6 |
| 1 cup | 2% milk | 250 mL |
| 2 tbsp | all-purpose flour | 25 mL |
| 1 tsp | chili powder | 5 mL |
| 1/2 tsp | ground cumin | 2 mL |
| 1/2 tsp | salt | 2 mL |
| | Paprika | |

**KITCHEN TIP**

Try replacing the carrots with shredded potato, leeks, zucchini, chopped broccoli or green peas.

1. Place one-half of cheese in prepared pan. Arrange carrots over cheese and top with remaining cheese.
2. In a bowl whisk together eggs, milk, flour, chili powder, cumin and salt. Pour over cheese in pan; sprinkle lightly with paprika.
3. Bake in preheated oven for 25 minutes or until a knife inserted in center comes out clean and top is golden brown. Let stand for 5 minutes before cutting into squares.

| NUTRITIONAL ANALYSIS | Energy | Protein | Carbohydrate | Fat | Calcium | Iron |
|---|---|---|---|---|---|---|
| per serving (6) | 429 kcal | 38.7 g | 9.5 g | 25.7 g | 113 % CDV | 17 % CDV |

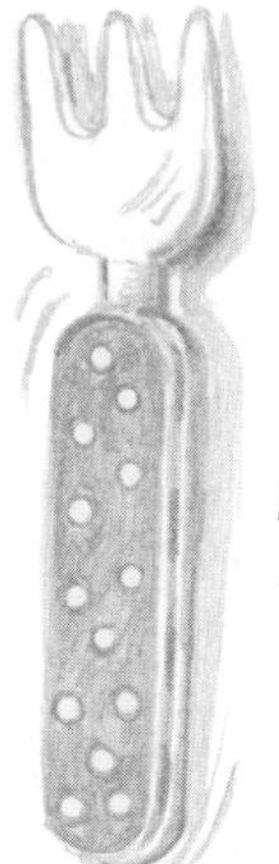

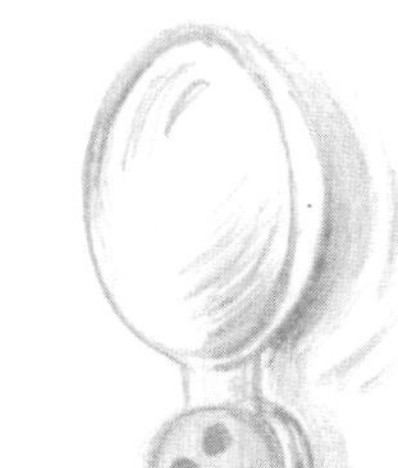

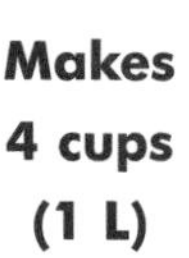

# Garden Pasta and Relish Salad

**Makes 4 cups (1 L)**

*Relish gives a marvelous flavor and moisture to this pasta salad. Add some vegetables and the taste is complete.*

| | | |
|---|---|---|
| 2 cups | fusilli or small shell pasta | 500 mL |
| 1/2 cup | frozen peas (see Tip, at left) | 125 mL |
| 1/2 cup | diced red or green bell pepper | 125 mL |
| 1 | green onion, finely chopped | 1 |
| 1/4 cup | sweet pickle relish | 50 mL |
| 1/4 cup | mayonnaise | 50 mL |
| 2 tbsp | plain yogurt | 25 mL |
| Pinch | salt | Pinch |
| Pinch | freshly ground black pepper | Pinch |

1. In a large saucepan, cook pasta in boiling water according to manufacturer's directions or until tender but firm. Drain. While pasta is still hot, stir in peas, red pepper and onion. Set aside.
2. In a small bowl, stir together relish, mayonnaise and yogurt. Stir mixture into pasta; add salt and pepper. Cover and refrigerate for several hours or until ready to serve.

### Kitchen Tip

Adding frozen peas to hot pasta allows them to thaw, yet still retain their bright green color.

| Nutritional Analysis | Energy | Protein | Carbohydrate | Fat | Calcium | Iron |
|---|---|---|---|---|---|---|
| per 1/2-cup (125 mL) serving | 161 kcal | 4.3 g | 24.3 g | 5.0 g | 2 % CDV | 7 % CDV |

# Strawberry Salad

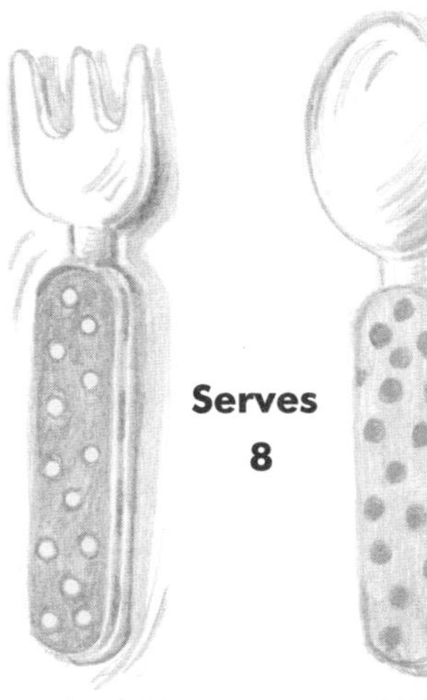

**Serves 8**

*Just the name of this salad is appealing to kids. They'll love it even more when they taste it!*

**Kitchen Tip**

Try replacing the strawberries with mandarin segments and add 1/4 cup (50 mL) mushrooms.

| | | |
|---|---|---|
| 1 | bunch fresh spinach (about 6 oz [150 g]), washed and torn into bite-sized pieces | 1 |
| 2 cups | lettuce, washed and torn into bite-sized pieces | 500 mL |
| 2 cups | sliced fresh strawberries | 500 mL |
| 2 tbsp | sesame seeds | 25 mL |
| **Dressing** | | |
| 2 tbsp | olive oil | 25 mL |
| 2 tbsp | vinegar | 25 mL |
| 1 tbsp | granulated sugar | 15 mL |
| Pinch | paprika | Pinch |

1. In a salad bowl, toss spinach and lettuce until combined. Add strawberries. Sprinkle with sesame seeds.
2. Dressing: In a small bowl, whisk together oil, vinegar, sugar and paprika. Just before serving, pour dressing over salad and toss lightly.

| Nutritional Analysis | Energy | Protein | Carbohydrate | Fat | Calcium | Iron |
|---|---|---|---|---|---|---|
| per 1-cup (250 mL) serving | 62 kcal | 1.4 g | 6.2 g | 4.1 g | 7 % CDV | 12 % CDV |

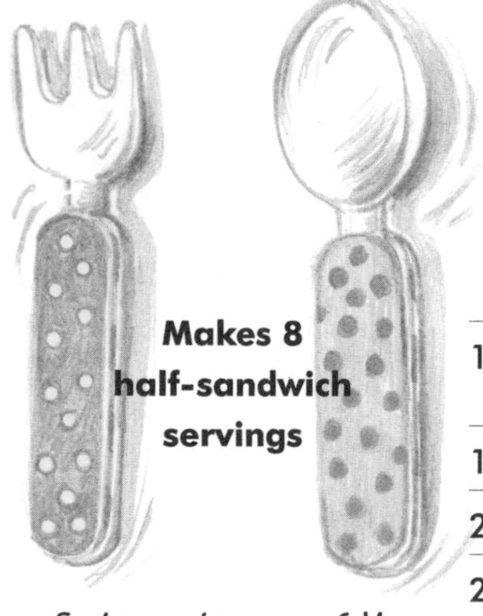

# Super Salmon Sandwiches

**Makes 8 half-sandwich servings**

*Salmon is one of the world's favorite sandwich fillings – and we think this version is one of the best. See if you agree.*

| | | |
|---|---|---|
| 1 | can (7.5 oz [213 g]) salmon, undrained | 1 |
| 1/4 cup | mayonnaise | 50 mL |
| 2 tbsp | finely chopped onion | 25 mL |
| 2 tsp | lemon juice | 10 mL |
| 1/4 tsp | salt | 1 mL |
| Pinch | freshly ground black pepper | Pinch |
| 4 | whole wheat English muffins split and toasted (see Tip, at left) | 4 |

1. In a small bowl, flake salmon. Remove and discard skin, but mash bones with salmon. Stir in mayonnaise, onion, lemon juice, salt and pepper.
2. Spread filling on one-half of toasted muffin and top with other half. Cut assembled sandwich into 2 pieces and serve.

### Kitchen Tip

Mashing the bones with the salmon (instead of discarding them) provides as much extra calcium as is contained in a small glass of milk.

We like the taste and texture of English muffins, but any bread will work with this filling.

If you have any filling left over, just cover and refrigerate for up to 2 days.

### Variation

**Oven-Toasted Cheese**: Broil each muffin half on a baking sheet until toasted; spread with salmon filling. Top each half with a slice of cheese, return to broiler and broil until cheese melts.

| Nutritional Analysis | Energy | Protein | Carbohydrate | Fat | Calcium | Iron |
|---|---|---|---|---|---|---|
| per 1/2-sandwich serving | 161 kcal | 7.9 g | 14.4 g | 7.6 g | 15 % CDV | 12 % CDV |

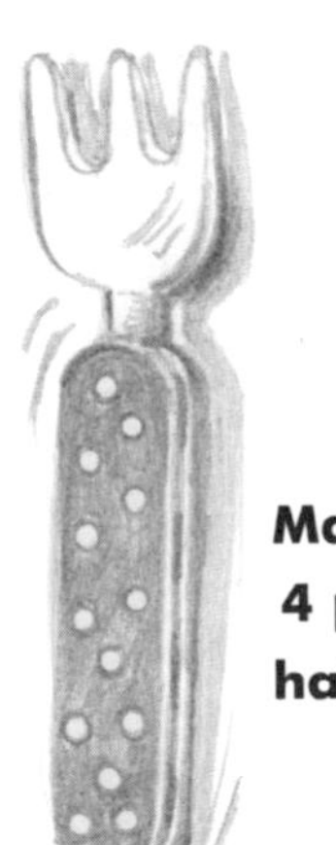
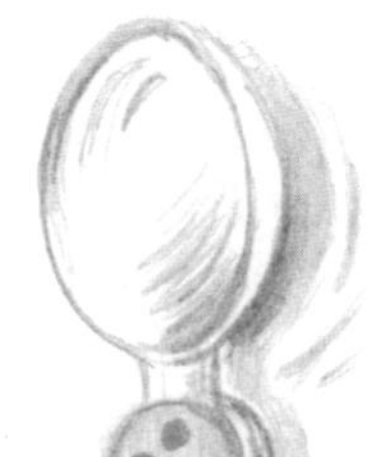
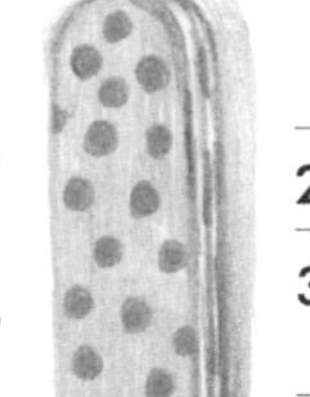

# Hasty Pita Lunch

*Preheat broiler*

**Makes 4 pita halves**

| | | |
|---|---|---|
| 2 | 7-inch (18 cm) whole wheat pitas | 2 |
| 3/4 cup | shredded Cheddar cheese (see Tip, at left) | 175 mL |
| 1 | green onion, finely chopped | 1 |
| 1 | medium tomato, diced | 1 |
| 1/4 tsp | dried basil | 1 mL |
| 1/4 tsp | dried oregano | 1 mL |

*This lunch can be made in the proverbial "blink of an eye" – or close to it! Keep the necessary ingredients on hand and you'll always be ready with an instant meal.*

1. With kitchen scissors, cut around edge of each pita to separate it into 2 rounds. Place cut-side up on baking sheet and broil for 2 minutes or until lightly golden.
2. Divide cheese between rounds, being careful to spread evenly to their edges. Sprinkle with green onion and tomato, then with basil and oregano. Return to oven and broil for 3 minutes or until cheese starts to melt.

### Kitchen Tip

For added convenience, look for pre-shredded cheese in the dairy case of your supermarkets. Typically, these are available in a number of varieties, including Cheddar, mozzarella, Monterey Jack – or a combination of cheeses.

| Nutritional Analysis | Energy | Protein | Carbohydrate | Fat | Calcium | Iron |
|---|---|---|---|---|---|---|
| per half pita | 158 kcal | 8.3 g | 21.7 g | 5.1 g | 14 % CDV | 3 % CDV |

# Tex-Mex Turkey Wraps

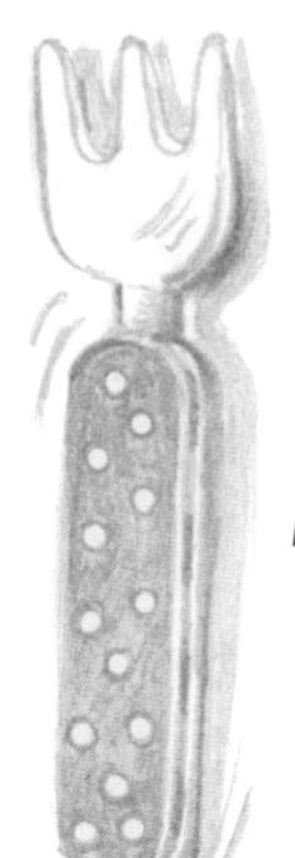

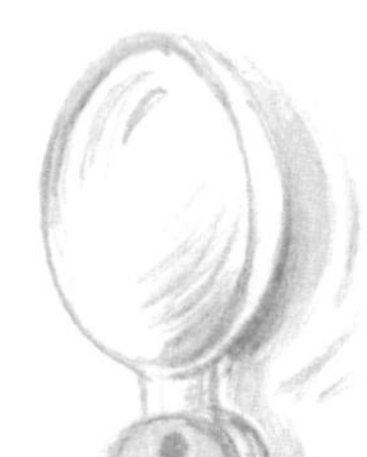

**Makes 12 wraps**

*Mexican dishes are zesty but simple – often requiring only everyday ingredients you already have in your refrigerator. These wraps are a great way to use up leftover turkey.*

### Kitchen Tip

If desired, spread additional salsa over cheese before baking.

*Preheat oven to 350° F (180° C)*
*Large baking pan*

| | | |
|---|---|---|
| 1 tbsp | vegetable oil | 15 mL |
| 2 | small onions, finely chopped | 2 |
| 2 | cloves garlic, minced | 2 |
| 4 cups | chopped cooked turkey | 1 L |
| 2 cups | medium or mild salsa (see Tip, at left) | 500 mL |
| 1 tsp | chili powder | 5 mL |
| 12 | large (10-inch [25 cm]) flour tortillas | 12 |
| 2 cups | shredded Cheddar cheese, divided | 500 mL |

1. In a nonstick skillet, heat oil over medium-high heat. Add onions and garlic; sauté for 5 minutes or until softened but not browned. Stir in turkey, salsa and chili powder; cook until warmed through.
2. Place tortillas on a flat surface. Divide turkey mixture between tortillas, spreading evenly over each. Divide 1 1/2 cups (375 mL) of the cheese over the tortillas. Roll tortillas and place in a single layer on baking pan. Top with remaining cheese and bake in preheated oven until cheese is melted.

| Nutritional Analysis | Energy | Protein | Carbohydrate | Fat | Calcium | Iron |
|---|---|---|---|---|---|---|
| per serving | 412 kcal | 28.9 g | 28.7 g | 19.8 g | 43 % CDV | 23 % CDV |

# Focaccia Pizza Squares

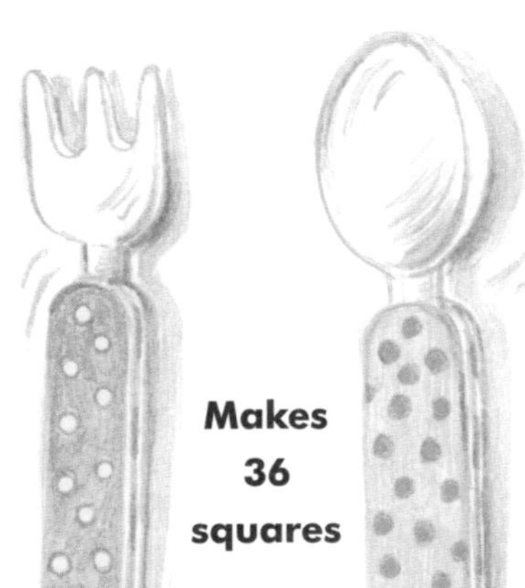

**Makes 36 squares**

*Focaccia is a type of Italian flatbread that is widely available in grocery stores today. It makes an ideal base for various toppings, and an easy pizza lunch or snack.*

*Preheat oven to 425° F (220° C)*
*Large baking pan*

| | | |
|---|---|---|
| 1 | focaccia or Italian-style flatbread (about 14 oz [400 g]) | 1 |
| 1 | can (7 1/2 oz [213 mL]) tomato sauce | 1 |
| 1/2 tsp | dried basil | 2 mL |
| 1/2 tsp | dried oregano | 2 mL |
| 1/2 cup | finely minced ham | 125 mL |
| 1/4 cup | diced green or red bell pepper | 50 mL |
| 1 cup | shredded Cheddar cheese | 250 mL |

1. Place flatbread on baking pan. In a bowl combine tomato sauce, basil and oregano. Spread sauce mixture evenly over bread. Sprinkle with ham, green pepper and cheese.
2. Bake in preheated oven for 15 minutes or until crust is golden and cheese has melted. Remove from oven and cut into 36 small pieces.

| Nutritional Analysis | Energy | Protein | Carbohydrate | Fat | Calcium | Iron |
|---|---|---|---|---|---|---|
| per square | 50 kcal | 2.2 g | 6.8 g | 1.5 g | 3 % CDV | 4 % CDV |

# Cheese Pizza Muffins

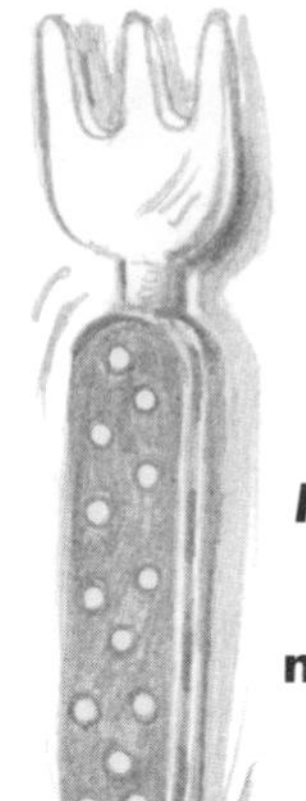

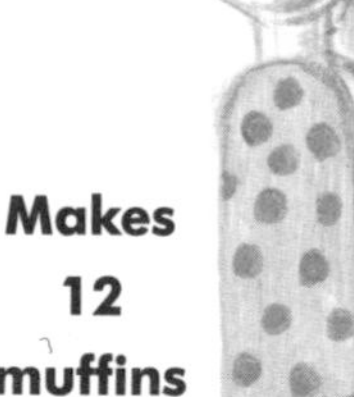

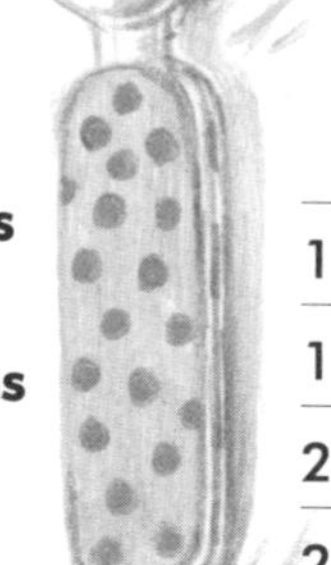

**Makes 12 muffins**

*These tasty muffins are ideal to have tucked away in the freezer for those days when you need lunch (or breakfast) in a hurry. Served with a glass of milk, they also make an ideal snack.*

*Preheat oven to 375° F (190° C)*
*12-cup muffin pan, greased or paper-lined*

| | | |
|---|---|---|
| 1 1/2 cups | all-purpose flour | 375 mL |
| 1 cup | whole wheat flour | 250 mL |
| 2 tbsp | granulated sugar | 25 mL |
| 2 tsp | baking powder | 10 mL |
| 1 tsp | dried basil | 5 mL |
| 1/2 tsp | dried oregano | 2 mL |
| 1/2 tsp | baking soda | 2 mL |
| 1/2 tsp | salt | 2 mL |
| 2 cups | shredded Cheddar cheese | 500 mL |
| 1 | egg | 1 |
| 1 1/2 cups | buttermilk | 375 mL |
| 1/3 cup | vegetable oil | 75 mL |

1. In a bowl combine all-purpose flour, whole wheat flour, sugar, baking powder, basil, oregano, baking soda, salt and cheese.
2. In another bowl, whisk together egg, buttermilk and oil. Add to dry ingredients. stir just until moistened.
3. Spoon batter into prepared muffin pan. Bake in preheated oven for 25 minutes or until muffins are firm to the touch. Cool 10 minutes before removing from pan to wire rack to cool completely.

| NUTRITIONAL ANALYSIS | Energy | Protein | Carbohydrate | Fat | Calcium | Iron |
|---|---|---|---|---|---|---|
| per muffin | 349 kcal | 15.6 g | 24.1 g | 21.4 g | 46 % CDV | 15 % CDV |

# Cheese Tortilla Wedges

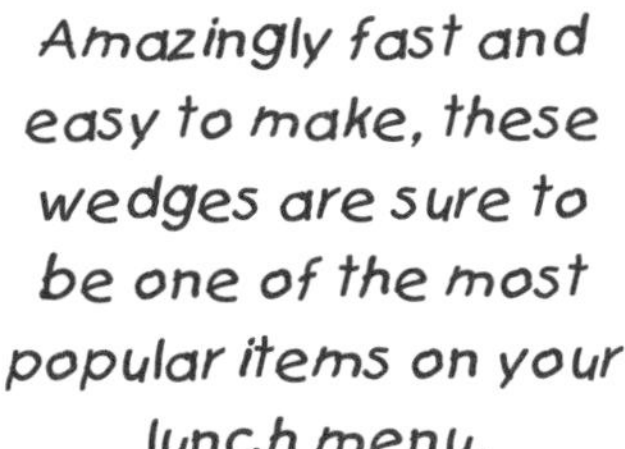

**Makes 8 wedges**

*Amazingly fast and easy to make, these wedges are sure to be one of the most popular items on your lunch menu.*

*Preheat oven to 400° F (200° C)*
*Baking sheet*

| | | |
|---|---|---|
| 4 | 8-inch (20 cm) flour tortillas | 4 |
| 3/4 cup | shredded mozzarella cheese | 175 mL |
| 1 | green onion, finely chopped | 1 |
| 1/2 tsp | dried oregano | 2 mL |
| 1 tsp | vegetable oil | 5 mL |

1. Place 2 tortillas on baking sheet. Distribute cheese evenly over each tortilla. Sprinkle with onion and oregano. Press remaining 2 tortillas on top. Brush tops with oil.
2. Bake in preheated oven for 5 minutes or until cheese is melted. Remove from oven and cut each stack into 4 wedges.

| NUTRITIONAL ANALYSIS | Energy | Protein | Carbohydrate | Fat | Calcium | Iron |
|---|---|---|---|---|---|---|
| per wedge | 128 kcal | 7.8 g | 10.2 g | 6.1 g | 22 % CDV | 5 % CDV |

# Antiijitos

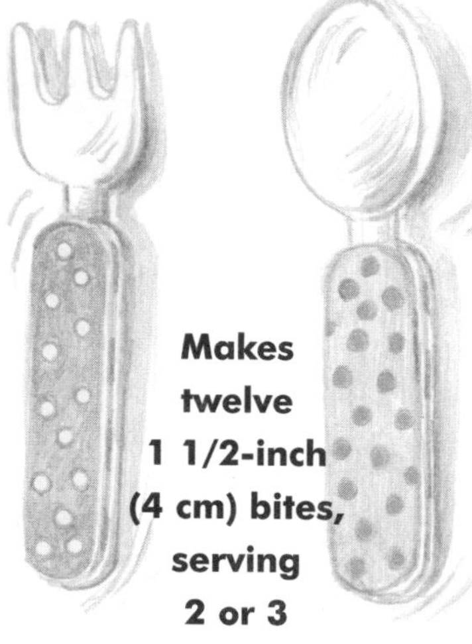

**Makes twelve 1 1/2-inch (4 cm) bites, serving 2 or 3**

| | | |
|---|---|---|
| 2 | large (10-inch [25 cm]) tortillas | 2 |
| 1/4 cup | spreadable cream cheese | 50 mL |
| 1/4 cup | salsa | 50 mL |

1. On each tortilla, thinly spread 2 tbsp (25 mL) each cream cheese and salsa. Roll each tortilla up tightly and cut the roll into 1 1/2-inch slices. Serve cold or bake in a preheated 350° F (180° C) oven for 5 minutes or until warmed through.

*Another speedy lunchtime treat, antijitos (pronounced "an-te-hee-toes") are a favorite with kids and adults alike.*

### Kitchen Tip

Antijitos make great appetizers for entertaining. For grown-up palates who prefer a little extra spice, add 1 tsp (5 mL) chopped jalapeño peppers to each tortilla before rolling.

| Nutritional Analysis | Energy | Protein | Carbohydrate | Fat | Calcium | Iron |
|---|---|---|---|---|---|---|
| per "bite" | 41 kcal | 0.9 g | 4.7 g | 2.1 g | 1 % CDV | 2 % CDV |

# Black Bean Burritos

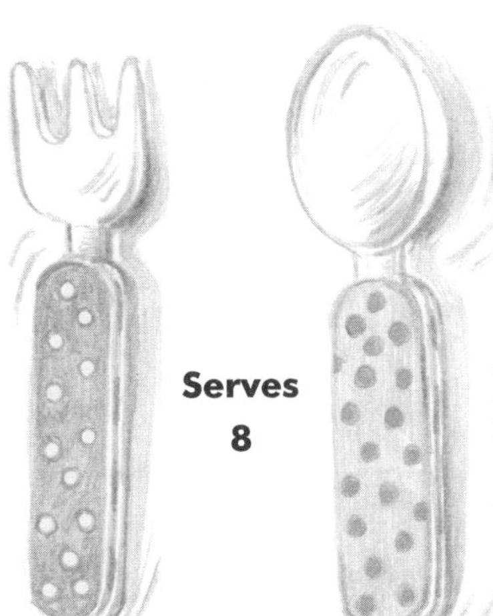

**Serves 8**

**KITCHEN TIP**

These burritos are excellent when topped with 1 to 2 tsp (5 to 10 mL) sour cream.

If your children are not accustomed to spicy food, you may wish to use only 1 tbsp (15 mL) chili powder.

| | | |
|---|---|---|
| 2 tbsp | vegetable oil | 25 mL |
| 1 | clove garlic, minced | 1 |
| Half | medium red onion, chopped | Half |
| 1 | green pepper, chopped | 1 |
| 1 | red bell pepper, chopped | 1 |
| 1 cup | canned black beans, rinsed and drained | 250 mL |
| 3 | carrots, shredded | 3 |
| 1/2 cup | chopped broccoli | 125 mL |
| 2 tbsp | chili powder (see Tip, at left) | 25 mL |
| 1 tbsp | ground cumin | 15 mL |
| 1/4 cup | water | 50 mL |
| 1/4 cup | red wine vinegar | 50 mL |
| 1 tbsp | brown sugar | 15 mL |
| 8 | soft tortilla shells, medium (8-inch [20 cm]) size | 8 |

1. In a large saucepan, heat oil over medium-high heat. Add garlic, onion, and peppers; sauté for about 5 minutes or until softened. Stir in beans, carrots, broccoli, chili powder, cumin, vinegar, water and brown sugar. Increase heat to high and cook for 5 minutes or until vegetables are tender.
2. In microwave, heat tortilla shells, 2 at a time, on High for 20 to 30 seconds.
3. Assembly: Place 1/2 cup (125 mL) bean mixture into middle of tortilla and fold all sides over to enclose.

| NUTRITIONAL ANALYSIS | Energy | Protein | Carbohydrate | Fat | Calcium | Iron |
|---|---|---|---|---|---|---|
| per burrito | 205 kcal | 5.7 g | 32.0 g | 6.5 g | 5 % CDV | 25 % CDV |

# Cheese and Tomato Macaroni

**Makes 4 cups (1 L)**

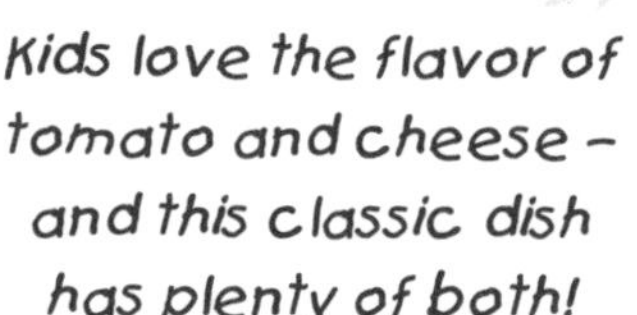

*Kids love the flavor of tomato and cheese – and this classic dish has plenty of both!*

| | | |
|---|---|---|
| 2 cups | elbow macaroni | 500 mL |
| 1 tbsp | butter or margarine | 15 mL |
| 3 tbsp | all-purpose flour | 45 mL |
| 2 cups | 2% milk, warmed to room temperature | 500 mL |
| 1 1/2 cups | shredded Cheddar cheese | 375 mL |
| 1 | can (19 oz [398 mL]) tomatoes, drained | 1 |
| 1/2 tsp | salt | 2 mL |
| Pinch | freshly ground black pepper | Pinch |

1. In a large saucepan, cook pasta in boiling water according to manufacturer's directions or until tender but firm. Drain.
2. In a second large saucepan, melt butter over medium heat. Add flour and cook, stirring, until it starts to bubble. Gradually add milk, whisking constantly, and cook until thickened. Add shredded cheese; stir until melted. Stir in drained tomatoes, salt and pepper.
3. Pour sauce over macaroni and toss to coat.

| NUTRITIONAL ANALYSIS | Energy | Protein | Carbohydrate | Fat | Calcium | Iron |
|---|---|---|---|---|---|---|
| per 1/2-cup (125 mL) serving | 259 kcal | 12.0 g | 28.9 g | 10.6 g | 33 % CDV | 11 % CDV |

# Pasta with Vegetables and Asian Peanut Sauce

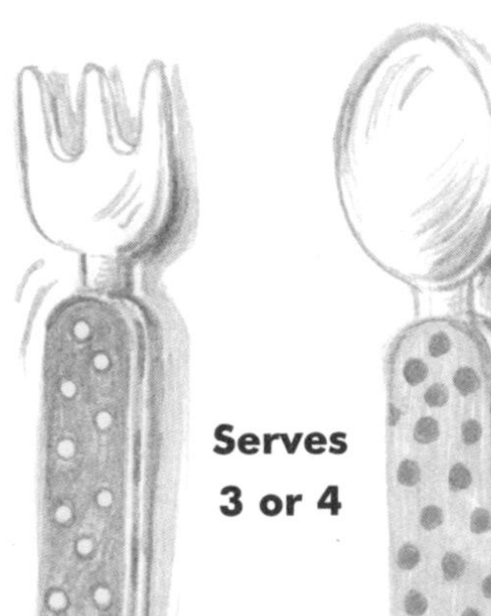
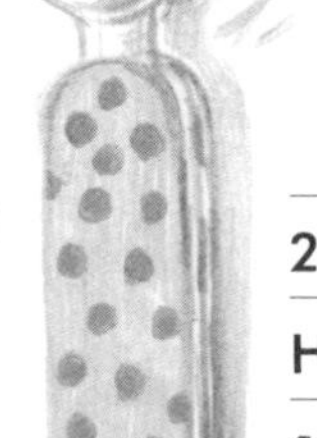

**Serves 3 or 4**

*For children and parents who love the flavor of peanuts (and are not allergic to them), here's a great combination of pasta, vegetables and sauce.*

| | | |
|---|---|---|
| 2 cups | short pasta (such as fusilli) | 500 mL |
| Half | red bell pepper, cut into thin strips | Half |
| 1 | large carrot, peeled and cut into thin strips | 1 |
| 1 | clove garlic | 1 |
| 1/2 cup | cilantro leaves (optional) | 125 mL |
| 1/2 cup | creamy peanut butter | 125 mL |
| 1/4 cup | soy sauce | 50 mL |
| 1 tbsp | lemon juice | 15 mL |
| 2 tsp | sesame oil | 10 mL |
| 1 cup | diced cucumber | 250 mL |
| 1 | green onion, sliced | 1 |
| Pinch | salt | Pinch |
| Pinch | freshly ground black pepper | Pinch |

1. In a large saucepan, cook pasta in boiling water according to manufacturer's directions or until tender but firm. A few minutes before the end of cooking time, add red pepper and carrot. Drain well and return to saucepan.
2. Meanwhile, in a food processor, process garlic and cilantro with on/off turns until chopped. Transfer to a bowl. Stir in peanut butter, soy sauce, lemon juice and sesame oil.
3. When pasta and vegetables are cooked and drained, add peanut sauce. Toss to coat. Stir in cucumber and green onions, and season with salt and pepper.

| Nutritional Analysis | Energy | Protein | Carbohydrate | Fat | Calcium | Iron |
|---|---|---|---|---|---|---|
| per serving (4) | 455 kcal | 17.2 g | 54.6 g | 20.1 g | 5 % CDV | 22 % CDV |

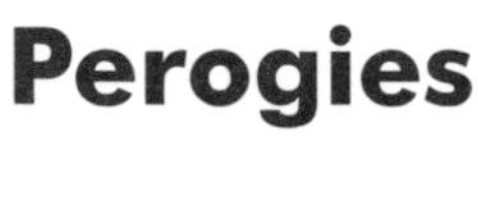

# Perogies

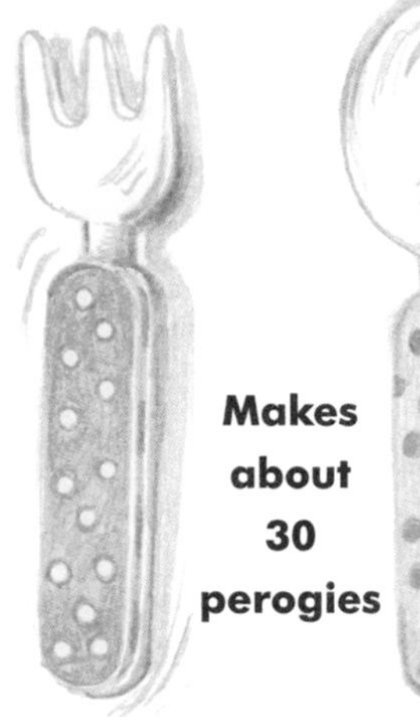


*This authentic East European dish makes great use of leftover mashed potatoes.*

| | | |
|---|---|---|
| 2 cups | all-purpose flour | 500 mL |
| 1 tsp | salt | 5 mL |
| 1 | egg, beaten | 1 |
| 2/3 cup | cold water | 150 mL |
| 1 cup | mashed potatoes | 250 mL |
| 1/2 cup | shredded Cheddar cheese | 125 mL |
| | Salt and freshly ground pepper to taste | |
| | Plain yogurt or sour cream | |

1. In a large bowl, combine flour, salt, egg and water. Mix together to form dough. Cover bowl and set aside.
2. In another bowl, combine mashed potatoes, cheese, salt and pepper.
3. Assembly: On a lightly floured surface, roll out dough. Cut circles out of dough using a 3-inch (7.5 cm) round cookie cutter or drinking glass. Place about 1 tsp (5 mL) potato mixture in center of each circle and fold over, pinching edges to seal.
4. In a large pot of boiling water, cook perogies 8 to 12 at a time for 4 to 5 minutes or until they float. Serve with yogurt or sour cream.

### Kitchen Tip

Cook perogies in boiling water or, for a change, pan-fry with a little butter and sliced onion.

Perogies freeze extremely well. Place assembled (uncooked) perogies on a baking sheet and freeze. Once frozen, transfer perogies to freezer bags and store in freezer. Cook perogies from frozen, adding about 3 minutes to boiling time.

| Nutritional Analysis | Energy | Protein | Carbohydrate | Fat | Calcium | Iron |
|---|---|---|---|---|---|---|
| per 3 perogie serving | 162 kcal | 5.7 g | 27.9 g | 3.0 g | 6 % CDV | 15 % CDV |

# Lentil Patties

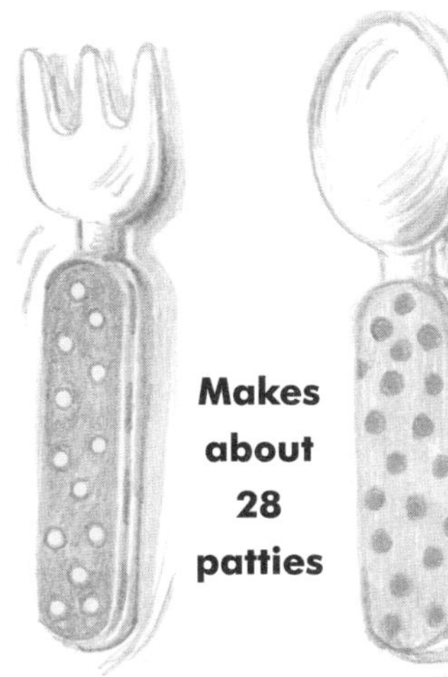

**Makes about 28 patties**

*If you're going to try just one lentil recipe, this is the one to make. Your kids and the rest of the family will love the flavor of these patties. They're also great as a snack, since they don't need to be reheated.*

**KITCHEN TIP**

Serve plain or with dip (Ranch-style is good) or try plum sauce.

These patties take a bit of time to prepare, so you may want to make them ahead and freeze until needed. When ready to serve, just thaw in the microwave.

| | | |
|---|---|---|
| 1 cup | red lentils | 250 mL |
| 2 tsp | olive oil | 10 mL |
| 2 | small onions, chopped | 2 |
| 2 | large tomatoes, chopped | 2 |
| 1 | small apple, peeled and chopped | 1 |
| 2 1/4 cups | bread crumbs, divided | 550 mL |
| 1 tsp | dried sage | 5 mL |
| Pinch | salt | Pinch |
| Pinch | freshly ground black pepper | Pinch |
| 1 | egg, lightly beaten | 1 |
| 4 tbsp | olive oil, divided | 50 mL |

1. Rinse lentils and transfer to a saucepan. Add 3 cups (750 mL) water. Bring to a boil; cook for about 30 minutes or until soft. Drain and set aside.
2. In a skillet heat 2 tsp (10 mL) olive oil over medium-high heat. Add onions, tomatoes and apples; cook for about 10 minutes or until soft. Transfer mixture to saucepan containing lentils, along with 1/4 cup (50 mL) of the bread crumbs, sage, salt and pepper. Add egg and mix well.
3. Wipe skillet clean and heat 1 tbsp (15 mL) of the olive oil over medium-high heat. Using your hands, form lentil mixture into patties. Roll each patty in remaining bread crumbs and cook for about 5 minutes per side or until crisp. Cook remaining patties, adding oil as required, 1 tbsp (15 mL) at a time.

| NUTRITIONAL ANALYSIS | Energy | Protein | Carbohydrate | Fat | Calcium | Iron |
|---|---|---|---|---|---|---|
| per patty | 84 kcal | 3.5 g | 11.9 g | 2.7 g | 2 % CDV | 11 % CDV |

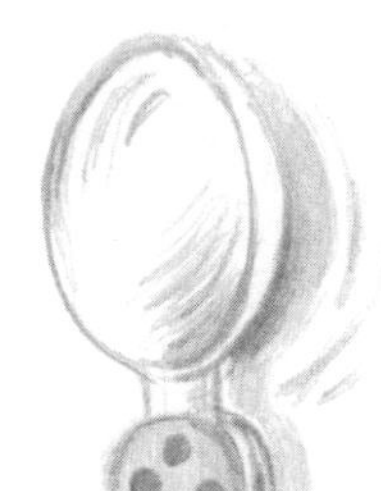

# Eggs Baked in Cheese

**Serves 4**

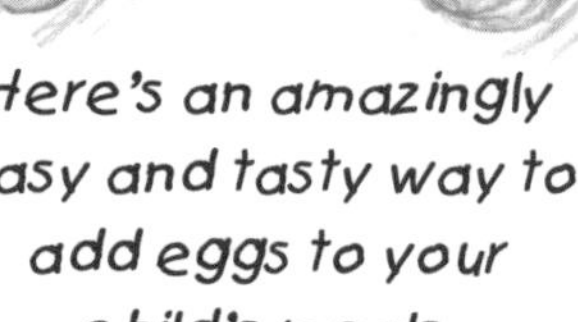

*Here's an amazingly easy and tasty way to add eggs to your child's meals.*

*Preheat oven to 350° F (180° C)*
*8-inch (2 L) baking pan, greased*

| | | |
|---|---|---|
| 2/3 cup | shredded Cheddar cheese | 150 mL |
| 4 | eggs | 4 |
| 1/2 cup | whole milk or light (10%) cream | 125 mL |
| 1/4 tsp | salt | 1 mL |
| Pinch | freshly ground black pepper | Pinch |
| Pinch | paprika | Pinch |
| | Finely chopped parsley (optional) | |

1. Sprinkle cheese over bottom of prepared pan. Break eggs over cheese.
2. In a bowl whisk together milk, salt and pepper. Pour over eggs. Sprinkle lightly with paprika.
3. Bake in preheated oven for 20 minutes or until eggs are just set. Sprinkle with parsley, if desired.

| Nutritional Analysis | Energy | Protein | Carbohydrate | Fat | Calcium | Iron |
|---|---|---|---|---|---|---|
| per serving | 167 kcal | 11.6 g | 2.4 g | 12.1 g | 25 % CDV | 12 % CDV |

# Quiche Lorraine

*Preheat oven to 400° F (200° C)*

**Serves 6**

*This classic quiche is a perennial lunchtime favorite. Feel free to experiment with ingredients (see Variations, below).*

| | | |
|---|---|---|
| 1 | 9-inch (23 cm) frozen pastry shell, thawed | 1 |
| 4 | eggs | 4 |
| 1 1/2 cups | light (10%) cream or whole milk | 375 mL |
| 1/2 tsp | salt | 2 mL |
| Pinch | ground nutmeg | Pinch |
| Pinch | freshly ground black pepper | Pinch |
| 1 cup | grated Swiss cheese | 250 mL |
| 6 | slices cooked bacon, crumbled | 6 |
| 2 | green onions, finely chopped | 2 |

1. Prick bottom of pastry shell with a fork; partially bake in preheated oven for 8 minutes. Remove from oven; reduce heat to 350° F (180° C).
2. In a small bowl, lightly beat eggs. Stir in cream, salt, nutmeg and pepper.
3. Spread cheese, bacon and onions in pastry shell. Pour in egg mixture. Bake for 35 minutes or until knife inserted in center comes out clean. Remove from oven and let stand for 10 minutes before cutting into 6 pieces.

### Variations

**Cheddar Cheese and Ham**: Replace Swiss cheese with Cheddar and bacon with 1/2 cup (125 mL) diced ham. Replace nutmeg with a pinch of dry mustard or Dijon mustard added to egg mixture.

**Savory Leek**: Replace green onion with 1 leek, sliced, washed and blanched for 5 minutes.

**Smoked Salmon**: Replace bacon with 1/2 cup (125 mL) diced smoked salmon. Use Swiss cheese or replace with an equal quantity of Cheddar.

| Nutritional Analysis | Energy | Protein | Carbohydrate | Fat | Calcium | Iron |
|---|---|---|---|---|---|---|
| per serving | 423 kcal | 20.8 g | 18.0 g | 29.5 g | 59 % CDV | 16 % CDV |

# Salmon Puff

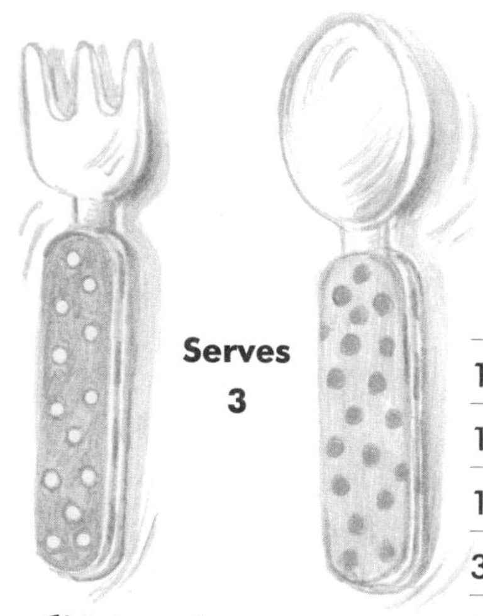

**Serves 3**

*This is actually a soufflé – we just thought "puff" sounds less intimidating! There's no reason to be worried about making this dish. It's easy enough for anyone to prepare.*

*Preheat oven to 375° F (190° C)*
*4-cup (1 L) casserole, greased*

| | | |
|---|---|---|
| 1 | can (7.5 oz [213 g]) salmon | 1 |
| 1/2 cup | 2% milk | 125 mL |
| 1 | slice white bread, crust removed | 1 |
| 3 | eggs, separated | 3 |
| 1/2 tsp | salt | 2 mL |
| 1/4 tsp | freshly ground black pepper | 1 mL |
| | Toast triangles as accompaniment | |

1. Drain liquid from salmon into a small saucepan. Transfer salmon to a bowl; flake salmon with a fork and set aside. Add milk to saucepan and warm gently over low heat.
2. In another bowl, cover bread slice with milk mixture. Allow to sit in a warm location until soft, then break apart with a fork. Add flaked salmon, egg yolks, salt and pepper; stir until smooth.
3. In a bowl with an electric mixer, beat egg whites until stiff. Fold into salmon mixture. Gently transfer mixture into prepared casserole or 3 individual dishes. Bake in preheated oven for about 20 minutes or until puffed and golden. Serve with toast triangles.

| Nutritional Analysis | Energy | Protein | Carbohydrate | Fat | Calcium | Iron |
|---|---|---|---|---|---|---|
| per serving | 247 kcal | 22.7 g | 7.5 g | 13.3 g | 34 % CDV | 22 % CDV |

# Zucchini Pudding

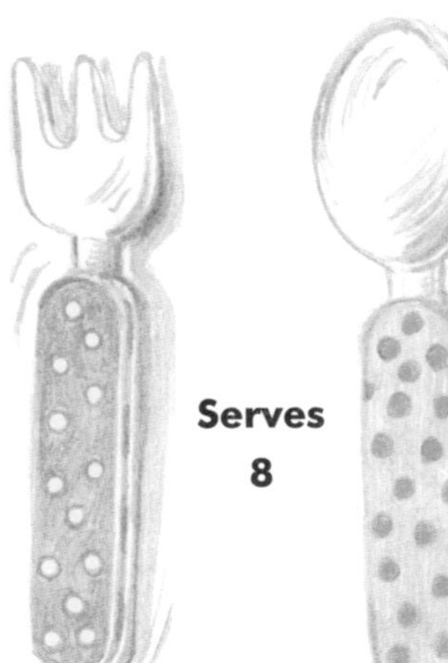

**Serves 8**

*This recipe sounds a little weird, we admit, but it makes a delicious side dish with chicken, beef or fish – or, served with French bread and cheese, as a meal in itself!*

### Kitchen Tip

To make individual puddings, bake in a lightly greased 12-cup muffin tin.

*Preheat oven to 350° F (180° C)*
*8-cup (2 L) casserole, lightly greased*

| | | |
|---|---|---|
| 3 cups | grated zucchini, rinsed and drained (about 2 medium zucchini) | 750 mL |
| Half | medium onion, chopped | Half |
| 4 | eggs | 4 |
| 1/2 cup | vegetable oil | 125 mL |
| 1/4 tsp | freshly ground pepper | 1 mL |
| Pinch | salt | Pinch |
| 2 tsp | chopped fresh parsley | 10 mL |
| 1 cup | bread crumbs | 250 mL |

1. Squeeze zucchini to remove any excess moisture. Set aside
2. In a bowl combine onion and eggs. Add zucchini and oil; mix well. Add pepper, salt, parsley and bread crumbs. Stir until well mixed. Transfer to casserole and bake for 45 minutes or until firm.

| Nutritional Analysis | Energy | Protein | Carbohydrate | Fat | Calcium | Iron |
|---|---|---|---|---|---|---|
| per serving | 236 kcal | 5.4 g | 14.1 g | 17.9 g | 6 % CDV | 14 % CDV |

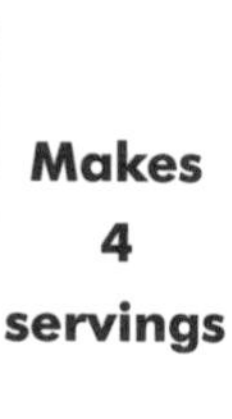
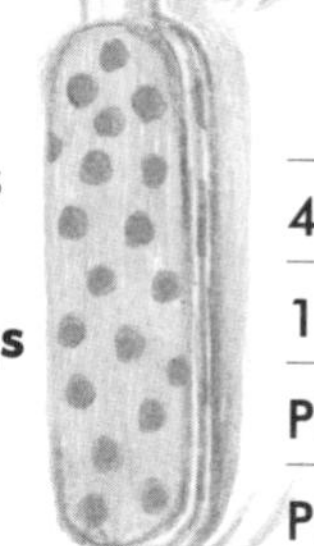

**Makes 4 servings**

*Here's the perfect way to add extra protein to baked potatoes. Try it for lunch or dinner.*

# Potatoes with Cheese and Egg Filling

*Preheat oven to 350° F (180° C)*

| | | |
|---|---|---|
| 4 | medium baking potatoes | 4 |
| 1 tbsp | butter or margarine | 15 mL |
| Pinch | paprika | Pinch |
| Pinch | salt | Pinch |
| Pinch | freshly ground black pepper | Pinch |
| 2 | slices processed cheese, halved | 2 |
| 4 | eggs | 4 |

1. Bake potatoes in preheated oven for 45 minutes or until tender. When cool enough to handle, use a sharp knife to cut a slice from the end of each potato. Using a spoon, scoop out most of cooked potato into a bowl. Set shells aside. Mash potato in bowl with butter, paprika, salt and pepper.
2. Place one half cheese slice in potato shell. Add 1 egg and one-quarter mashed potato mixture. Repeat with remaining potato shells. Bake for 15 minutes or until egg is cooked and potato is heated through.

| Nutritional Analysis | Energy | Protein | Carbohydrate | Fat | Calcium | Iron |
|---|---|---|---|---|---|---|
| per serving | 292 kcal | 11.6 g | 35.4 g | 11.7 g | 13 % CDV | 18 % CDV |

# Maria's Colorful French Fries

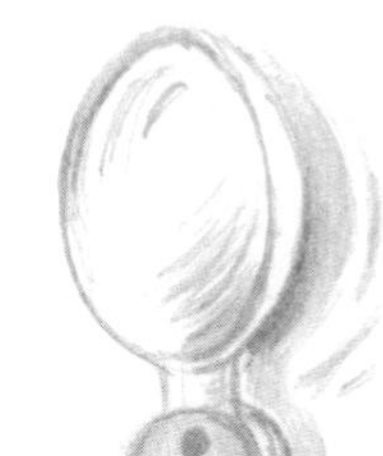

**Serves 12**

*Kids love french fries, and here we serve them up using two different types of potatoes. Serve plain or with ketchup.*

| | | |
|---|---|---|
| 2/3 cup | vegetable oil (see Tip, at left) | 150 mL |
| 2 | medium white (or Yukon gold) potatoes, peeled and cut into 1/2- by 2-inch (1 by 5 cm) pieces | 2 |
| Half | large sweet potato, peeled and cut into 1/2- by 2-inch (1 by 5 cm) pieces | Half |
| 1/2 tsp | salt | 2 mL |

1. In a large frying pan, heat oil over medium heat.
2. Meanwhile, in a bowl, toss together white and sweet potatoes. When oil is hot (test with a water drop), add one-third of potatoes to pan. Reduce heat to medium-high and cook, stirring occasionally, for 5 minutes or until golden and slightly browned. With a slotted spoon, transfer fries to a paper towel-lined plate to drain. Repeat procedure with remaining potatoes.
3. Allow potatoes to cool before serving (they will be very hot) and sprinkle with salt, if desired.

### Kitchen Tip

These french fries cook with only a small amount of oil. Canola or sunflower oil are good choices.

### Safety Tip

Make sure frying pan is placed on back burner while cooking. And, as always when cooking with young children around, never leave pan unattended – not even for a minute.

| Nutritional Analysis | Energy | Protein | Carbohydrate | Fat | Calcium | Iron |
|---|---|---|---|---|---|---|
| per serving | 54 kcal | 0.5 g | 4.7 g | 3.9 g | 1 % CDV | 2 % CDV |

# Zucchini Sticks

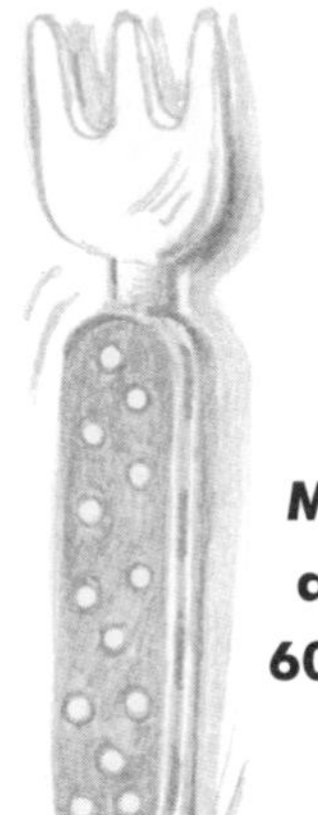

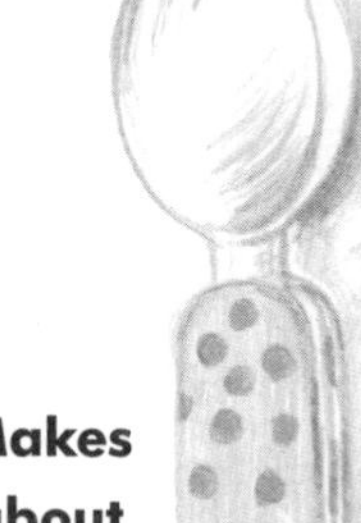

**Makes about 60 sticks**

*These unusual sticks are delicious hot or cold.*

**KITCHEN TIP**

Serve with sour cream or other creamy dressing.

*Preheat oven to 400° F (200° C)*
*Baking sheet, lightly greased*

| | | |
|---|---|---|
| 3/4 cup | bread crumbs | 175 mL |
| 1/4 cup | grated Parmesan cheese | 50 mL |
| 1/2 tsp | garlic powder | 2 mL |
| 1/2 tsp | dried sage | 2 mL |
| 1/4 tsp | salt | 1 mL |
| 1/4 tsp | freshly ground black pepper | 1 mL |
| 2 | eggs | 2 |
| 3 | medium zucchini, cut into 3- by 1/2-inch (8 by 1 cm) sticks | 3 |
| 1/4 cup | vegetable oil | 50 mL |

1. In a bowl combine bread crumbs, Parmesan, garlic powder, sage, salt and pepper; mix well.
2. In another bowl, beat eggs lightly.
3. Dip zucchini sticks in eggs, then in the bread crumb mixture; transfer to prepared baking sheet. Drizzle sticks with oil and bake for 20 minutes or until lightly browned, turning sticks over once halfway through baking time.

| NUTRITIONAL ANALYSIS | Energy | Protein | Carbohydrate | Fat | Calcium | Iron |
|---|---|---|---|---|---|---|
| per stick | 17 kcal | 0.5 g | 1.3 g | 1.1 g | 1 % CDV | 1 % CDV |

# Spaghetti Squash and Cheese

**Serves 12**

*Delicious on its own, with a slice of bread, or as a side dish with any meat, chicken or fish – this is a wonderful way to enjoy squash.*

| | | |
|---|---|---|
| 1 | spaghetti squash (about 3 lbs [1.5 kg]), well scrubbed and rinsed | 1 |
| 1 | clove garlic, crushed | 1 |
| 2 tbsp | butter | 25 mL |
| 1 cup | shredded Gruyere cheese | 250 mL |

1. With a sharp knife, cut spaghetti squash in half. Scoop out and discard seeds. Place squash halves cut-side down on a heatproof glass plate and microwave on High for 15 minutes or until flesh is soft. Allow to cool.
2. Using a fork, scoop out flesh into a large bowl while pulling "spaghetti strings" apart. Discard skin.
3. In a small bowl, combine garlic and butter. Microwave on High for 1 minute. Pour mixture over spaghetti squash. Add cheese and toss to coat.

**KITCHEN TIP**

For a change of taste, omit the cheese and garlic butter and mix plain spaghetti squash with 1 cup (250 mL) tomato sauce and sprinkle with 1 tbsp (15 mL) olive oil.

| NUTRITIONAL ANALYSIS | Energy | Protein | Carbohydrate | Fat | Calcium | Iron |
|---|---|---|---|---|---|---|
| per serving | 141 kcal | 7.2 g | 8.0 g | 9.3 g | 31 % CDV | 4 % CDV |

# Microwave Two-Cheese Rice

**Serves 8**

**KITCHEN TIP**

Try replacing both types of rice with equal quantities of cooked macaroni or other pasta.

Add 1 cup (250 mL) chopped cooked ham for additional protein and flavor!

For more cheese flavor, increase sauce ingredients (everything except rice) by one-half.

| | | |
|---|---|---|
| 2 tsp | butter | 10 mL |
| Half | clove garlic, minced | Half |
| 1/4 tsp | ground nutmeg | 1 mL |
| 2 tbsp | all-purpose flour | 25 mL |
| Half | can (6.5 oz [385 mL]) 2% evaporated milk | Half |
| 2/3 cup | shredded Cheddar cheese | 150 mL |
| 2/3 cup | crumbled feta cheese | 150 mL |
| 1 cup | cooked white rice | 250 mL |
| 1 cup | cooked brown rice | 250 mL |

1. Melt butter in microwave on High for 15 seconds. Add garlic and nutmeg; microwave on High for 15 seconds. Add flour and microwave on High for 1 minute.
2. Stir in evaporated milk and microwave on High for 5 to 8 minutes until thickened. Stir in cheeses and microwave on High for 1 minute until sauce thickened and cheese melted. Pour over cooked rice and serve.

| NUTRITIONAL ANALYSIS | Energy | Protein | Carbohydrate | Fat | Calcium | Iron |
|---|---|---|---|---|---|---|
| per 1/2-cup (125 mL) serving | 175 kcal | 8.2 g | 16.4 g | 8.4 g | 30 % CDV | 5 % CDV |

# Rice and Tofu

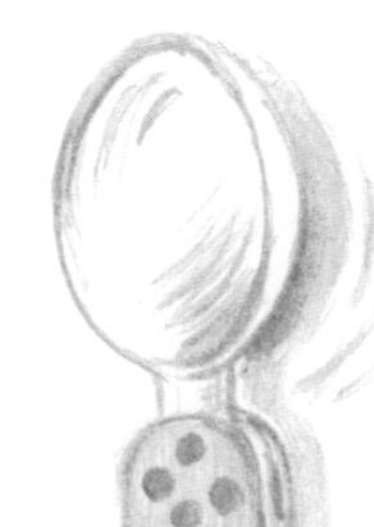

**Serves 8**

*Delicious as a complete meal, or as a tasty accompaniment to chicken or fish, this dish makes tofu into something special. In fact, it's so good, you may want to double the recipe!*

| | | |
|---|---|---|
| 2 tbsp | butter, divided | 25 mL |
| 2 cups | cooked rice | 500 mL |
| 1 | egg, lightly beaten | 1 |
| 4 oz | firm tofu, drained and cubed | 125 g |
| Third | medium onion, diced | Third |
| 1/2 cup | cooked diced carrots | 125 mL |
| 1/2 cup | cooked green peas | 125 mL |

1. In a saucepan melt 1 tbsp (15 mL) butter over medium-high heat. Add rice and cook, stirring, for 3 minutes or until cooked through. Transfer to a bowl and set aside.
2. Using same pan, melt 1 tsp (5 mL) butter. Add egg and scramble until cooked. Transfer to another bowl and set aside.
3. Wipe pan clean, and melt another 1 tsp (5 mL) butter. Add tofu and cook, stirring, for 2 minutes or until lightly browned. Transfer to another bowl and set aside.
4. Wipe pan clean, and melt remaining 1 tsp (5 mL) butter. Add onion and cook for 2 minutes or until softened. Add reserved rice, egg and tofu. Stir in carrots and peas. Cook mixture until heated through. Serve immediately.

**Kitchen Tip**

For flavor variety, sprinkle with light soy sauce or teriyaki sauce.

Try different vegetables, such as zucchini, corn, spinach. Diced cooked chicken or beef can also replace the tofu.

| Nutritional Analysis | Energy | Protein | Carbohydrate | Fat | Calcium | Iron |
|---|---|---|---|---|---|---|
| per 1/2-cup (125 mL) serving | 119 kcal | 4.8 g | 15.1 g | 4.5 g | 6 % CDV | 21 % CDV |

# Tasty Tofu

**Serves 8**

**KITCHEN TIP**

For young children who don't like the strong taste of garlic, omit this ingredient from Step 2. If you wish, once the child has been served, you can season the remaining sauce with garlic powder.

Serve this dish on its own or over rice. For added flavor and texture, try adding snow peas at end of cooking.

| | | |
|---|---|---|
| 12 oz | extra-firm tofu, patted dry and cut into 1/2-inch (1 cm) cubes | 350 g |
| 1 tbsp | vegetable oil | 15 mL |
| 1 | clove garlic, minced (see Tip, at left) | 1 |
| 1 tsp | ground ginger | 5 mL |
| 1/3 cup | teriyaki sauce | 75 mL |
| 2 tbsp | brown sugar | 25 mL |
| 2 tsp | molasses | 10 mL |
| 1 tbsp | sesame oil | 15 mL |
| 1 | green onion, chopped | 1 |

1. In a saucepan heat oil over medium-high heat. Add tofu and sauté for 10 minutes or until browned on all sides. (Cubes should be crispy.) Transfer to a bowl and set aside.
2. Add the garlic and ginger to pan; cook, stirring, for about 15 seconds. Add teriyaki sauce, brown sugar, molasses, sesame oil and onions. Bring to a boil, stirring occasionally. Add tofu and cook for 3 minutes, tossing cubes gently until thoroughly glazed and sauce is syrupy in texture.

| NUTRITIONAL ANALYSIS | Energy | Protein | Carbohydrate | Fat | Calcium | Iron |
|---|---|---|---|---|---|---|
| per serving | 118 kcal | 7.6 g | 7.3 g | 7.3 g | 13 % CDV | 52 % CDV |

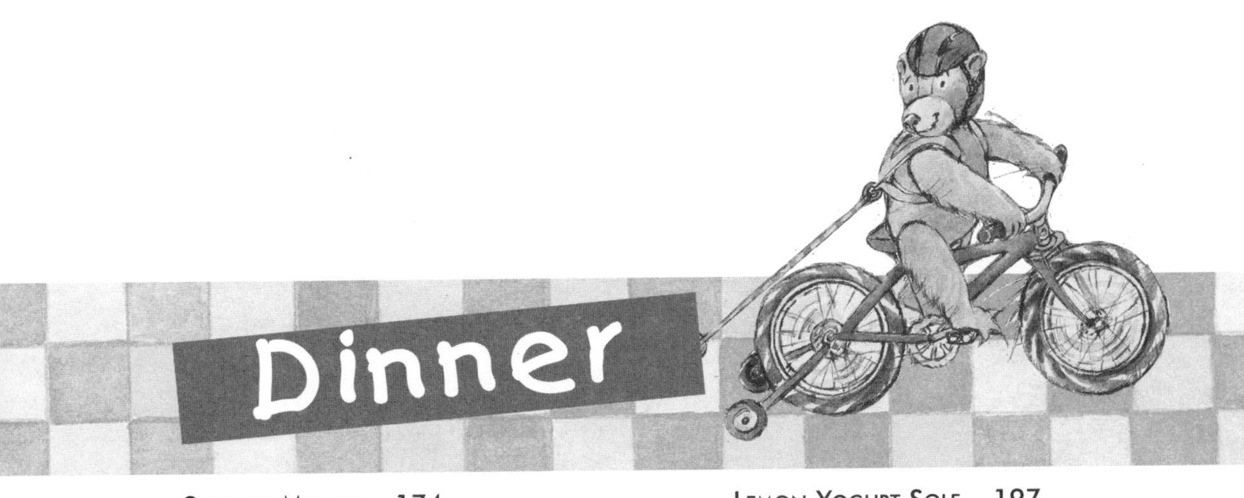

# Dinner

# Sopa de Mexico

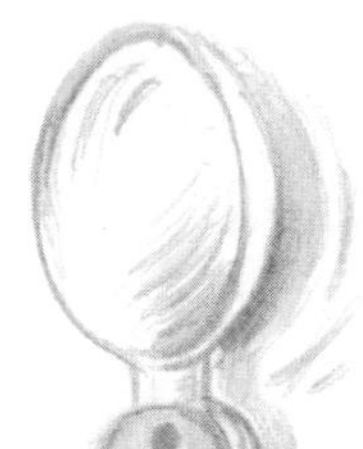

**Makes 6 cups (1.5 L)**

*Beans, corn, chili, Mexican seasonings and tomatoes give this soup its authentic flavors. It works well as a vegetarian dish or with meat added.*

**Kitchen Tip**

If your children are not accustomed to spicy food, you may wish to use only 1 tsp (5 mL) chili powder.

| | | |
|---|---|---|
| 1/2 cup | dried pinto or kidney beans | 125 mL |
| 2 tsp | vegetable oil | 10 mL |
| 1/2 cup | chopped onion | 125 mL |
| 2 | cloves garlic, crushed | 2 |
| 2 tsp | chili powder | 10 mL |
| 1/2 tsp | ground cumin | 2 mL |
| 1/2 tsp | ground oregano | 2 mL |
| Pinch | freshly ground black pepper | Pinch |
| 3 cups | beef stock or vegetable stock | 750 mL |
| 1 | large carrot, peeled and sliced | 1 |
| 1 cup | frozen corn kernels | 250 mL |
| | Garnishes: sour cream, corn tortilla chips, shredded cheese, chopped avocado, tomato, green onions and cilantro | |

1. In a saucepan combine beans with 1 1/2 cups (375 mL) cold water. Cover and bring to a boil; reduce heat and cook for 5 minutes. Remove from heat and let stand for 1 hour. Drain and discard liquid. Transfer to a bowl and set aside.
2. In same pan, heat oil over medium-high heat. Add onion and garlic; sauté for 5 minutes or until softened. Stir in chili powder, cumin, oregano and pepper. Add broth and reserved beans. Cover and bring to a boil; reduce heat and simmer, stirring occasionally, for 1 1/2 hours or until beans are tender.
3. Add carrots and corn; cook for 10 minutes or until vegetables are tender. Serve with a variety of garnishes at the table. You may need to assist younger children with their choices.

| Nutritional Analysis | Energy | Protein | Carbohydrate | Fat | Calcium | Iron |
|---|---|---|---|---|---|---|
| per 1-cup (250 mL) serving | 122 kcal | 6.0 g | 20.8 g | 2.6 g | 6 % CDV | 20 % CDV |

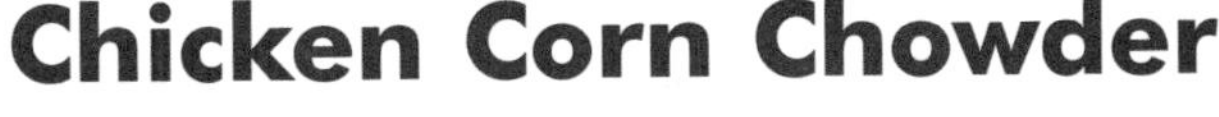

# Chicken Corn Chowder

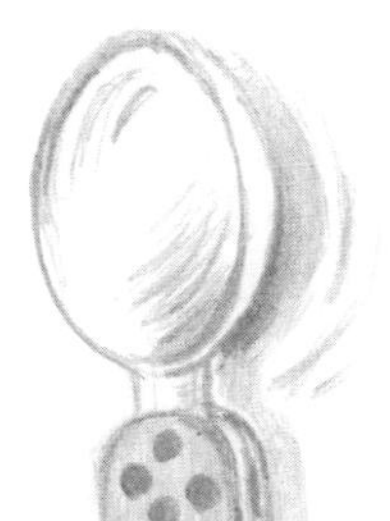

**Makes 6 cups (1.5 L)**

*Here's an easy way to make a comforting thick chowder for dinner.*

| | | |
|---|---|---|
| 2 | boneless skinless chicken breasts | 2 |
| 2 cups | water | 500 mL |
| 1/2 tsp | salt | 2 mL |
| Pinch | freshly ground black pepper | Pinch |
| 1 | stalk celery, finely chopped | 1 |
| Half | small onion, finely chopped | Half |
| 1 | large potato, peeled and cubed | 1 |
| 1 | large carrot, peeled and sliced | 1 |
| 1 | can (14 oz [341 mL]) creamed corn | 1 |
| 1 cup | 2% milk | 250 mL |

1. In a large saucepan, bring chicken, water, salt and pepper to a boil. Reduce heat, cover and cook for about 20 minutes or until chicken is no longer pink. Remove chicken from cooking liquid and, when cool enough to handle, cut into cubes. Set aside.
2. Add celery, onion, potato, and carrot to cooking liquid. Bring to a boil, reduce heat and simmer for 10 minutes or until vegetables are tender. Add corn, milk and reserved chicken. Reheat to serving temperature.

| **Nutritional Analysis** | Energy | Protein | Carbohydrate | Fat | Calcium | Iron |
|---|---|---|---|---|---|---|
| per 1-cup (250 mL) serving | 232 kcal | 21.1 g | 40.6 g | 2.6 g | 14 % CDV | 16 % CDV |

# Macaroni and Beef with Cheese

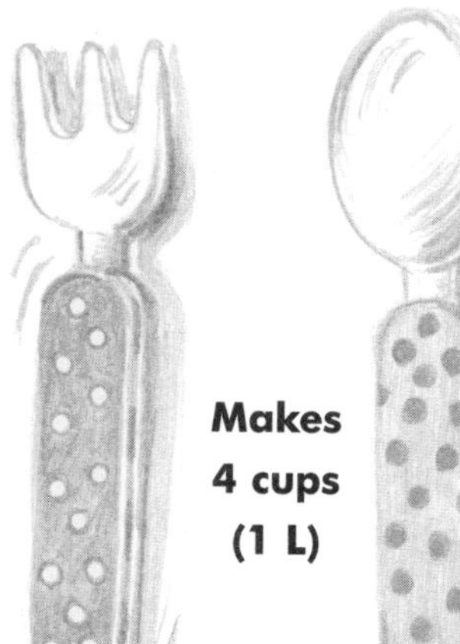

Makes 4 cups (1 L)

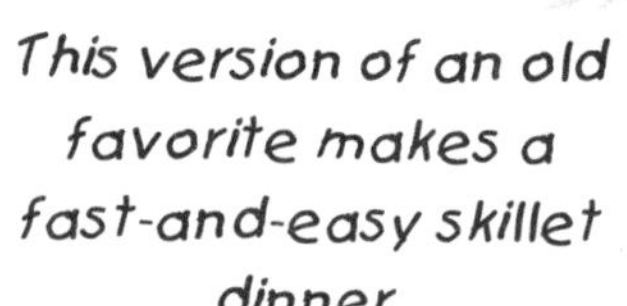

*This version of an old favorite makes a fast-and-easy skillet dinner.*

| | | |
|---|---|---|
| 8 oz | ground beef | 250 g |
| 1 | small onion, finely chopped | 1 |
| 1 | can (14 oz [398 mL]) tomatoes, with juice | 1 |
| 1/3 cup | elbow macaroni | 75 mL |
| 1/2 cup | shredded Cheddar cheese | 125 mL |
| 1/4 tsp | dried basil | 1 mL |
| 1/4 tsp | dried oregano | 1 mL |
| 1/4 tsp | chili powder | 1 mL |

1. In a large nonstick skillet over medium heat, combine beef and onion; cook, stirring frequently to break up meat, for 5 minutes or until browned. Drain fat. Add tomatoes and macaroni. Bring to a boil, cover and cook for 10 minutes or until macaroni is tender. (If mixture becomes too thick, add a little water.)
2. Remove skillet from heat. Stir in cheese, basil, oregano and chili powder. Cover and allow to sit for 5 minutes or until cheese has melted.

| Nutritional Analysis | Energy | Protein | Carbohydrate | Fat | Calcium | Iron |
|---|---|---|---|---|---|---|
| per 1/2-cup (125 mL) serving | 160 kcal | 10.0 g | 13.1 g | 7.5 g | 10 % CDV | 13 % CDV |

# Speedy Fettuccine Alfredo

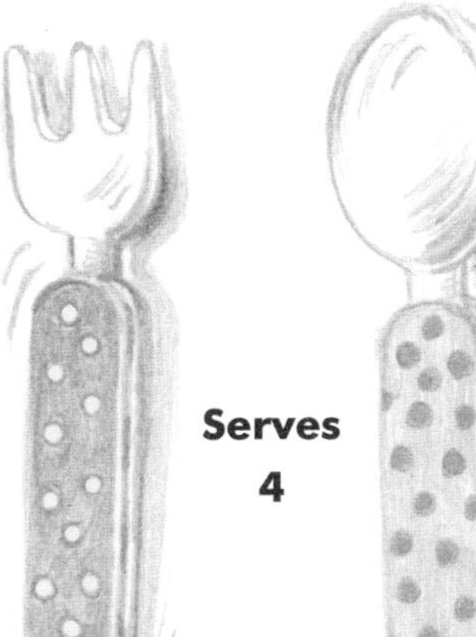

**Serves 4**

**Kitchen Tip**

Try adding sautéed vegetables or grilled chicken – or whatever you have available in your refrigerator.

For a lighter version of this dish, use whole milk instead of light cream.

| | | |
|---|---|---|
| 8 oz | fettuccine | 250 g |
| 3 tbsp | butter | 45 mL |
| 3/4 cup | grated Parmesan cheese | 175 mL |
| 2/3 cup | light (10%) cream | 150 mL |
| | Salt and freshly ground black pepper | |

1. In a large saucepan, cook pasta in boiling water according to manufacturer's directions or until tender but firm. Drain.
2. In another saucepan, melt butter over medium heat. Add Parmesan and cream; bring to a boil, stirring constantly. Reduce heat and simmer for 10 minutes or until sauce has thickened slightly. Season to taste with salt and pepper. Pour sauce over pasta and toss to coat.

| Nutritional Analysis | Energy | Protein | Carbohydrate | Fat | Calcium | Iron |
|---|---|---|---|---|---|---|
| per serving | 266 kcal | 10.1 g | 15.6 g | 18.2 g | 34 % CDV | 6 % CDV |

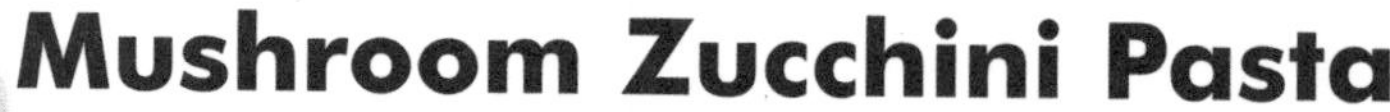

# Mushroom Zucchini Pasta

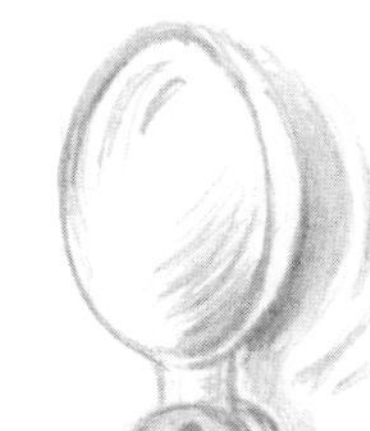

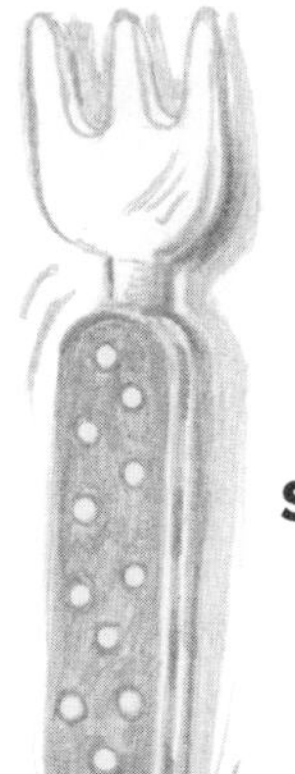

**Serves 4**

**Kitchen Tip**

For a burst of tomato flavor, serve this dish drizzled with cream of tomato soup.

| | | |
|---|---|---|
| 8 oz | rotini or other short pasta | 250 g |
| 2 tbsp | butter or margarine, divided | 25 mL |
| 2 | cloves garlic, minced, divided | 2 |
| 6 oz | mushrooms, sliced | 175 g |
| 2 tsp | lemon juice | 10 mL |
| 6 oz | zucchini, unpeeled, diced | 175 g |
| 1 tbsp | minced fresh parsley, divided | 15 mL |
| 1/2 tsp | crushed dried basil | 2 mL |
| Pinch | salt and freshly ground black pepper | Pinch |

1. In a large saucepan, cook pasta in boiling water according to manufacturer's directions or until tender but firm. Drain.
2. In a large skillet, melt 1 tbsp (15 mL) butter over medium heat. Add one-half of the minced garlic and cook for 3 minutes. Add mushrooms and lemon juice; toss well. Stir in zucchini, 2 tsp (10 mL) of the parsley, basil, salt and pepper. Cover and cook, stirring often, for 3 to 5 minutes or until the vegetables are tender-crisp.
3. In a large bowl, place remaining butter, garlic and parsley. Add hot pasta and toss well. Add vegetables and toss again.

| Nutritional Analysis | Energy | Protein | Carbohydrate | Fat | Calcium | Iron |
|---|---|---|---|---|---|---|
| per serving | 295 kcal | 9.2 g | 51.7 g | 5.8 g | 4 % CDV | 19 % CDV |

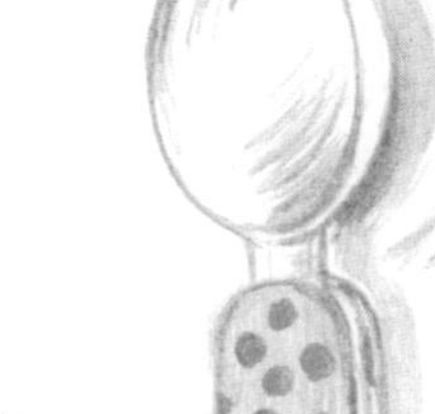

# Creamy Salmon Fettuccine

**Serves 4**

*Not nearly as high in fat as it sounds, this dish gets its creamy taste from evaporated milk.*

| | | |
|---|---|---|
| 12 oz | fettuccine | 375 g |
| 1 tbsp | butter or margarine | 15 mL |
| 1 | small onion, finely chopped | 1 |
| 1 tbsp | all-purpose flour | 15 mL |
| 1 | can (14 oz [385 mL]) 2% evaporated milk | 1 |
| 1 | can (7.5 oz [213 g]) salmon | 1 |
| 1 tbsp | lemon juice | 15 mL |
| 1 tsp | grated lemon zest | 5 mL |
| | Chopped fresh parsley | |

1. In a large saucepan, cook pasta in boiling water according to manufacturer's directions or until tender but firm. Drain.
2. In another saucepan, melt butter over medium heat. Add onion and cook for 5 minutes or until soft. Stir in flour and cook for 1 minute. Gradually whisk in milk. Cook, stirring constantly, for 5 minutes or until sauce has thickened.
3. Drain salmon. Remove and discard skin, but mash bones (for extra calcium). Flake salmon with a fork and add to sauce; cook just until heated through. Stir in lemon juice and zest. Pour sauce over cooked pasta and toss to coat. Serve with chopped parsley.

| Nutritional Analysis | Energy | Protein | Carbohydrate | Fat | Calcium | Iron |
|---|---|---|---|---|---|---|
| per serving | 591 kcal | 30.9 g | 82.4 g | 14.3 g | 57 % CDV | 3 % CDV |

# Noodle Casserole

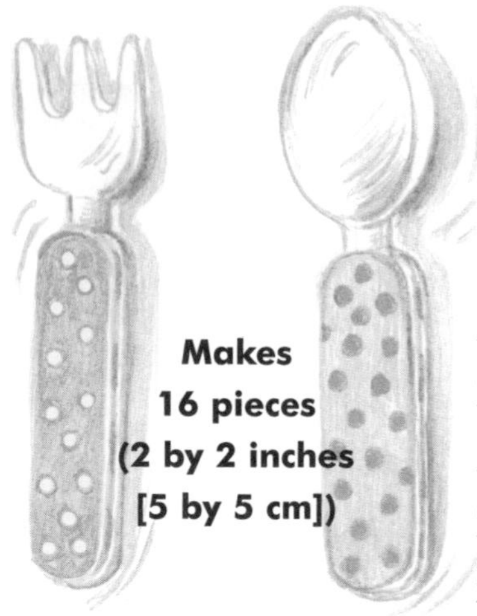

**Makes 16 pieces (2 by 2 inches [5 by 5 cm])**

*Preheat oven to 350° F (180° C)*
*8-inch (2 L) square baking dish, greased*

| | | |
|---|---|---|
| 8 oz | medium-wide egg noodles | 250 g |
| 1 lb | white Cheddar cheese, shredded | 500 g |
| 8 oz | cottage cheese | 250 g |
| 2 | eggs, beaten | 2 |
| 1/4 cup | chopped parsley | 50 mL |
| 2 tbsp | butter or margarine | 25 mL |

*This traditional Armenian dish is similar to Italian lasagna, but without the tomato sauce.*

1. In a large saucepan, cook noodles in boiling water according to manufacturer's directions or until tender but firm. Drain and rinse with cold water.
2. In a large bowl, combine Cheddar, cottage cheese and eggs; mix well. Divide mixture into 2 equal portions. Add parsley to one of the portions, stirring until thoroughly combined.
3. Place half of the noodles in prepared baking dish. Pour parsley-added portion of cheese mixture over. Add remaining noodles and cover with plain cheese mixture. Top with dabs of butter.
4. Bake in preheated oven for 30 minutes or until brown. Allow to sit for 10 minutes, then cut into squares and serve.

**KITCHEN TIP**

This dish freezes well. Package in serving-portions for individual meals in a hurry.

| NUTRITIONAL ANALYSIS | Energy | Protein | Carbohydrate | Fat | Calcium | Iron |
|---|---|---|---|---|---|---|
| per square | 182 kcal | 11.2 g | 4.6 g | 13.2 g | 30 % CDV | 5 % CDV |

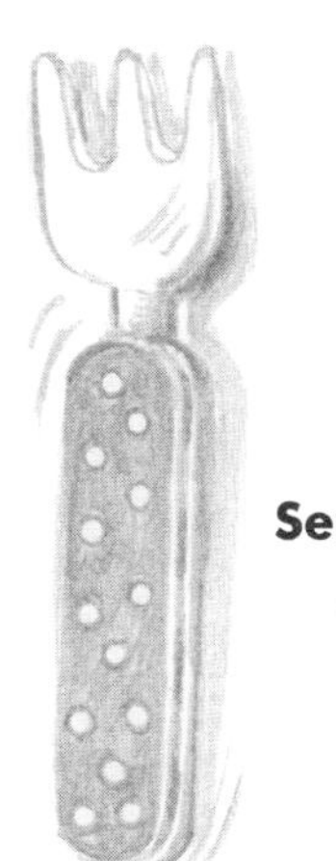
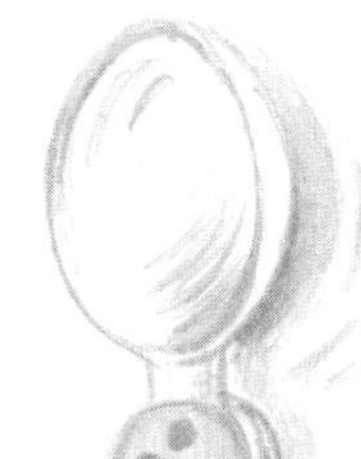

# Orzo Summer Vegetable

**Serves 8**

*Kids love pasta of all types, including the rice-shaped orzo used in this dish. It makes an ideal accompaniment to the bounty of summer vegetables.*

**Kitchen Tip**

If you are using frozen corn, there's no need to thaw it first; just add it directly to the hot orzo.

| | | |
|---|---|---|
| 2 cups | orzo | 500 mL |
| 2 cups | snow peas or sugar-snap peas, trimmed and halved | 500 mL |
| 1/4 cup | olive oil, divided | 50 mL |
| 1 cup | corn kernels, fresh or frozen (see Tip, at left) | 250 mL |
| 1 1/2 cups | diced tomatoes | 375 mL |
| 1 cup | diced seedless cucumber | 250 mL |
| 1/2 cup | finely chopped red onion | 125 mL |
| 1/4 cup | chopped fresh mint (optional) | 50 mL |
| 1 tsp | grated lemon zest | 5 mL |
| 1/4 cup | lemon juice | 50 mL |
| 1/2 tsp | salt | 2 mL |
| 1/2 tsp | freshly ground black pepper | 2 mL |

1. In a large saucepan of boiling water, cook orzo for 6 minutes. Add snow peas and cook for 2 minutes or until peas and orzo are just tender. Drain well.
2. In a large bowl, combine orzo, peas and 1 tbsp (15 mL) olive oil. Stir in corn, tomato, cucumber, onion, mint (if using) and lemon zest.
3. In a small bowl, whisk together remaining oil, lemon juice, salt and pepper. Add to orzo mixture and toss to coat. Serve warm or allow to cool.

| Nutritional Analysis | Energy | Protein | Carbohydrate | Fat | Calcium | Iron |
|---|---|---|---|---|---|---|
| per serving | 203 kcal | 5.8 g | 31.7g | 6.4 g | 4 % CDV | 17 % CDV |

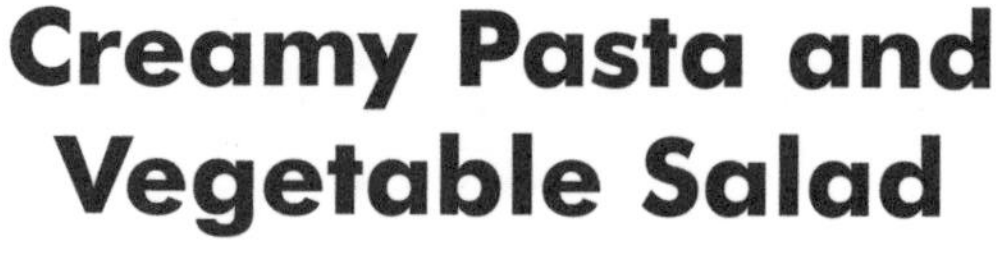

# Creamy Pasta and Vegetable Salad

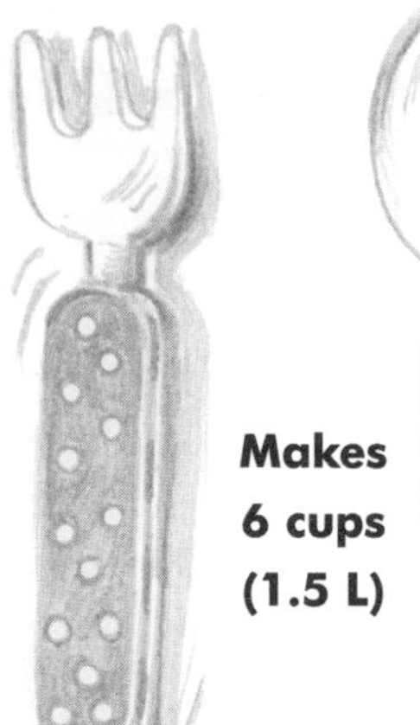

**Makes 6 cups (1.5 L)**

*This recipe is wonderful served as a warm entrée or as a cold pasta salad.*

**Kitchen Tip**

If desired, replace snow peas with frozen peas.

Add or substitute your favorite vegetables for those called for in the recipe.

Try this dish topped with slivers of grilled chicken breast.

| | | |
|---|---|---|
| 1/4 cup | parsley sprigs | 50 mL |
| 1/4 cup | fresh basil leaves (or 1 tbsp [15 mL] dried) | 50 mL |
| 1 | green onion, cut into chunks | 1 |
| 1/2 cup | 2% milk | 125 mL |
| 1/4 cup | mayonnaise | 50 mL |
| 1 tbsp | lemon juice | 15 mL |
| 1/2 tsp | dry mustard | 2 mL |
| 1/2 tsp | granulated sugar | 2 mL |
| Pinch | salt | Pinch |
| Pinch | freshly ground black pepper | Pinch |
| 2 cups | rotini | 500 mL |
| 1 cup | slivered carrot strips | 250 mL |
| 1 cup | diagonally sliced snow peas (see Tip, at left) | 250 mL |
| 1/4 cup | finely chopped green or red bell pepper (optional) | 50 mL |

1. In a food processor or by hand, finely chop parsley, basil and green onion.
2. In a bowl whisk together milk, mayonnaise and lemon juice until smooth. Stir in herb-onion mixture. Add mustard, sugar, salt and pepper; stir to blend.
3. In a large pot of boiling water, cook pasta for 10 minutes. Add carrots and snow peas; cook for 2 minutes or until pasta is tender but firm and vegetables are tender-crisp. Drain well.
4. If serving warm, immediately add mayonnaise mixture to pasta while still hot and toss to coat.
5. If serving cold, rinse pasta and vegetables under running water until cool. Drain and toss with mayonnaise mixture. Serve at once or cover and refrigerate for several hours until needed.

| Nutritional Analysis | Energy | Protein | Carbohydrate | Fat | Calcium | Iron |
|---|---|---|---|---|---|---|
| per 1/2-cup (125 mL) serving | 75 kcal | 1.9 g | 8.9 g | 3.6 g | 4 % CDV | 7 % CDV |

# Family Cheese Fondue

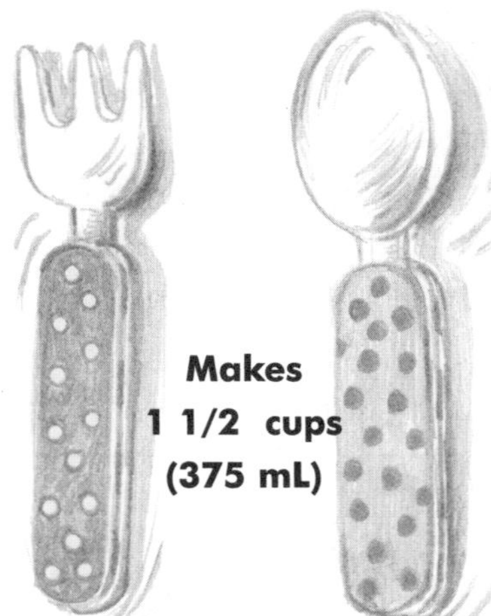

**Makes 1 1/2 cups (375 mL)**

*Warm, gooey and great-tasting – what more could a child want from a meal? Fondues can be a little messy, but they're great fun for the whole family.*

| | | |
|---|---|---|
| 2 tbsp | butter or margarine | 25 mL |
| 2 tbsp | all-purpose flour | 25 mL |
| 2/3 cup | chicken broth (see Tip) | 150 mL |
| 1 lb | shredded Swiss or Cheddar cheese | 500 g |
| 1/2 tsp | ground nutmeg | 2 mL |
| Pinch | salt | Pinch |
| Pinch | freshly ground black pepper | Pinch |
| 3 cups | cubed French bread | 750 mL |

1. In a saucepan or fondue pot, melt butter over medium heat. Whisk in flour and cook for 1 minute or until bubbly. Gradually whisk in broth, stirring constantly until smooth and thickened.
2. Reduce heat to low. Add cheese and cook, stirring constantly, for 3 minutes or until cheese is melted. Stir in nutmeg, salt and pepper. Remove from heat.
3. Spoon fondue into individual small bowls and serve with bread cubes for dipping. Be sure that the child's portion has cooled to a safe temperature before serving.

### Kitchen Tip

For a grown-up version, replace chicken stock with white wine. Vegetarians can substitute vegetable stock.

Cheese fondue thickens as it cools, which makes it less likely to drip, and therefore easier for a child to eat. If you wish a thinner consistency, however, just whisk in a little more milk or stock.

Instead of (or in addition to) bread cubes, dippers can include blanched vegetables or apple slices.

You can prepare fondues in the microwave. Set power to Medium and stir frequently, making sure the container is microwave-safe, of course!

| Nutritional Analysis | Energy | Protein | Carbohydrate | Fat | Calcium | Iron |
|---|---|---|---|---|---|---|
| per 1/4-cup (50 mL) serving | 377 kcal | 21.5 g | 2.9 g | 31.1 g | 76 % CDV | 7 % CDV |

# Moroccan Chicken Breasts

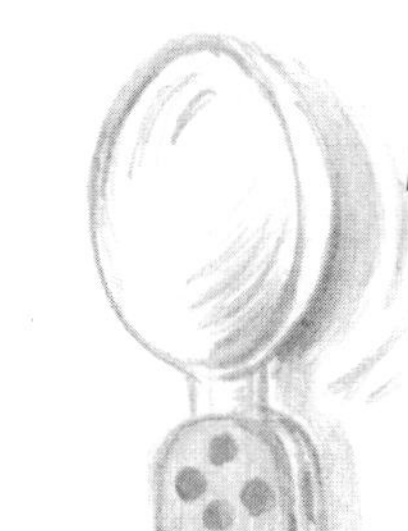

**Serves 4**

*This moist and delicious chicken dish combines everyday ingredients to create North African flavors that are unusual – but still enjoyable for children.*

*Preheat oven to 400° F (200° C)*
*Baking sheet, greased*

| | | |
|---|---|---|
| 1/2 cup | plain yogurt | 125 mL |
| 2 tbsp | orange juice | 25 mL |
| 2 | cloves garlic, crushed | 2 |
| 1 tsp | grated orange zest | 5 mL |
| 1/2 tsp | salt | 2 mL |
| 1/2 tsp | ground cinnamon | 2 mL |
| 1/2 tsp | ground cumin | 2 mL |
| 1/4 tsp | ground cloves | 1 mL |
| 1/4 tsp | ground ginger | 1 mL |
| 4 | boneless skinless chicken breasts | 4 |
| 2/3 cup | dried whole wheat bread crumbs | 150 mL |

1. In a small bowl, stir together yogurt, orange juice, garlic, zest, salt, cinnamon, cumin, cloves and ginger.
2. Place chicken in a shallow baking dish. Pour yogurt mixture over and turn chicken to coat. Cover and refrigerate for at least 4 hours, turning chicken occasionally.
3. Remove chicken from marinade and dredge in bread crumbs until thoroughly coated. Place on prepared baking sheet and bake in preheated oven for 20 minutes or until chicken is no longer pink and juices run clear when pierced with a fork.

### Kitchen Tip

Instead of roasting in the oven, chicken can be grilled on a preheated barbecue. Cook for about 8 minutes per side over medium-high heat with barbecue lid down.

### Food Safety Tip

To minimize the risk of bacterial contamination, be sure that you thoroughly wash hands, utensils, cutting boards and all work surfaces before, during and after handling raw meat – especially poultry.

| Nutritional Analysis | Energy | Protein | Carbohydrate | Fat | Calcium | Iron |
|---|---|---|---|---|---|---|
| per serving | 373 kcal | 56.7 g | 14.9 g | 8.0 g | 12 % CDV | 27 % CDV |

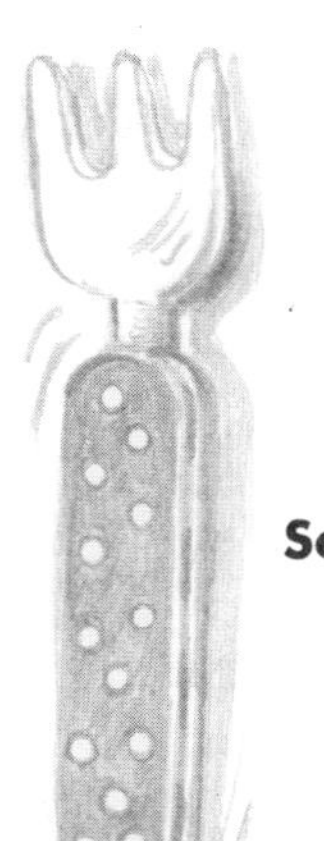
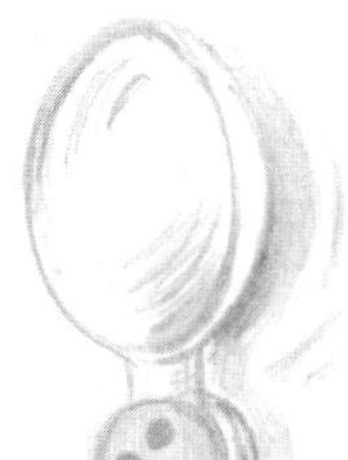

# Tomato Herbed Chicken

**Serves 4**

*The tangy sauce in this recipe really perks up the mild flavors of chicken to make it something special. It also helps to keep the chicken wonderfully moist.*

**Kitchen Tip**

Serve with orzo or any shell pasta to soak up all the wonderful sauce.

When draining canned mushroom, save the liquid to add flavor to soup or when cooking rice or other vegetables.

| | | |
|---|---|---|
| 2 tbsp | vegetable oil | 25 mL |
| 4 | boneless skinless chicken breasts | 4 |
| 1 tbsp | all-purpose flour | 15 mL |
| 1 | small onion, finely chopped | 1 |
| 1 | stalk celery, sliced | 1 |
| Half | green pepper, chopped | Half |
| 1 tsp | dried oregano | 5 mL |
| 1/4 tsp | dried thyme | 1 mL |
| 1/4 tsp | salt | 1 mL |
| 1 | can (19 oz [540 mL]) tomatoes, crushed, with juice | 1 |
| 1 | can (10 oz [284 mL]) sliced mushrooms, drained (see Tip, at left) | 1 |
| | Cooked pasta (see Tip, at left) | |

1. In a skillet heat oil over medium heat. Sprinkle chicken with flour and add to skillet. Cook, turning, until brown on all sides. Transfer chicken to a plate and set aside.
2. Add onion, celery and green pepper to skillet; sauté for 5 minutes or until softened. Add oregano, thyme, salt, tomatoes and mushrooms. Bring to a boil. Reduce heat and simmer, uncovered, for 10 minutes or until liquid is reduced and thickened. Add reserved chicken; cover and simmer for 20 minutes or until chicken is cooked and no longer pink.
3. Serve chicken and sauce over cooked pasta.

| Nutritional Analysis | Energy | Protein | Carbohydrate | Fat | Calcium | Iron |
|---|---|---|---|---|---|---|
| per serving | 247 kcal | 29.3 g | 11.6 g | 9.4 g | 7 % CDV | 26 % CDV |

# Chicken and Dumplings

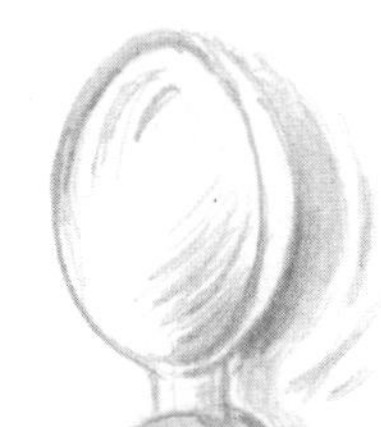

**Serves 4**

*Kids love the mild flavor and soft texture of dumplings. They're what Margaret's youngest son, Andrew, used to call "those other kind of potatoes" when asked what he'd like for dinner.*

| | | |
|---|---|---|
| 4 | chicken breasts or drumsticks | 4 |
| 3 cups | chicken stock (see Tip, at left) | 750 mL |
| 2 | onions, quartered | 2 |
| 2 | large carrots, cut into chunks | 2 |
| 2 | stalks celery, cut into chunks | 2 |
| 1 | bay leaf | 1 |
| 1/4 tsp | salt | 1 mL |
| 1/4 tsp | freshly ground black pepper | 1 mL |
| 2 cups | variety (tea biscuit) baking mix (see Tip, at left) | 500 mL |
| 2/3 cup | 2% milk | 150 mL |
| 4 | sprigs parsley, finely chopped | 4 |

1. In a large saucepan with a lid, combine chicken, stock, onions, carrots, celery, bay leaf, salt and pepper. Bring to a boil over high heat. Reduce heat to medium and cook, covered, for about 20 minutes.
2. In a bowl combine baking mix, milk and parsley; stir to blend. Drop large spoonfuls of batter over simmering chicken. Tightly cover pan and cook for another 15 minutes or until dumplings are firm and chicken is cooked through.

### Kitchen Tip

If you don't have any homemade chicken stock, use tinned chicken broth or 3 chicken bouillon cubes dissolved in 3 cups (750 mL) water.

If you prefer, make your own tea biscuits rather than using a mix.

| Nutritional Analysis | Energy | Protein | Carbohydrate | Fat | Calcium | Iron |
|---|---|---|---|---|---|---|
| per serving | 335 kcal | 36.5 g | 10.5 g | 15.5 g | 13 % CDV | 21 % CDV |

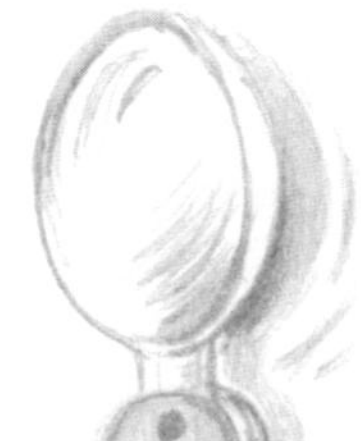

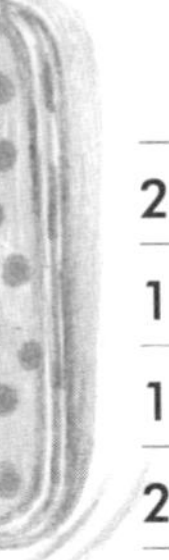

# Lemon Mustard Chicken

*Shallow baking dish*

**Serves 4**

| 2 tbsp | Dijon mustard | 25 mL |
|---|---|---|
| 1 tbsp | lemon juice | 15 mL |
| 1 tbsp | vegetable oil | 15 mL |
| 2 | green onions, chopped | 2 |
| 4 | boneless skinless chicken breasts | 4 |

*Here's a deliciously tangy chicken dish that requires just a few minutes of preparation time. Dinner's ready in half an hour!*

1. In a small bowl, whisk together mustard, lemon juice, oil and green onions. Pour marinade into a sealable plastic bag and add chicken, making sure it is thoroughly coated. Seal bag and refrigerate for at least 2 hours or up to 8 hours.
2. Preheat oven to 375° F (190° C). Remove chicken from lemon mixture and transfer to a shallow baking dish. Bake for 30 minutes or until chicken is no longer pink and juices run clear when pierced with a fork.

### Kitchen Tip

Instead of roasting in the oven, chicken can be grilled on a preheated barbecue. Cook for about 8 minutes per side over medium-high heat with barbecue lid down.

| Nutritional Analysis | Energy | Protein | Carbohydrate | Fat | Calcium | Iron |
|---|---|---|---|---|---|---|
| per serving | 168 kcal | 27.7 g | 0.7 g | 5.4 g | 3 % CDV | 10 % CDV |

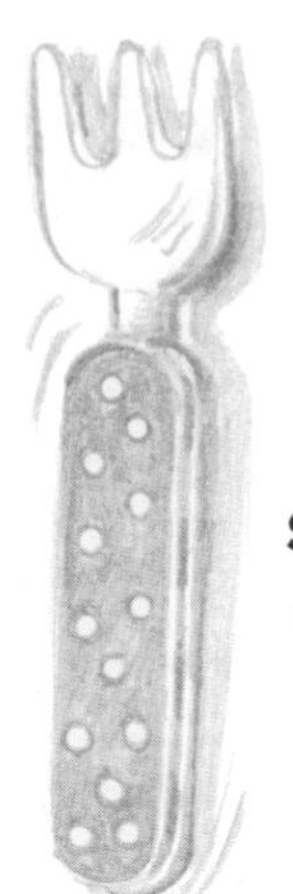

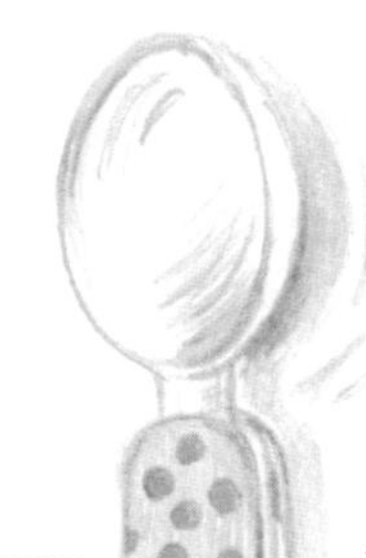

# Yogurt Chicken

*Preheat oven to 350° F (180° C)*
*8-inch (2 L) square baking dish, ungreased*

**Serves 4 to 6**

*In this traditional Greek recipe, yogurt makes the chicken incredibly tender! Serve with a side of rice pilaf or roasted potatoes.*

| | | |
|---|---|---|
| 8 | chicken pieces (drumsticks, thighs, breasts), rinsed and patted dry | 8 |
| 2 cups | plain yogurt | 500 mL |
| 1 | egg, beaten | 1 |
| 1 tbsp | all-purpose flour | 15 mL |
| 1 tsp | salt | 5 mL |
| 1/2 tsp | freshly ground black pepper | 2mL |
| 1/2 tsp | ground nutmeg | 2mL |
| 2 tbsp | butter | 25 mL |
| 2 | cloves garlic, minced | 2 |
| 1 cup | chicken stock | 250 mL |

### Kitchen Tip

If you don't have any homemade chicken stock, use tinned chicken broth, preferably a low-sodium variety.

1. Place chicken in baking dish and add sufficient cold water to cover by 1 inch (2.5 cm). Bake in preheated oven for 45 minutes.
2. Meanwhile, in a bowl combine yogurt, egg, flour, salt, pepper and nutmeg. Set aside.
3. In a saucepan, melt butter over medium-high heat. Add garlic and sauté for 5 minutes or until just golden. (Be careful not to burn.) Add stock and bring to a boil. Gradually add reserved yogurt mixture, stirring continuously. Return to a boil and remove from heat. Pour over baked chicken. Reduce oven temperature to to 300° F (160° C). Cover chicken and bake for another 30 minutes or until no longer pink and juices run clear when pierced with a fork.

| Nutritional Analysis | Energy | Protein | Carbohydrate | Fat | Calcium | Iron |
|---|---|---|---|---|---|---|
| per serving (4) | 399 kcal | 35.8 g | 8.7 g | 23.6 g | 24 % CDV | 22 % CDV |

# Fruity Chicken

*Preheat oven to 400° F (200° C)*
*Roasting pan with lid*

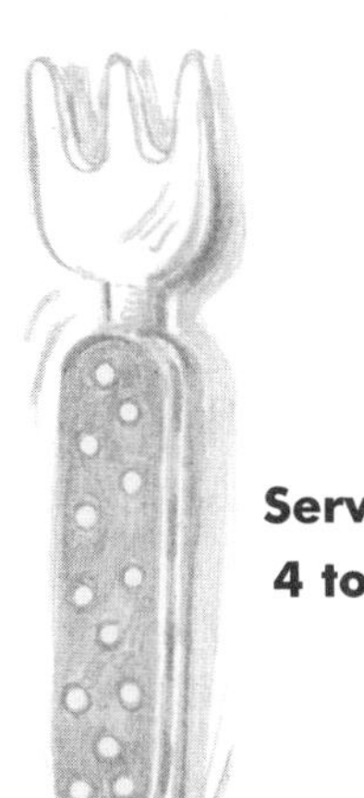
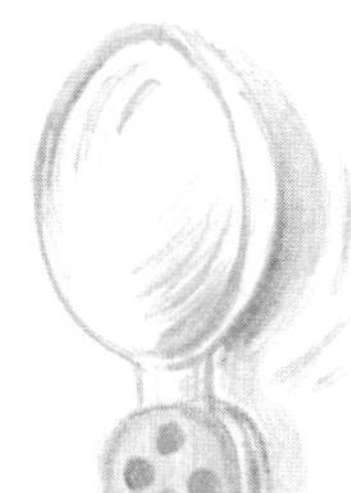

**Serves 4 to 6**

*Kids love the flavor and sweetness of dried fruit – and its a good source of iron, too!*

| | | |
|---|---|---|
| 1 | whole chicken (about 5 lbs [2.5 kg]) | 1 |
| 1 tsp | paprika | 5 mL |
| 1/2 tsp | salt | 2 mL |
| 1/4 tsp | freshly ground black pepper | 1 mL |
| Half | pkg (9 oz [275 g]) pitted prunes | Half |
| Half | pkg (9 oz [275 g]) dried apricots | Half |
| 1/2 cup | dried cranberries | 125 mL |
| 2 tbsp | honey | 25 mL |
| 1/2 cup | orange juice | 125 mL |
| 1/2 cup | water | 125 mL |

1. Season chicken with the paprika, salt and pepper.
2. In a bowl, toss together prunes, apricots and raisins until well mixed. Stuff chicken cavity with fruit and place in roasting pan. (Place any extra fruit around chicken in pan.)
3. In a small bowl, whisk together honey, juice and water. Drizzle over chicken.
4. Bake uncovered for 1 hour, then remove from oven, cover and bake for another 30 minutes or until chicken is no longer pink and juices run clear when pierced with a fork.

| Nutritional Analysis | Energy | Protein | Carbohydrate | Fat | Calcium | Iron |
|---|---|---|---|---|---|---|
| per serving (6) | 510 kcal | 30.5 g | 47.1 g | 23.5 g | 7 % CDV | 35 % CDV |

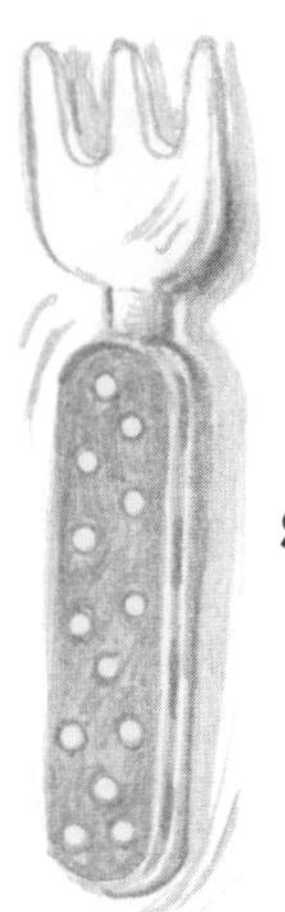

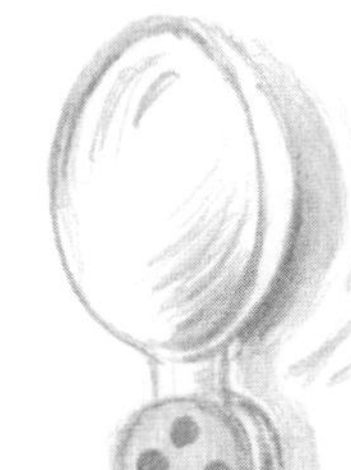

# Crispy Chicken

*Preheat oven to 375° F (190° C)*
*Baking sheet, lightly greased*

**Serves 12**

*This dish is so quick and easy, the kids can help to prepare it!*

| | | |
|---|---|---|
| 1/2 cup | plain low-fat yogurt | 125 mL |
| 1/2 tsp | dried tarragon (optional) | 2 mL |
| 1/4 tsp | salt | 1 mL |
| 1/4 tsp | freshly ground black pepper | 1 mL |
| 1 1/2 cups | finely crushed corn flake cereal | 375 mL |
| 1/4 cup | grated Parmesan cheese | 50 mL |
| 12 | boneless skinless chicken thighs (about 28 oz [800 g] total), rinsed and patted dry | 12 |

**Kitchen Tip**

Serve plain or with plum sauce for dipping

1. In a bowl combine yogurt, tarragon, salt and pepper; stir to mix well. In another bowl, combine corn flakes and Parmesan.
2. Roll chicken in yogurt mixture to coat, then roll in crumb mixture. Place on prepared baking sheet and bake in preheated oven for 45 to 50 minutes or until chicken is no longer pink and juices run clear when pierced with a fork.

| Nutritional Analysis | Energy | Protein | Carbohydrate | Fat | Calcium | Iron |
|---|---|---|---|---|---|---|
| per serving | 106 kcal | 15.0 g | 3.5 g | 3.2 g | 6 % CDV | 12 % CDV |

# Tuna Burgers

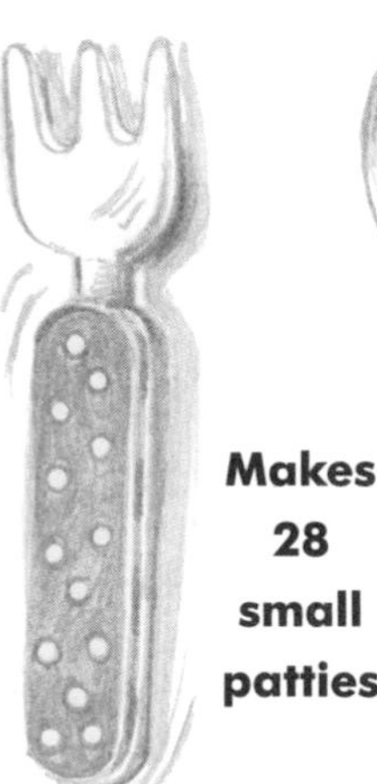
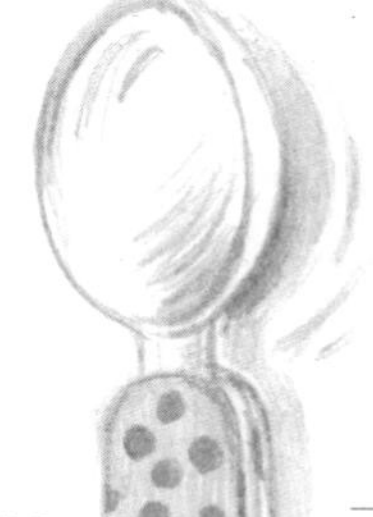

**Makes 28 small patties**

| | | |
|---|---|---|
| 1 | carrot, finely chopped | 1 |
| 1 | small onion, finely chopped | 1 |
| 3 tbsp | green peas | 45 mL |
| 2 | cans (each 6 oz [184 g]) tuna, drained | 2 |
| 2 | eggs | 2 |
| 3 tbsp | light mayonnaise | 45 mL |
| 1 1/2 cups | bread crumbs | 375 mL |
| Pinch | salt | Pinch |
| Pinch | freshly ground black pepper | Pinch |
| 3 tbsp | vegetable oil | 45 mL |

1. In a food processor combine carrot, onion, peas, tuna, eggs, mayonnaise, bread crumbs, salt and pepper. Process until mixture is well blended and binds together. Using your hands, form into small (2 1/2-inch [7 cm]) patties.
2. In a skillet heat oil over medium-high heat. Add patties in batches and cook for about 10 minutes on each side or until golden.

**Kitchen Tip**

Serve these patties with a fresh whole wheat roll and sliced tomatoes.

| Nutritional Analysis | Energy | Protein | Carbohydrate | Fat | Calcium | Iron |
|---|---|---|---|---|---|---|
| per patty | 68 kcal | 5.0 g | 5.1 g | 2.9 g | 2 % CDV | 6 % CDV |

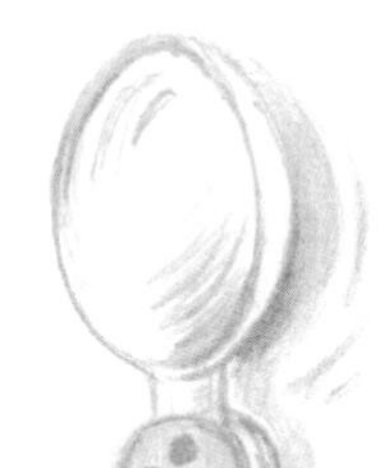

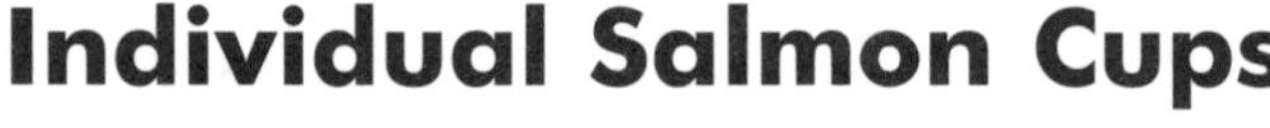

# Individual Salmon Cups

*3 ovenproof custard cups*

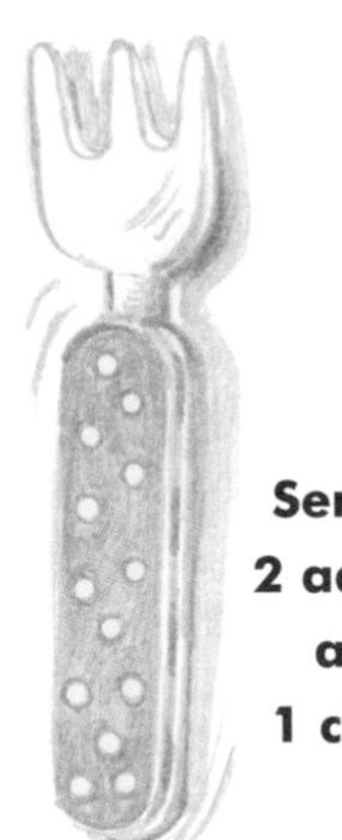

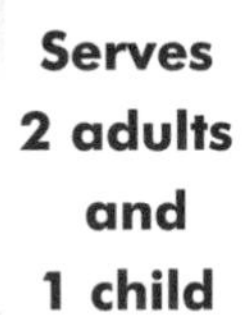

**Serves 2 adults and 1 child**

*A can of salmon and a microwave oven are the main requirements for this quick and easy recipe. The light lemon sauce adds a nice highlight to the salmon.*

| | | |
|---|---|---|
| 1 | can (7.5 oz [213 g]) salmon, drained | 1 |
| 1/2 cup | finely chopped carrots | 125 mL |
| 1/2 cup | fresh bread crumbs | 125 mL |
| 1 | egg | 1 |
| 1/4 tsp | dried thyme | 1 mL |
| 1/4 tsp | salt | 1 mL |
| **SAUCE** | | |
| 1/2 cup | 2% milk | 125 mL |
| 1 tbsp | all-purpose flour | 15 mL |
| 1 tbsp | butter or margarine, melted | 15 mL |
| 2 tsp | lemon juice | 10 mL |
| Pinch | freshly ground black pepper | Pinch |

### KITCHEN TIP

The child's cup cooks faster than the 2 larger adult portions, so you will need to remove it from the microwave before the full 3 minutes of cooking time.

1. In a bowl remove skin from salmon, flake salmon and mash bones. Add carrots, bread crumbs, egg, thyme and salt; mix well.
2. Spoon mixture into 3 custard cups, dividing mixture to make the child's portion smaller than those of the 2 adults. Arrange cups in a circle in microwave and cook on High for 3 minutes, slightly less for child's portion (see Tip, at left) or until almost set. Let stand for 2 minutes before serving.
3. Sauce: In a small microwave-safe bowl or glass measure, whisk together milk, flour, butter, lemon juice and pepper. Microwave on High for 1 minute. Stir, then cook for another 45 seconds or until mixture comes to a boil and thickens. Spoon a small amount of sauce over each salmon cup.

| NUTRITIONAL ANALYSIS | Energy | Protein | Carbohydrate | Fat | Calcium | Iron |
|---|---|---|---|---|---|---|
| per serving | 292 kcal | 20.6 g | 19.5 g | 14.1 g | 35 % CDV | 22 % CDV |

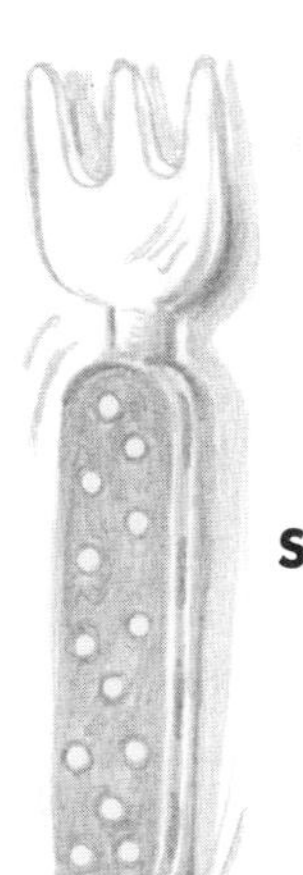

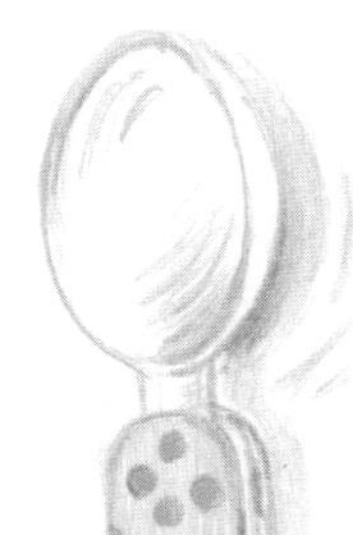

# Baked Salmon

**Serves 4**

*Preheat oven to 425° F (220° C)*
*Baking sheet*

| | | |
|---|---|---|
| 1 lb | salmon fillet | 500 g |
| 2 tbsp | olive oil | 25 mL |
| 3 tbsp | honey garlic sauce | 50 mL |

1. Cover baking sheet with a length of foil. Place salmon on foil and drizzle with oil and honey garlic sauce. Wrap foil around fish and bake in preheated oven for 10 minutes per 1 inch (2.5 cm) thickness or until fish flakes easily with a fork.

*Kids love eating fish when it's prepared as simply and easily as it is here.*

**Kitchen Tip**

This recipe is also delicious using trout instead of salmon.

If you wish, you can make this recipe with frozen fish. Just increase cooking time to 30 minutes.

| Nutritional Analysis | Energy | Protein | Carbohydrate | Fat | Calcium | Iron |
|---|---|---|---|---|---|---|
| per serving | 194 kcal | 24.0 g | 0.2 g | 10.2 g | 20 % CDV | 10 % CDV |

# Salmon and Veggies

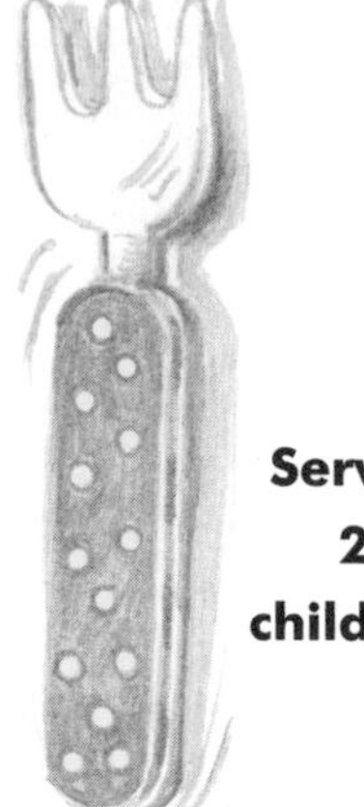
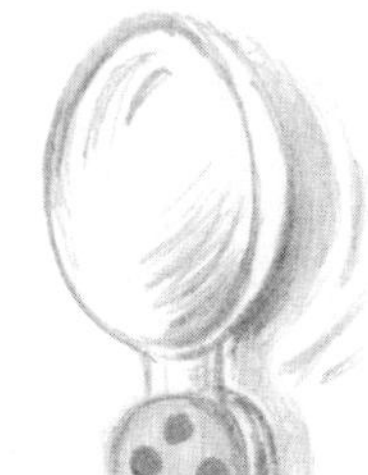

**Serves 2 children**

*Here's a colorful kid-sized recipe that's packed with nutrition.*

**KITCHEN TIP**

Serve this dish with whole grain pita bread to scoop up vegetables.

*Preheat oven to 425° F (220° C)*
*Baking sheet*

| | | |
|---|---|---|
| Half | medium potato, diced | Half |
| 1/2 tsp | olive oil | 2 mL |
| 4 oz | salmon fillet | 125 g |
| 1 | green onion, chopped | 1 |
| 1 | slice tomato, diced | 1 |
| 3 or 4 | strips yellow or red bell pepper, diced | 3 or 4 |
| 1/2 tsp | lemon juice | 2 mL |
| 1/2 tsp | chopped fresh parsley | 2 mL |
| Pinch | salt | Pinch |

1. In a pot of boiling water, cook potato for about 5 minutes. Drain.
2. Tear off a square of aluminum foil and place on baking sheet. Brush center of foil with olive oil. Place fish fillet on oiled area. Top fish with potato, onion, tomato and pepper strips. Drizzle with lemon juice and sprinkle with parsley and salt.
3. Fold edges of foil up to enclose fish tightly. Bake in preheated oven for 15 minutes or until fish flakes easily with a fork.

| NUTRITIONAL ANALYSIS | Energy | Protein | Carbohydrate | Fat | Calcium | Iron |
|---|---|---|---|---|---|---|
| per child's serving | 169 kcal | 14.0 g | 9.1 g | 8.4 g | 12 % CDV | 14 % CDV |

# Rolled Fish Filets with Salmon Filling

*Preheat oven to 350° F (180° C)*
*8-cup (2 L) baking dish, greased*

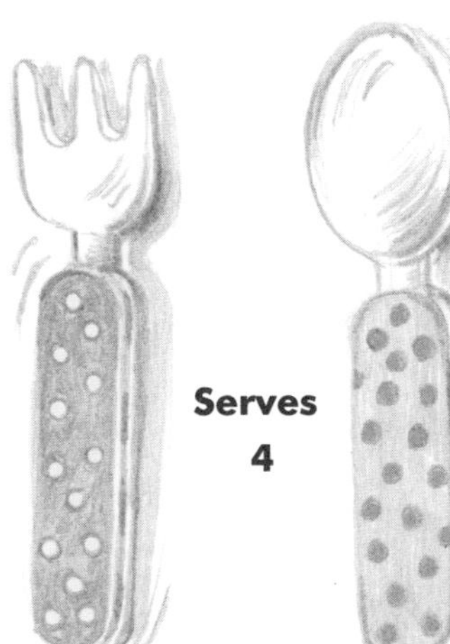

**Serves 4**

*Here's a special fish recipe that kids enjoy, but is elegant enough to serve to dinner guests. The combination of textures and colors makes a very attractive entrée.*

| | | |
|---|---|---|
| 4 | fish fillets (about 1 lb [500 g]) (see Tip, at left) | 4 |
| | Salt and freshly ground black pepper | |
| 1 | can (7.5 oz [213 g]) salmon, drained | 1 |
| 1/4 cup | finely chopped celery | 50 mL |
| 2 tbsp | finely chopped parsley | 25 mL |
| 2 tbsp | tomato sauce or ketchup | 25 mL |
| 1/2 cup | chicken stock (see Tip) | 125 mL |
| 2 tbsp | butter or margarine | 25 mL |
| 2 tbsp | all-purpose flour | 25 mL |
| 1/4 cup | light (10%) cream or 2% milk | 50 mL |

1. Pat fish dry with paper towels; sprinkle lightly with salt and pepper.
2. Place salmon in a bowl. Remove and discard skin; mash salmon and bones with a fork. Add celery, parsley and tomato sauce; stir until combined. Divide mixture evenly over fillets; roll and fasten with toothpicks. Transfer to prepared baking dish.
3. Pour stock over fish. Cover and bake in preheated oven for 20 minutes or until fish flakes easily with a fork. With a slotted spoon, transfer fish to a warm serving plate, leaving juices in dish.
4. Pour fish juices into a small saucepan. Whisk in butter and flour; cook over medium heat, stirring constantly, until sauce thickens. Stir in cream and heat until warmed through. Pour sauce over rolled fish and serve.

### Kitchen Tip

Choose a firm white fish such as sole, haddock or whitefish.

If serving adults, you can replace chicken stock with white wine.

### Safety Tip

For small children, remove toothpicks before serving.

| Nutritional Analysis | Energy | Protein | Carbohydrate | Fat | Calcium | Iron |
|---|---|---|---|---|---|---|
| per serving | 260 kcal | 33.3 g | 4.1 g | 11.3 g | 22 % CDV | 21 % CDV |

# Fish Fillets Florentine

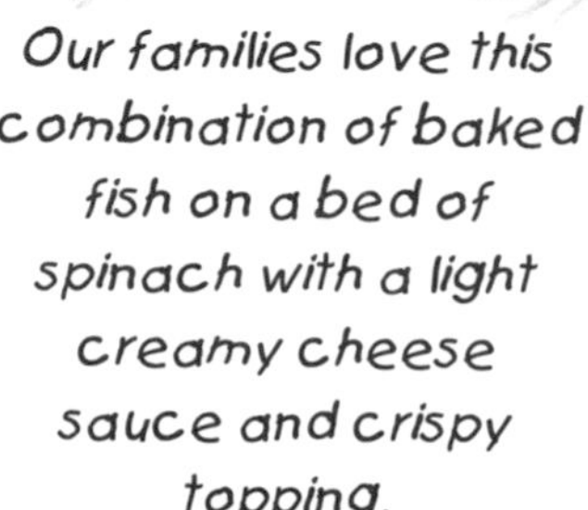

**Serves 4**

*Our families love this combination of baked fish on a bed of spinach with a light creamy cheese sauce and crispy topping.*

*Preheat oven to 400° F (200° C)*
*8-inch (2 L) square baking pan, greased*

| | | |
|---|---|---|
| 1 | pkg (10 oz [300 g]) frozen chopped spinach, thawed | 1 |
| 1 tbsp | butter or margarine | 15 mL |
| 1 | small onion, finely chopped | 1 |
| 1 lb | fish fillets, such as sole or cod | 500 g |
| 2/3 cup | 2% milk | 150 mL |
| 1/2 cup | processed Cheddar cheese (see Tip, at left) | 125 mL |
| 2 tbsp | dry bread crumbs | 25 mL |
| 2 tbsp | grated Parmesan cheese | 25 mL |

### Kitchen Tip

Don't try making the sauce with regular cheese; the processed type provides a much smoother result.

1. In a sieve, drain spinach, pressing with a spoon to remove as much moisture as possible.
2. In a small skillet, melt butter over medium heat. Add onion and cook for 5 minutes or until translucent. Add spinach and cook, stirring frequently, for 5 minutes or until moisture has evaporated. Transfer mixture to prepared pan, spreading evenly. Place fish on top of spinach.
3. In a saucepan over medium heat, stir together milk and processed cheese until smooth and melted. Pour sauce over fish; top with bread crumbs and Parmesan cheese.
4. Bake in preheated oven for 10 minutes or until fish is almost opaque. Turn on broiler and place pan 3 inches (7.5 cm) under heat; broil for 3 minutes or until crumbs are golden and fish flakes easily with a fork.

| Nutritional Analysis | Energy | Protein | Carbohydrate | Fat | Calcium | Iron |
|---|---|---|---|---|---|---|
| per serving | 298 kcal | 32.2 g | 12.2 g | 13.4 g | 43 % CDV | 31 % CDV |

# Lemon Yogurt Sole

**Serves 8**

*For speed, simplicity, flavor, and lasting kid appeal, this recipe is an absolute must!*

*Preheat broiler*
*Baking sheet lined with foil*

| | | |
|---|---|---|
| 2 tbsp | light mayonnaise | 25 mL |
| 2 tbsp | plain yogurt | 25 mL |
| 1 tsp | all-purpose flour | 5 mL |
| 1 tsp | lemon juice | 5 mL |
| 1/2 tsp | dried thyme | 2 mL |
| 14 oz | frozen sole fillets, thawed and thoroughly patted dry | 400 g |

1. In a bowl combine mayonnaise, yogurt, flour, lemon juice and thyme; mix well.
2. Arrange sole fillets in a single layer on baking sheet. Spread mayonnaise-yogurt over fish. Broil for about 8 minutes or until fish flakes easily with a fork.

### Kitchen Tip

For a complete meal, serve with green beans or broccoli and a slice of fresh bread.

| Nutritional Analysis | Energy | Protein | Carbohydrate | Fat | Calcium | Iron |
|---|---|---|---|---|---|---|
| per serving | 51 kcal | 8.5 g | 0.7 g | 1.4 g | 1 % CDV | 5 % CDV |

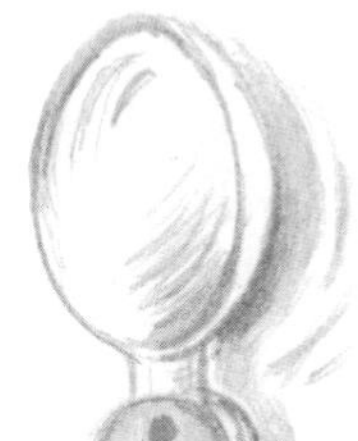

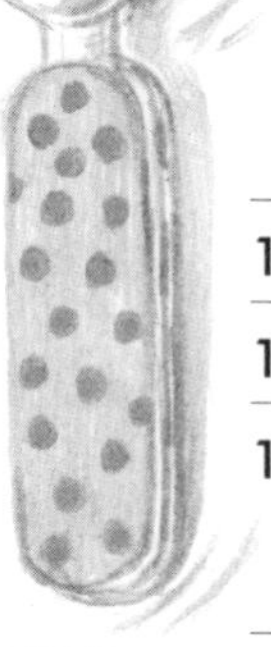

# Savory Sole Fingers

**Serves 8**

*Commercially prepared fish sticks can't compare with these. Kids love to dip them.*

| | | |
|---|---|---|
| 1 cup | bread crumbs | 250 mL |
| 1/2 cup | grated Parmesan cheese | 125 mL |
| 14 oz | frozen sole fillets, thawed, thoroughly patted dry, and cut into strips | 400 g |
| 3 tbsp | olive oil, divided | 45 mL |
| 2 tbsp | butter or margarine, divided | 25 mL |

1. In a bowl combine bread crumbs and Parmesan; stir to mix well. Dredge fish strips in crumbs to coat completely and transfer to a plate.
2. In a skillet heat half of the oil and half of the butter over medium heat. In batches, add fish and cook for 5 minutes on one side; turn over and cook for another 2 minutes or until lightly browned.

**KITCHEN TIP**

Serve with rice or potatoes.

Ranch-style dressing makes a great dip for these sticks.

| NUTRITIONAL ANALYSIS | Energy | Protein | Carbohydrate | Fat | Calcium | Iron |
|---|---|---|---|---|---|---|
| per serving | 187 kcal | 12.2 g | 9.9 g | 10.7 g | 12 % CDV | 10 % CDV |

# Basic Beef Mixture

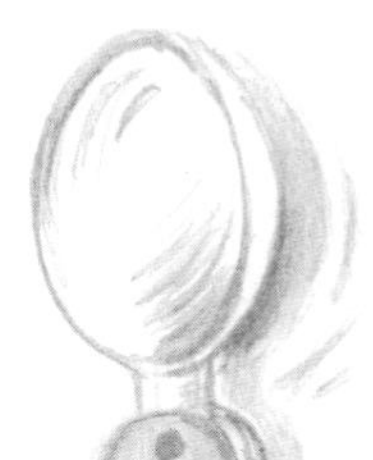

**Makes 6 cups (1.5 L)**

*Ground beef forms the basis of many dishes that kids love – including Sloppy Joes, pizza, shepherds pie, chili, or just as as a topping for baked or mashed potatoes. Make a big batch of this recipe and freeze in smaller amounts. The recipe originated from The Beef Information Centre.*

| | | |
|---|---|---|
| 2 lbs | lean or medium ground beef | 1 kg |
| 4 | cloves garlic, minced | 4 |
| 2 | medium onions, finely chopped | 2 |
| 2 cups | tomato sauce or pasta sauce | 500 mL |
| 2 tsp | dried basil | 10 mL |
| 2 tsp | dried oregano | 10 mL |
| 1/2 tsp | salt | 2 mL |
| 1/4 tsp | freshly ground black pepper | 1 mL |

1. In a large skillet over medium-high heat, cook beef, garlic and onion, using a spoon to break up the meat, for 10 minutes or until beef is no longer pink. Drain fat.
2. Add tomato sauce, basil, oregano, salt and pepper. Bring to a boil; reduce heat and simmer for 5 minutes. Divide beef mixture into 1-cup (250 mL) portions. Refrigerate for up to 2 days or freeze for up to 3 months.

## Variations

**Sloppy Joes:** In a saucepan combine 1 cup (250 mL) Basic Beef Mixture , 2 tbsp (25 mL) finely chopped green pepper and 2 tbsp (25 mL) finely chopped celery. Heat thoroughly and serve over cooked rice, toasted bun or bread. Makes 1 1/4 cups (300 mL).

**Pizza:** Spread 1 cup (250 mL) Basic Beef Mixture over a 12-inch (30 cm) pre-baked pizza shell or flat-bread crust. Top with 1/2 cup (125 mL) shredded Cheddar and 1/2 cup (125 mL) Mozzarella cheese. Place pizza on a baking sheet; broil until cheese is melted. Makes one 12-inch (30 cm) pizza.

**Baked Potato Topping:** Bake or microwave 1 potato. Cut a cross in top of potato; squeeze to open. Top with 1/4 cup (50 mL) heated Basic Beef Mixture and serve. Makes 1 serving.

**Shepherd's Pie:** In a shallow ovenproof casserole, combine 1 cup (250 mL) Basic Beef Mixture, 1/2 cup (125 mL) frozen mixed vegetables and 1/2 cup (125 mL) sliced canned mushrooms. Top with 2 cups (500 mL) cooked mashed potatoes. Bake in 350° F (180° C) oven for 15 minutes. Makes 3 to 4 servings.

**Last-Minute Chili:** In a small saucepan, combine 1 cup (250 mL) Basic Beef Mixture, 1/2 cup (125 mL) tomato sauce, 1/2 cup (125 mL) drained kidney beans and 1 tsp (5 mL) chili powder. Makes 2 cups (500 mL).

| Nutritional Analysis | Energy | Protein | Carbohydrate | Fat | Calcium | Iron |
|---|---|---|---|---|---|---|
| per 1/2-cup (125 mL) serving | 204 kcal | 16.6 g | 5.6 g | 12.7 g | 4 % CDV | 23 % CDV |

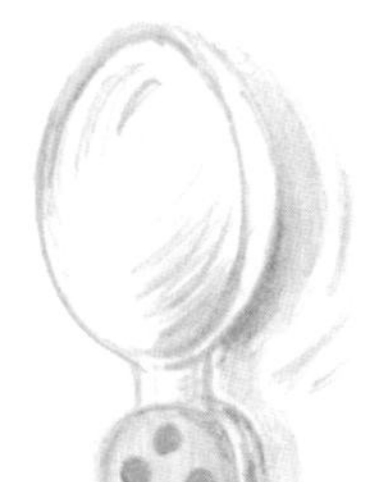

# Pizza-Style Hamburgers

*Preheat barbecue or broiler*

**Makes 6 burgers**

*Ask kids to name their favorite foods and chances are that pizza and hamburgers will rank near the top of the list. Here's a dish that combines the best of both.*

| | | |
|---|---|---|
| 1 lb | ground beef (see Tip, at left) | 500 g |
| 1 | egg, beaten | 1 |
| 1/4 cup | finely chopped green pepper | 50 mL |
| 2 tbsp | finely chopped onion | 25 mL |
| 1/4 cup | dry bread crumbs or small-flake rolled oats | 50 mL |
| 1/2 cup | pizza sauce or tomato sauce | 125 mL |
| 1/2 tsp | dried basil | 2 mL |
| 1/2 tsp | dried oregano | 2 mL |
| 6 | slices mozzarella cheese | 6 |
| 6 | hamburger buns, split and warmed | 6 |

### Kitchen Tip

Regular ground beef is less expensive than the lean or extra-lean variety, and actually makes juicier burgers. Broiling or grilling allows some of the fat to drip away.

1. In a bowl combine beef, egg, green pepper, onion, bread crumbs, pizza sauce, basil and oregano. Do not overmix. With moistened hands, shape mixture into 6 evenly shaped flat patties. (For younger children, you may wish to make a larger number of smaller burgers.)
2. Grill on a preheated barbecue or under the broiler for about 5 minutes per side or until well done and center is no longer pink. During last few minutes of cooking time, top each burger with cheese; cook until cheese starts to melt. Serve on warm buns.

| Nutritional Analysis | Energy | Protein | Carbohydrate | Fat | Calcium | Iron |
|---|---|---|---|---|---|---|
| per burger | 441 kcal | 26.1 g | 26.7 g | 24.8 g | 28 % CDV | 31 % CDV |

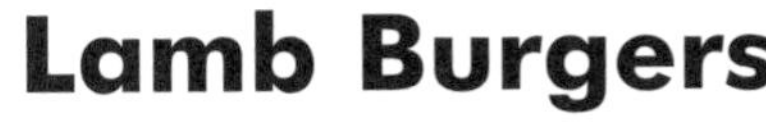

# Lamb Burgers

*Preheat barbecue or broiler*

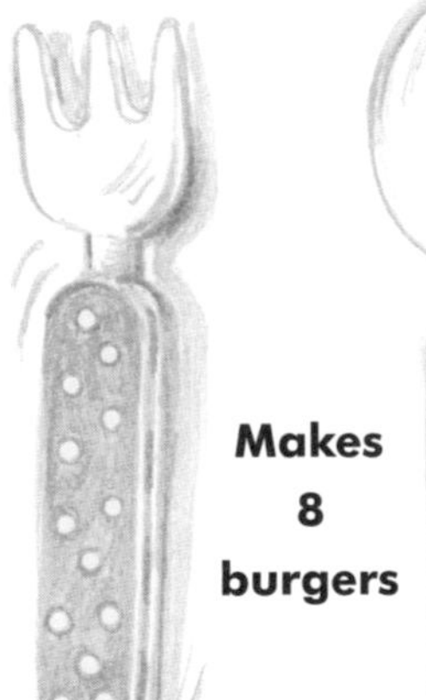


*Try this recipe when you feel like a change from the traditional beef burgers. For an extra flavor sensation, serve with a fresh fruit salsa.*

**Food Safety Tip**

Unlike beef burgers, which should be completely cooked through to destroy any harmful bacteria, lamb burgers can be served with some pink remaining at the center.

| | | |
|---|---|---|
| 2 lbs | lean ground lamb (see Tip) | 1 kg |
| 8 oz | goat cheese | 250 g |
| 2 to 4 | cloves garlic, mashed | 2 to 4 |
| 1/4 cup | chopped fresh parsley or mint | 50 mL |
| 1/2 tsp | ground cumin | 2 mL |
| 1/2 tsp | red pepper flakes | 2 mL |
| 1/2 tsp | salt | 2 mL |
| 1/2 tsp | freshly ground black pepper | 2 mL |

1. In a large bowl, combine lamb, cheese, garlic, parsley and seasonings. With moistened hands, shape meat into 8 patties. (For younger children, you may wish to make a larger number of smaller burgers.) Place patties on a plate, cover and chill until ready to cook.
2. Grill on a preheated barbecue or under the broiler. Cook until meat is brown on the outside but still slightly pink at the center.

| Nutritional Analysis | Energy | Protein | Carbohydrate | Fat | Calcium | Iron |
|---|---|---|---|---|---|---|
| per burger | 451 kcal | 25.4 g | 1.4 g | 37.7 g | 14 % CDV | 21 % CDV |

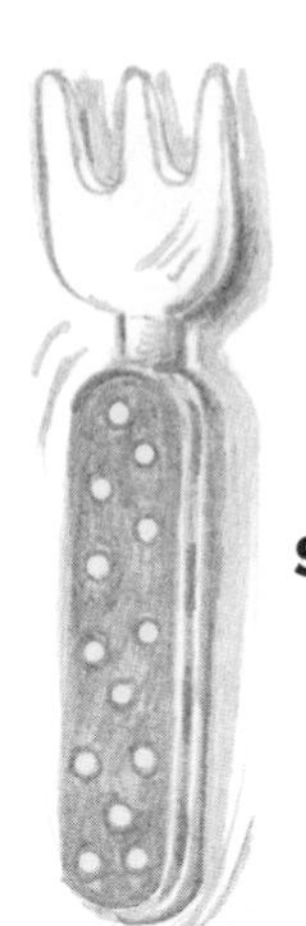
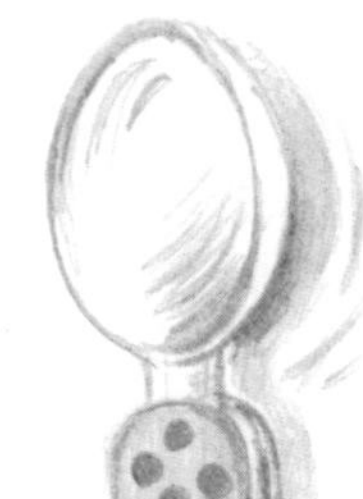

# Beef Satays

*Baking sheet lined with foil*

**Serves 8**

*Don't be discouraged by the long list of ingredients in this recipe – it's really fast and easy to make. Serve as an appetizer or a main meal.*

| | | |
|---|---|---|
| **Satay Sauce** | | |
| 2 tsp | lime juice, divided | 10 mL |
| 1 | green onion, minced | 1 |
| 1/3 cup | unsweetened coconut milk | 75 mL |
| 1 tsp | granulated sugar | 5 mL |
| 1/2 tsp | soy sauce | 2 mL |
| 1/4 tsp | ground cumin | 1 mL |
| 1/4 tsp | ground coriander | 1 mL |
| 1/4 tsp | Chinese chili sauce | 1 mL |
| Pinch | ground turmeric | Pinch |
| **Marinade** | | |
| 1/4 cup | hoisin sauce | 50 mL |
| 1/4 cup | plum sauce | 50 mL |
| 2 tbsp | white vinegar | 25 mL |
| 1 tbsp | honey | 15 mL |
| 1/2 tsp | Chinese chili sauce | 2 mL |
| 1 | green onion, minced | 1 |
| 1 tbsp | minced cilantro | 15 mL |
| 1 lb | top sirloin or beef filet, cut into 4- by 1/2- by 1/8-inch (10 cm by 1 cm by 2 mm) strips | 500 g |

### Kitchen Tip

For a lower-fat version, replace beef with boneless skinless chicken breasts. (You'll also get less iron, however.)

Hot pepper sauce can replace the Chinese chili sauce.

This recipe is peanut-free, but if you'd like a traditional peanut flavor in the sauce, add 2 tsp (10 mL) peanut butter.

You may want to use less chili sauce, and a smaller amount of cilantro, if your kids are encountering these ingredients for the first time.

| Nutritional Analysis | Energy | Protein | Carbohydrate | Fat | Calcium | Iron |
|---|---|---|---|---|---|---|
| per serving | 147 kcal | 13.3 g | 10.8 g | 5.6 g | 1 % CDV | 21 % CDV |

1. Sauce: In a small saucepan, combine 1 tsp (5 mL) of the lime juice with the green onion, coconut milk, sugar, soy sauce, cumin, coriander, chili sauce and turmeric. Bring to a slow boil and cook for about 1 minute. Remove from heat and allow to cool to room temperature. Stir in remaining lime juice. (Sauce can be made up to a day ahead and refrigerated.)
2. Marinade: In a bowl combine hoisin sauce, plum sauce, vinegar, honey, chili sauce, green onion and cilantro. Add beef strips and toss to coat. Cover and refrigerate for at least 1 hour.
3. Remove beef from marinade, and transfer to prepared baking sheet. Preheat broiler. Place sheet as close to heat as possible and broil for about 5 minutes or until beef is cooked.

# Meatball Medley

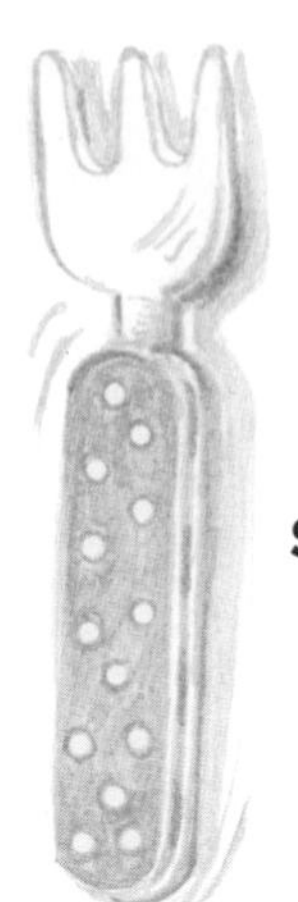
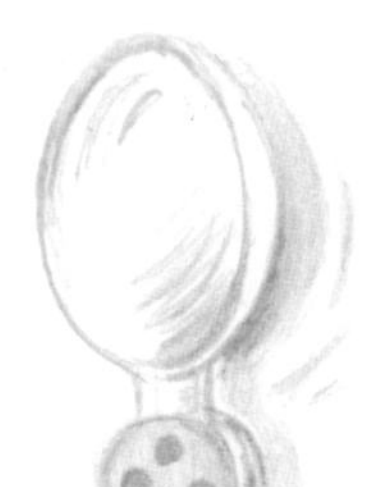
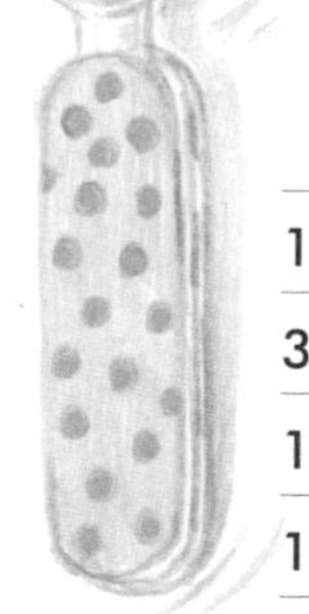

**Serves 12**

*Great on their own or enjoy with spaghetti or other thin pasta. Serve with a sprinkling of freshly grated Parmesan.*

| | | |
|---|---|---|
| 1 1/2 lbs | lean ground beef | 750 g |
| 3 tbsp | water | 45 mL |
| 1 | small onion, diced | 1 |
| 1 | egg | 1 |
| 2 tbsp | grated Parmesan cheese | 25 mL |
| 1 tsp | dried basil | 5 mL |
| 1/2 tsp | salt | 2 mL |
| 1/4 tsp | freshly ground black pepper | 1 mL |
| 1/4 tsp | dried sage | 1 mL |
| 4 tsp | vegetable oil | 20 mL |
| **SAUCE** | | |
| 1 | large onion, chopped | 1 |
| 4 | cloves garlic, minced | 4 |
| 2 1/4 cups | sliced mushrooms | 550 mL |
| 2 tsp | dried basil | 10 mL |
| 3/4 tsp | dried sage | 4 mL |
| 1/4 tsp | red pepper flakes | 1 mL |
| 4 tsp | all-purpose flour | 20 mL |
| 3 cups | beef stock | 750 mL |
| 3 tbsp | tomato paste | 45 mL |
| 1 tbsp | red wine vinegar | 15 mL |
| 1 | bay leaf | 1 |
| 3 | carrots, sliced | 3 |
| 1/2 tsp | salt | 2 mL |
| 1 | red bell pepper, chopped | 1 |
| 1 | yellow bell pepper, chopped | 1 |
| 1 | medium zucchini, chopped | 1 |
| 1 cup | frozen peas | 250 mL |

#### KITCHEN TIP

This is a good opportunity for older children to help with preparing the dish.

To freeze, prepare recipe up to the end of Step 4. Freeze, then thaw when ready to use. Warm meatball mixture over low heat, then proceed with Step 5.

1. Meatballs: In a large bowl, combine beef, water, onion, egg, cheese, basil, salt, pepper and sage. Mix well. With moistened hands, shape meat mixture into about 24 meatballs.
2. In a large skillet, heat oil over medium heat. In batches, if necessary, cook meatballs, turning often, for about 10 minutes. Transfer cooked meatballs to a plate and set aside.
3. Sauce: In the same skillet, combine onion, garlic, mushrooms, basil, sage and red pepper flakes. Cook, stirring, for about 3 minutes or until the onions are tender. Sprinkle with flour and cook, continuing to stir frequently, for another 3 minutes.
4. Increase heat to high and gradually pour in the stock. Bring to a boil, scraping up any brown bits from the bottom and sides of the skillet. Stir in tomato paste, vinegar, bay leaf, carrots and salt. Reduce heat to low. Add reserved meatballs and simmer for 30 minutes or until the carrots are tender.
5. Stir in red and yellow peppers; cook for 3 minutes. Add zucchini and peas; simmer for about 8 minutes or until heated throughout. Remove and discard bay leaf before serving.

| NUTRITIONAL ANALYSIS | Energy | Protein | Carbohydrate | Fat | Calcium | Iron |
|---|---|---|---|---|---|---|
| per serving | 207 kcal | 15.3 g | 9.4 g | 12.2 g | 7 % CDV | 26 % CDV |

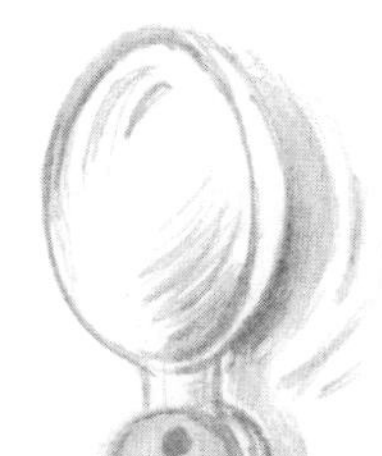

# Speedy Beef Strogonoff

**Serves 4**

*This easy meal is perfect for busy weeknight suppers – it's ready in about 20 minutes.*

**Kitchen Tip**

For speediest cooking, use instant-type rice.

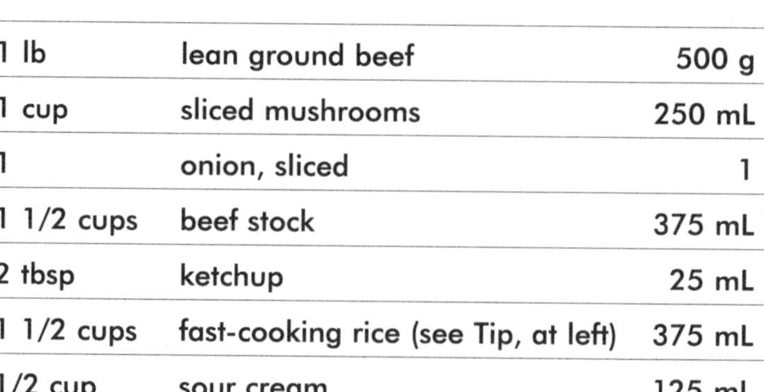

| | | |
|---|---|---|
| 1 lb | lean ground beef | 500 g |
| 1 cup | sliced mushrooms | 250 mL |
| 1 | onion, sliced | 1 |
| 1 1/2 cups | beef stock | 375 mL |
| 2 tbsp | ketchup | 25 mL |
| 1 1/2 cups | fast-cooking rice (see Tip, at left) | 375 mL |
| 1/2 cup | sour cream | 125 mL |

1. In a skillet over medium-high heat, cook ground beef, breaking up meat with a spoon, until browned and crumbly. Drain fat. Add mushrooms and onion; cook for 5 minutes. Stir in broth and ketchup. Bring to a boil. Add rice and sour cream. Remove from heat, cover and let stand for 5 minutes.

| Nutritional Analysis | Energy | Protein | Carbohydrate | Fat | Calcium | Iron |
|---|---|---|---|---|---|---|
| per serving | 615 kcal | 31.3 g | 65.8 g | 24.0 g | 10 % CDV | 36 % CDV |

# Family Beef Pot Roast with Vegetables

**Serves 6**

*Pot roast makes a hearty traditional family meal – and it's an easy way to satisfy hungry appetites.*

**Kitchen Tip**

Cheaper cuts of meat may be tougher, but are often more flavorful. In this recipe, just about any cut of meat becomes fork tender after cooking slowly in liquid. Blade, chuck, rump or cross-rib are all good choices.

| | | |
|---|---|---|
| 1 | 4-lb (2 kg) beef pot roast (see Tip, at left) | 1 |
| 1/3 cup | all-purpose flour | 75 mL |
| 1/4 tsp | salt | 1 mL |
| 1/4 tsp | freshly ground black pepper | 1 mL |
| 1/4 tsp | garlic powder | 1 mL |
| 2 tbsp | vegetable oil | 25 mL |
| 1 cup | beef stock or vegetable stock (or tomato juice), divided | 250 mL |
| 6 | small potatoes, peeled | 6 |
| 3 | onions, quartered | 3 |
| 6 | small carrots, thickly sliced | 6 |
| 1/4 cup | water | 50 mL |

1. Wipe beef dry with paper towels. In a large plastic bag, combine flour, salt, pepper and garlic powder. Place roast in bag and shake to coat. Remove from bag; reserve extra flour.
2. In a large heavy-bottomed saucepan with a lid, heat oil over medium-high. Add roast and brown well on all sides. Reduce heat. Add 1/2 cup (125 mL) of the stock; cover and simmer for 1 1/2 hours. (Or bake in a preheated 325° F [160° C] oven.) Add vegetables and remaining stock. Continue cooking for another 1 hour or until tender. Add extra liquid, if necessary, during cooking time.
3. Transfer beef and vegetables to a serving plate. In a bowl, whisk together reserved flour and water until smooth. Whisk mixture into juices remaining in pan; cook, stirring constantly, until smooth.

| Nutritional Analysis | Energy | Protein | Carbohydrate | Fat | Calcium | Iron |
|---|---|---|---|---|---|---|
| per serving | 626 kcal | 72.4 g | 35.7 g | 20.1 g | 8 % CDV | 78 % CDV |

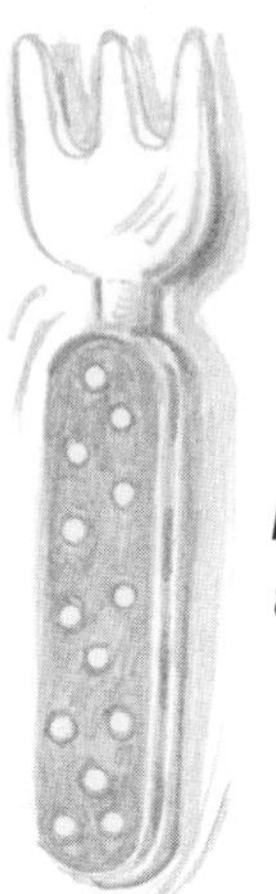
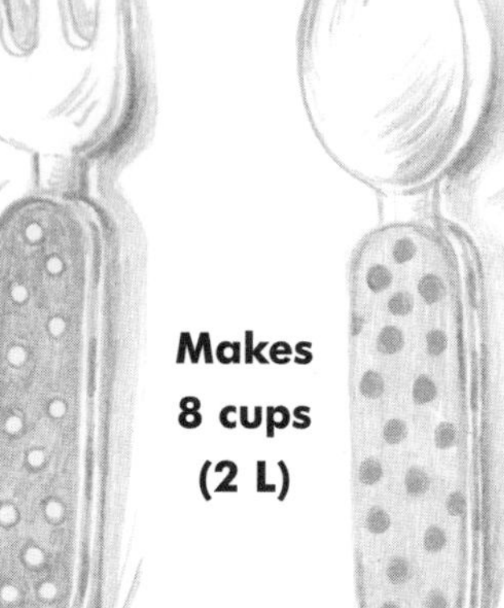

# Beef and Vegetable Stew

**Makes 8 cups (2 L)**

| | | |
|---|---|---|
| 1 1/2 tbsp | vegetable oil | 22 mL |
| 1 lb | stewing beef, cubed | 500 g |
| 4 cups | beef stock | 1 L |
| 1/2 tsp | dried parsley | 2 mL |
| 1 | bay leaf | 1 |
| 1/2 tsp | dried thyme | 2 mL |
| 1/4 tsp | freshly ground black pepper | 1 mL |
| 1 | can (28 oz [796 mL]) diced tomatoes, drained | 1 |
| 2 | potatoes, peeled and cut into 1-inch (2.5 cm) cubes | 2 |
| 3 | carrots, peeled and sliced | 3 |
| 4 | stalks celery, sliced into 1-inch (2.5 cm) pieces | 4 |
| 2 cups | mushrooms, quartered | 500 mL |
| 1 | medium onion, chopped | 1 |
| 1/4 cup | cornstarch | 50 mL |
| 1/4 cup | cold water | 50 mL |

1. In a large stock pot, heat oil over medium-high heat. Add beef and sauté until meat is browned. Stir in beef stock. Add parsley, bay leaf, thyme and pepper. Reduce heat and simmer for 1 hour.
2. Stir in tomatoes, potatoes, carrots, celery, mushrooms and onion. In a small bowl, whisk together cornstarch and water until dissolved; whisk into tomato mixture. Cover and simmer for another 1 hour and 15 minutes

| Nutritional Analysis | Energy | Protein | Carbohydrate | Fat | Calcium | Iron |
|---|---|---|---|---|---|---|
| per 1-cup (250 mL) serving | 196 kcal | 17.8 g | 18.2 g | 6.0 g | 8 % CDV | 30 % CDV |

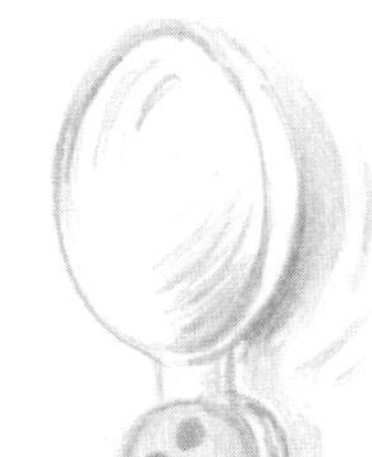

# Asian Tenderloin

**Serves 4**

*A few simple ingredients really perk up ordinary pork tenderloin in this dish. It's just a little spicy – not too much for young palates.*

| | | |
|---|---|---|
| 1/4 cup | plum sauce | 50 mL |
| 1/4 cup | hoisin sauce | 50 mL |
| 2 | cloves garlic, minced | 2 |
| 1/8 tsp | Tabasco sauce | 0.5 mL |
| 1/2 tsp | salt | 2 mL |
| 1/4 tsp | freshly ground black pepper | 1 mL |
| 1 lb | pork tenderloin | 500 g |

1. In a shallow dish, stir together plum sauce, hoisin sauce, garlic, Tabasco, salt and pepper. Add tenderloin and turn to coat well. Cover and marinate for about 1 hour.
2. Preheat barbecue or grill. Remove tenderloin from marinade and set aside. Transfer marinade to a small saucepan and bring to a boil; cook for 5 minutes.
3. Place tenderloin on barbecue and grill over high heat for about 3 minutes per side. Reduce heat to medium and cook for about 15 minutes or until juices run clear when pierced with a fork. Baste frequently with marinade throughout cooking.

### Kitchen Tip

Hoisin sauce is a traditional Asian ingredient that is widely available at most large grocery stores or Asian specialty food shops.

For a little more heat, adults may want to increase the amount of Tabasco sauce.

| Nutritional Analysis | Energy | Protein | Carbohydrate | Fat | Calcium | Iron |
|---|---|---|---|---|---|---|
| per serving | 182 kcal | 27.7 g | 9.2 g | 3.1 g | 2 % CDV | 21 % CDV |

# Braised Lamb

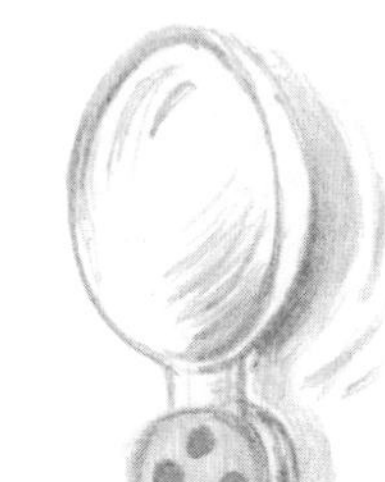

**Serves 5**

*Winter comfort food doesn't get much better than this! Use lamb or beef – either will make a great family dinner.*

| | | |
|---|---|---|
| 3 tbsp | olive oil | 45 mL |
| 2 lbs | lean lamb or beef, cut into cubes (see Tip, at left) | 1 kg |
| 3 | medium onions, chopped | 3 |
| 1 | large clove garlic, minced | 1 |
| 3 tbsp | all-purpose flour | 45 mL |
| 1 1/2 cups | apple juice | 375 mL |
| 1 cup | chicken stock or beef stock | 250 mL |
| 3 tbsp | tomato paste | 45 mL |
| 1/2 tsp | salt | 2 mL |
| 1/4 tsp | freshly ground black pepper | 1 mL |

**KITCHEN TIP**

If you use beef instead of lamb, cooking time may vary, depending on the cut of beef. Check frequently for tenderness. Beef will also create a slightly thinner sauce – although it's still delicious to sop up with pieces of crusty bread.

1. In a large saucepan, heat oil on medium-high heat. Add lamb in small batches; cook for 5 minutes or until browned on all sides, removing pieces as they brown. Reduce heat to medium. Add onions and garlic; cook, stirring, for 3 minutes or until softened (but not browned). Add flour and cook, stirring, for 1 minute. Stir in apple juice, stock and tomato paste.
2. Return lamb to saucepan. Bring to a boil; reduce heat, cover and cook for 1 1/2 hours or until meat is tender. Season with salt and pepper to taste.

| NUTRITIONAL ANALYSIS | Energy | Protein | Carbohydrate | Fat | Calcium | Iron |
|---|---|---|---|---|---|---|
| per serving | 761 kcal | 35.7 g | 21.6 g | 58.6 g | 7 % CDV | 37 % CDV |

# Braised Winter Vegetables

**Serves 6**

*Braised winter vegetables are a marvelous accompaniment to roasts of chicken, beef or pork.*

*Preheat oven to 400° F (200° C)*
*Large roasting pan*

| | | |
|---|---|---|
| 3 | carrots, peeled and cut into chunks | 3 |
| 3 | small white turnip, peeled and cut into chunks | 3 |
| Half | rutabaga peeled and cut into chunks | Half |
| 1 | large sweet potato, peeled and cut into chunks | 1 |
| 3 tbsp | olive oil | 45 mL |
| 1/2 tsp | salt | 2 mL |
| 1/4 tsp | freshly ground black pepper | 1 mL |
| | Chopped fresh parsley | |

1. Place carrots, turnip, rutabaga and sweet potato in roasting pan. Sprinkle with oil, salt and pepper. Cover pan and roast in preheated oven for 35 minutes or until vegetables are tender. Serve garnished with chopped parsley.

| Nutritional Analysis | Energy | Protein | Carbohydrate | Fat | Calcium | Iron |
|---|---|---|---|---|---|---|
| per serving | 157 kcal | 2.7 g | 22.3 g | 7.3 g | 11 % CDV | 11 % CDV |

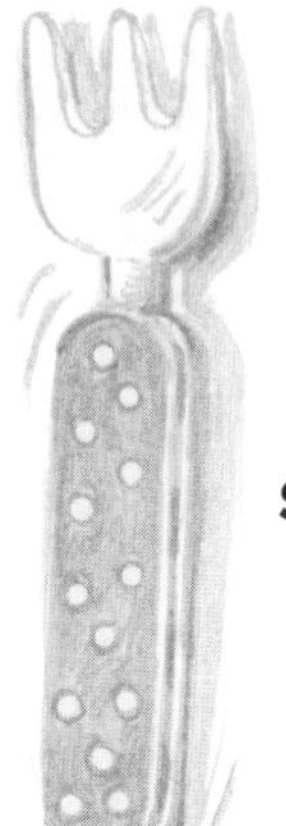

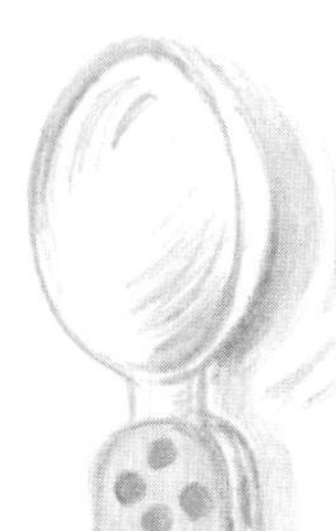

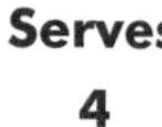


# Stuffed Baked Sweet Potatoes

*Preheat oven to 350° F (180° C)*
*Small baking pan*

| | | |
|---|---|---|
| 2 | sweet potatoes (medium size) | 2 |
| 1/4 cup | orange juice | 50 mL |
| 2 tbsp | butter or margarine | 25 mL |
| 1/4 tsp | grated orange zest | 1 mL |
| 1/4 tsp | ground nutmeg | 1 mL |
| 1/4 tsp | salt | 1 mL |
| Pinch | freshly ground pepper | Pinch |

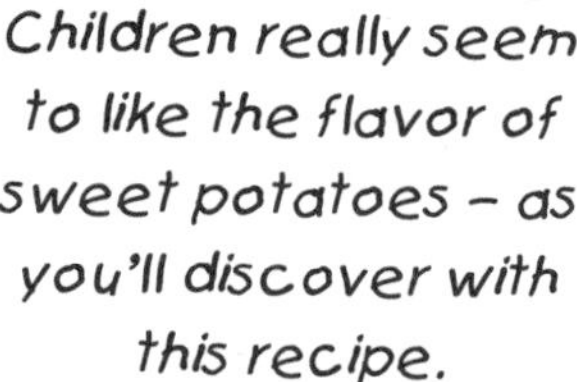


1. Wash potatoes and pierce with a fork in several places. Place on oven rack in preheated oven. Bake for 1 hour or until potatoes are tender.
2. When cool enough to handle, cut each potato in half. With a spoon, carefully remove pulp to a bowl, being sure not to damage shell. Mash pulp with orange juice, butter, orange zest, nutmeg, salt and pepper. Stuff shells with mixture and transfer to baking pan.
3. Bake stuffed shells for 10 minutes or until heated through. (Before serving to small children, test the stuffing to make sure it is not too hot inside. You may wish to remove filling from shell.)

### Kitchen Tip

These potatoes can be baked at the same time that you cook a roast.

| Nutritional Analysis | Energy | Protein | Carbohydrate | Fat | Calcium | Iron |
|---|---|---|---|---|---|---|
| per serving | 118 kcal | 1.2 g | 17.3 g | 5.1 g | 2 % CDV | 4 % CDV |

# Swedish Potatoes

*Preheat oven to 350° F (180° C)*
*8-cup (2 L) casserole, greased*

**Serves 8**

*Here's a simply wonderful, easily made casserole that's great for a crowd!*

| | | |
|---|---|---|
| 6 | large potatoes, peeled and cut into chunks | 6 |
| 3/4 cup | sour cream | 175 mL |
| Half | pkg (8 oz [250 g]) cream cheese, softened | Half |
| 2 tbsp | finely chopped onion | 25 mL |
| 1/2 tsp | salt | 2 mL |
| 1/4 tsp | freshly ground black pepper | 1 mL |
| 3/4 cup | fine dry breadcrumbs | 175 mL |

1. In a large saucepan, cook potatoes in boiling water until tender. Drain and mash.
2. In a small bowl, beat together sour cream, cream cheese, onion, salt and pepper. Add mixture to mashed potatoes and stir until smooth.
3. Spoon potato mixture into prepared casserole. Top with breadcrumbs. Bake in preheated oven for 30 minutes or until hot and golden brown.

**Kitchen Tip**

Double the recipe and freeze one portion to have on hand for surprise guests. It's easy to reheat.

| Nutritional Analysis | Energy | Protein | Carbohydrate | Fat | Calcium | Iron |
|---|---|---|---|---|---|---|
| per serving | 225 kcal | 5.6 g | 31.0 g | 9.1 g | 7 % CDV | 15 % CDV |

# Garlic Roasted Potatoes

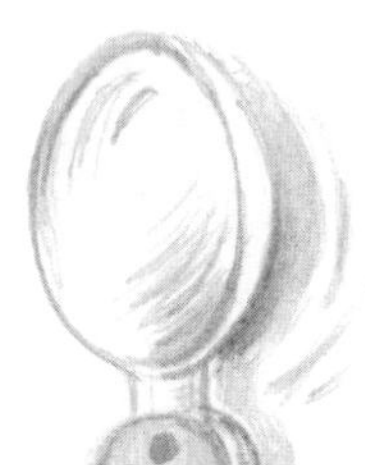

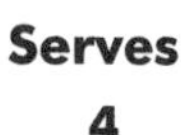

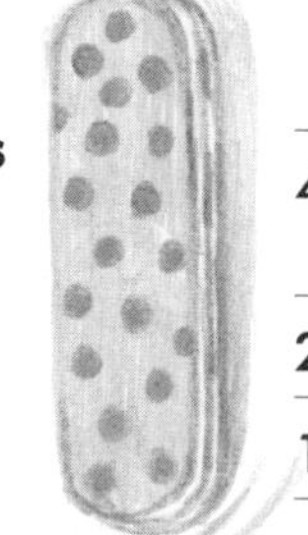

**Serves 4**

*These are absolutely the very best roasted crispy potatoes you will ever eat. They're our all-time favorite!*

*Preheat oven to 400° F (200° C)*
*Shallow baking pan, greased*

| | | |
|---|---|---|
| 4 | **Yukon Gold potatoes, cut into chunks** | 4 |
| 2 tbsp | **olive oil** | 25 mL |
| 1 or 2 | **cloves garlic, sliced** | 1 or 2 |
| | **Salt and freshly ground pepper** | |

1. Place potato chunks in a plastic bag. Add oil and garlic. Seal bag and toss until potatoes are coated. Transfer to prepared baking pan. Sprinkle with salt and pepper. Bake in preheated oven for 35 minutes or until potatoes are tender and golden brown.

| **Nutritional Analysis** | Energy | Protein | Carbohydrate | Fat | Calcium | Iron |
|---|---|---|---|---|---|---|
| per serving | 141 kcal | 2.4 g | 20.6 g | 5.8 g | 1 % CDV | 9 % CDV |

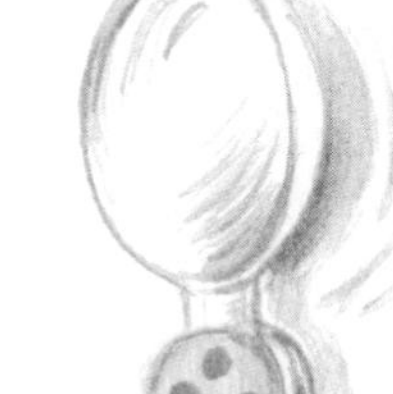

# Rice and Broccoli Casserole

**Serves 6**

*Assemble this vegetable casserole ahead, refrigerate and then bake just before serving. Everyone who's tried this recipe loves it!*

*Preheat oven to 350° F (180° C)*
*Shallow 8-cup (2 L) casserole, greased*

| | | |
|---|---|---|
| 2 cups | broccoli florets (see Tip, at left) | 500 mL |
| 2 cups | cooked rice | 500 mL |
| 1 | small onion, finely chopped | 1 |
| 2 | eggs | 2 |
| 1 1/2 cups | 2% milk | 375 mL |
| 1/2 tsp | salt | 2 mL |
| 1/4 tsp | freshly ground black pepper | 1 mL |
| 1/4 tsp | ground nutmeg | 1 mL |
| 1/4 cup | grated Parmesan cheese | 50 mL |

1. In a colander, blanch broccoli over boiling water for 2 minutes. Transfer to a bowl and combine with rice and onion. Transfer to prepared casserole.
2. In a small bowl, whisk together eggs, milk, salt, pepper and nutmeg. Pour over rice mixture. Sprinkle with cheese. Cover and refrigerate until ready to bake.
3. Bake in a preheated oven for 35 minutes or until mixture is bubbling and set in the center.

### Kitchen Tip

Instead of fresh broccoli, use an equal quantity of frozen chopped broccoli. It should be thawed before combining with the rice, but need not be blanched.

| Nutritional Analysis | Energy | Protein | Carbohydrate | Fat | Calcium | Iron |
|---|---|---|---|---|---|---|
| per serving | 153 kcal | 7.7 g | 21.1 g | 4.2 g | 19 % CDV | 9 % CDV |

# Parmesan Leeks

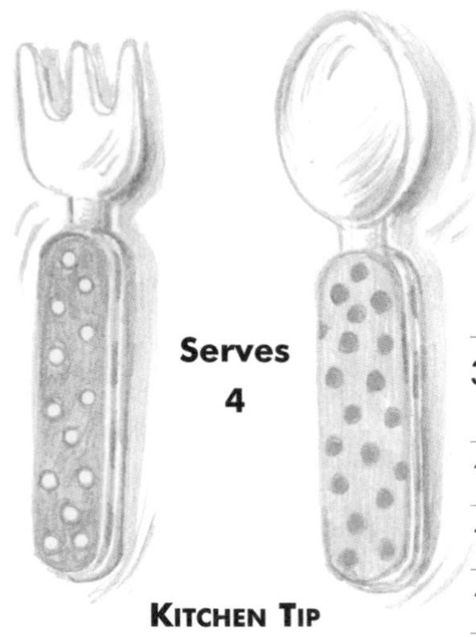

**Serves 4**

**Kitchen Tip**

A lot of dirt can hide between the layers of a leek, so be sure to trim and wash well before boiling.

*Preheat broiler*
*6-cup (1.5 L) casserole, greased*

| | | |
|---|---|---|
| 3 | leeks, trimmed, well washed, and cut into bite-size pieces | 3 |
| 1 tbsp | butter or margarine | 15 mL |
| 1 tbsp | all-purpose flour | 15 mL |
| 1/4 cup | 2% milk | 50 mL |
| 1/4 tsp | salt | 1 mL |
| Pinch | freshly ground black pepper | Pinch |
| 2 tbsp | grated Parmesan cheese | 25 mL |

1. In a large saucepan of boiling water, cook leeks for 5 to 10 minutes or until tender. Drain all but 1/4 cup (50 mL) cooking liquid; set aside. Transfer leeks to prepared casserole.
2. In a small saucepan, melt butter over medium heat. Whisk in flour, milk and reserved leek cooking liquid. Reduce heat to simmer; whisk until smooth. Add salt and pepper. Pour sauce mixture over the leeks. Sprinkle with Parmesan cheese. Broil until golden brown.

| Nutritional Analysis | Energy | Protein | Carbohydrate | Fat | Calcium | Iron |
|---|---|---|---|---|---|---|
| per serving | 108 kcal | 3.1 g | 15.4 g | 1.7 g | 13 % CDV | 11 % CDV |

# Deluxe Coleslaw

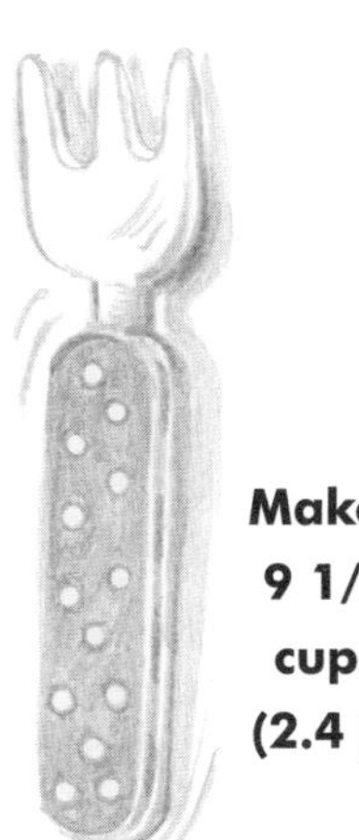

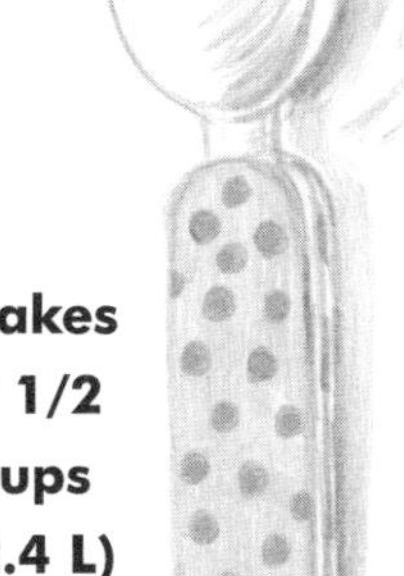

**Makes 9 1/2 cups (2.4 L)**

*This crunchy salad makes a nice change from plain iceberg lettuce. It's terrific in the summer with burgers and corn on the cob.*

| | | |
|---|---|---|
| 1 cup | mayonnaise | 250 mL |
| 2 tbsp | 2% milk | 25 mL |
| 2 tbsp | vinegar or lemon juice | 25 mL |
| 1 tsp | brown sugar | 5 mL |
| 1/2 tsp | salt | 2mL |
| 1/4 tsp | freshly ground black pepper | 1 mL |
| 1/4 tsp | paprika | 1 mL |
| 1 | medium head cabbage, shredded | 1 |
| 1 | large stalk celery, thinly sliced | 1 |
| 1 | large carrot, shredded | 1 |
| 2 tbsp | minced onion | 25 mL |

1. In a small bowl, mix together mayonnaise, milk, vinegar, brown sugar, salt, pepper and paprika.
2. In a large bowl, toss together the cabbage, celery, carrot, onion. Add mayonnaise mixture and combine well. Cover and refrigerate for at least 1 hour before serving.

| Nutritional Analysis | Energy | Protein | Carbohydrate | Fat | Calcium | Iron |
|---|---|---|---|---|---|---|
| per 1/2-cup (125 mL) serving | 94 kcal | 0.4 g | 1.6 g | 9.6 g | 2 % CDV | 2 % CDV |

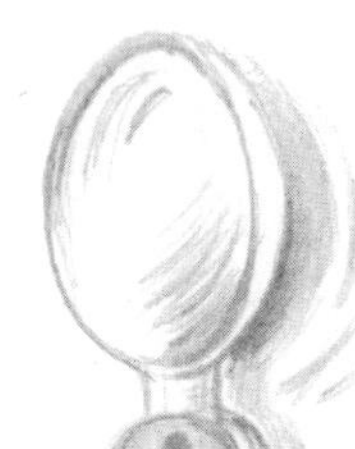

# Glazed Carrots

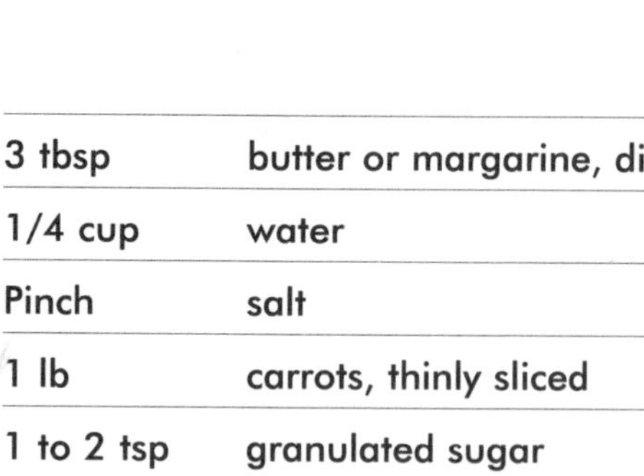

**Serves 4**

*Can't get your kids to eat their carrots? It's amazing what adding a light glaze can do. Your entire family will love it!*

| | | |
|---|---|---|
| 3 tbsp | butter or margarine, divided | 45 mL |
| 1/4 cup | water | 50 mL |
| Pinch | salt | Pinch |
| 1 lb | carrots, thinly sliced | 500 g |
| 1 to 2 tsp | granulated sugar | 5 to 10 mL |
| 2 tbsp | minced fresh basil | 25 mL |

1. In a large skillet, heat 1 tbsp (15 mL) of the butter over medium-low heat, along with water and salt. Once butter has melted, stir in carrots. Cook, covered, for 8 to 10 minutes or until tender. Drain carrots and set aside.
2. Using the same skillet, melt remaining butter. When butter begins to sizzle, add sugar. Shake pan a few times, then add carrots and basil; cook, tossing carrots gently, for 3 to 5 minutes or until glazed.

| Nutritional Analysis | Energy | Protein | Carbohydrate | Fat | Calcium | Iron |
|---|---|---|---|---|---|---|
| per 1/2-cup (125 mL) serving | 144 kcal | 1.7 g | 15.9 g | 9.1 g | 10 % CDV | 14 % CDV |

# Chinese Veggies

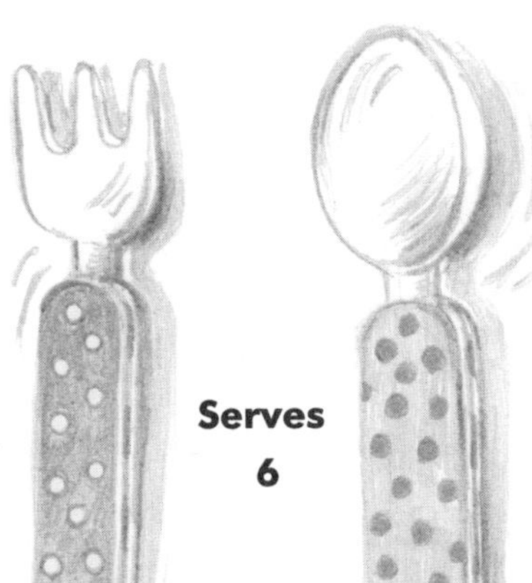

**Serves 6**

**KITCHEN TIP**

Adjust cooking time to prepare vegetables to desired softness.

If you don't have any homemade chicken stock, use tinned chicken broth, preferably a low-sodium variety.

| | | |
|---|---|---|
| 1 tbsp | vegetable oil | 15 mL |
| 1 lb | broccoli florets, chopped | 500 g |
| 1 | onion, thinly sliced | 1 |
| 1 tbsp | minced ginger root | 15 mL |
| 3 | baby bok choy | 3 |
| 4 oz | snow peas | 125 g |
| 3 | celery stalks, thinly sliced | 3 |
| 5 | green onions, thinly sliced | 5 |
| 3/4 cup | chicken stock | 175 mL |

1. In a wok or a large skillet, heat oil over high heat. Add bboccoli, onions and ginger; stir-fry for 1 minute. Add bok choy, snow peas, celery and green onions. Pour broth over. Toss vegetables until well coated. Bring to a boil, cover and cook for 2 to 3 minutes or until the vegetables are tender-crisp.

| NUTRITIONAL ANALYSIS | Energy | Protein | Carbohydrate | Fat | Calcium | Iron |
|---|---|---|---|---|---|---|
| per serving | 58 kcal | 3.0 g | 6.6 g | 2.8 g | 9 % CDV | 13 % CDV |

# Creamy Cheddar Sauce

**Makes 3/4 cup (175 mL)**

*This sauce is perfect with so many vegetables and is bound to make your little ones ask for more. Try it on cooked cauliflower, broccoli, carrots, green beans or anything else you think they will like.*

| | | |
|---|---|---|
| 1/3 cup | 2% milk | 75 mL |
| 1/3 cup | mayonnaise | 75 mL |
| 1 cup | shredded Cheddar cheese | 250 mL |
| Pinch | freshly ground black pepper | Pinch |
| Pinch | freshly grated nutmeg | Pinch |
| | Cooked vegetables | |

1. In a small saucepan over medium heat, whisk together milk and mayonnaise until smooth. Add cheese, pepper and nutmeg. Cook until cheese has melted. (Be sure the sauce does not boil.) Pour over vegetables. Toss and serve.

| NUTRITIONAL ANALYSIS | Energy | Protein | Carbohydrate | Fat | Calcium | Iron |
|---|---|---|---|---|---|---|
| per 1-tbsp (15 mL) serving | 88 kcal | 2.8 g | 0.6 g | 8.2 g | 10 % CDV | 1 % CDV |

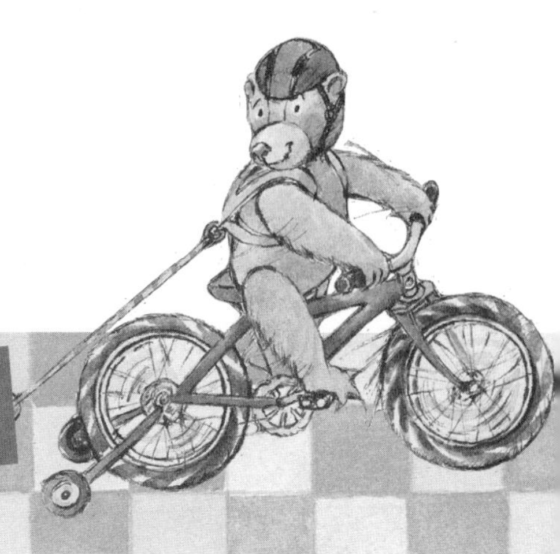

# Snacks

# Mild Salsa Cheese Dip

**Makes 1 cup (250 mL)**

*This easy dip is a treat for the whole family when served with vegetables or nachos.*

| | | |
|---|---|---|
| 1/2 cup | mild salsa | 125 mL |
| 1 cup | shredded Cheddar cheese | 250 mL |
| Half | pkg (8 oz [250 g]) cream cheese | Half |
| 1 to 2 tbsp | ketchup | 15 to 25 mL |
| | Assorted raw vegetables or corn nacho chips | |

1. In a small saucepan over medium heat, combine salsa, Cheddar cheese and cream cheese. Cook, stirring, until cheeses are melted. Stir in ketchup until mixture is smooth. Serve with vegetables or nachos.

| Nutritional Analysis | Energy | Protein | Carbohydrate | Fat | Calcium | Iron |
|---|---|---|---|---|---|---|
| per 1/4-cup (50 mL) serving | 249 kcal | 10.2 g | 4.6 g | 20.8 g | 31 % CDV | 8 % CDV |

# Ranch Dip for Kids

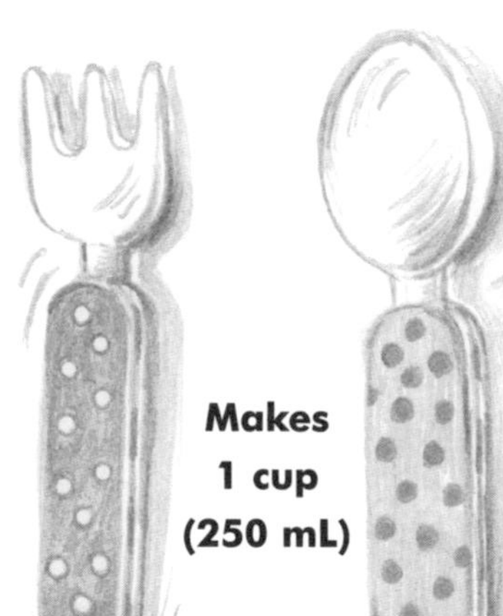

**Makes 1 cup (250 mL)**

*Want to make a big plate of veggies disappear? Just serve this dip – kids find it irresistible!*

| | | |
|---|---|---|
| 2/3 cup | sour cream | 150 mL |
| 1/3 cup | light mayonnaise | 75 mL |
| 1 tbsp | cider vinegar | 15 mL |
| 1 tsp | dried dill | 5 mL |
| 1 tsp | Dijon mustard | 5 mL |
| Pinch | salt | Pinch |
| Pinch | freshly ground black pepper | Pinch |

1. In a small bowl, whisk together sour cream, mayonnaise and vinegar until smooth. Add dill, mustard, salt and pepper. Whisk to blend. Cover and refrigerate for up to 1 week.

| Nutritional Analysis | Energy | Protein | Carbohydrate | Fat | Calcium | Iron |
|---|---|---|---|---|---|---|
| per 1/4 cup (50 mL) | 87 kcal | 1.0 g | 2.7 g | 8.3 g | 3 % CDV | <1 % CDV |

# Creamy Spinach Dip

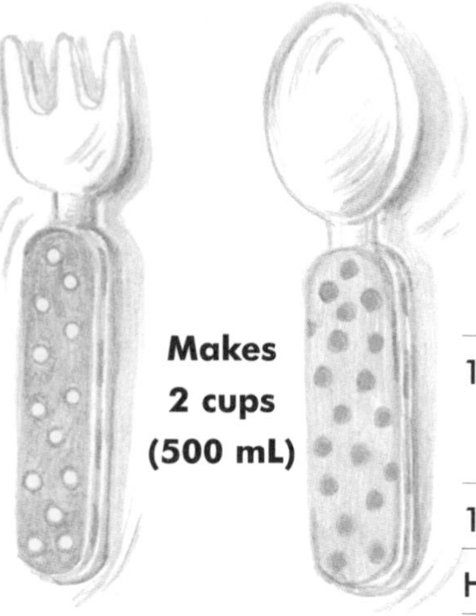

**Makes 2 cups (500 mL)**

*This dip is a perennial favorite with snackers young and old. Serve with torn pita pieces or raw vegetables.*

| | | |
|---|---|---|
| 1 | pkg (10 oz [284 g]) frozen chopped spinach, thawed, excess liquid squeezed out | 1 |
| 1/2 cup | plain yogurt | 125 mL |
| Half | pkg (8 oz [250 g]) cream cheese | Half |
| 2 tbsp | finely chopped onion | 25 mL |
| 1/2 tsp | Worcestershire sauce | 2 mL |
| Pinch | salt | Pinch |
| Pinch | freshly ground black pepper | Pinch |

1. In a food processor, combine spinach, yogurt, cream cheese and onion; process with on/off turns until smooth. Add Worcestershire sauce, salt and pepper; process to blend. Transfer dip to a bowl; cover and refrigerate for several hours or overnight to allow flavors to develop.

| Nutritional Analysis | Energy | Protein | Carbohydrate | Fat | Calcium | Iron |
|---|---|---|---|---|---|---|
| per 1/4-cup (50 mL) serving | 74 kcal | 2.8 g | 2.9 g | 6.1 g | 9 % CDV | 10 % CDV |

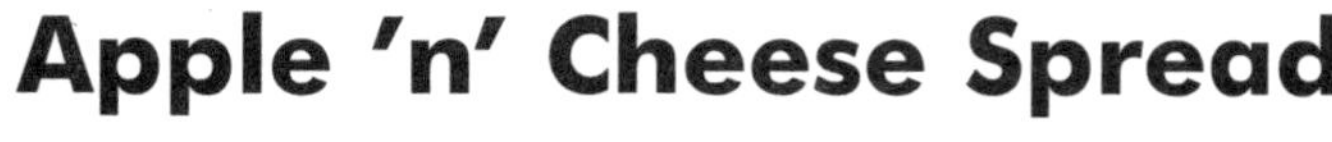

# Apple 'n' Cheese Spread

**Makes 1 cup (250 mL)**

*Serve this spread on crackers, toast or apple slices. It's a perfect snack (or breakfast) for enticing finicky young appetites.*

### Kitchen Tip

If your child is able to eat apple skin, then leave apples unpeeled to provide added fiber.

To prepare apple slices, core and peel (if desired; see above) as many apples as are needed for the meal. Cut into thin slices. Dip each slice in a mixture of lemon juice and water to prevent browning.

Store unused spread in refrigerator.

| | | |
|---|---|---|
| Half | pkg (8 oz [250 g]) cream cheese, at room temperature | Half |
| 1/2 cup | shredded mild Cheddar cheese | 125 mL |
| 2 tsp | lemon juice | 10 mL |
| 1/2 tsp | dry mustard | 2 mL |
| 1 | apple, peeled and grated (see Tip, at left) | 1 |
| | Crackers, toast or apple slices (see Tip, at left) | |

1. In a bowl with an electric mixer or in a food processor, blend cream cheese until smooth. Add Cheddar cheese, lemon juice and mustard; blend until creamy. Stir in grated apple; cover and refrigerate for 2 hours to allow flavors to blend. Before serving, bring dip to room temperature (for best spreading consistency).

| Nutritional Analysis | Energy | Protein | Carbohydrate | Fat | Calcium | Iron |
|---|---|---|---|---|---|---|
| per 1/4-cup (50 mL) serving | 230 kcal | 6.3 g | 16.7 g | 16.3 g | 17 % CDV | 6 % CDV |

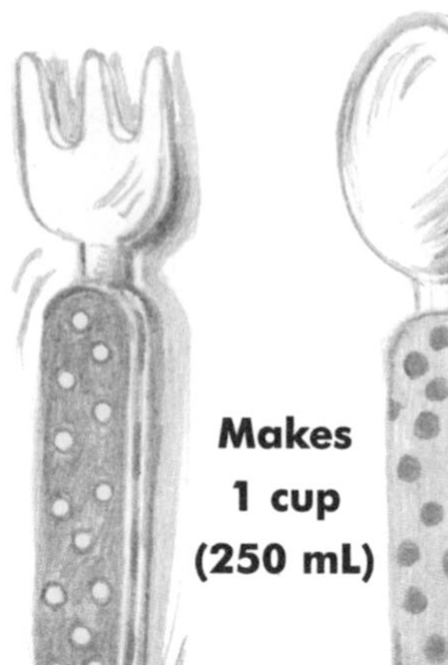

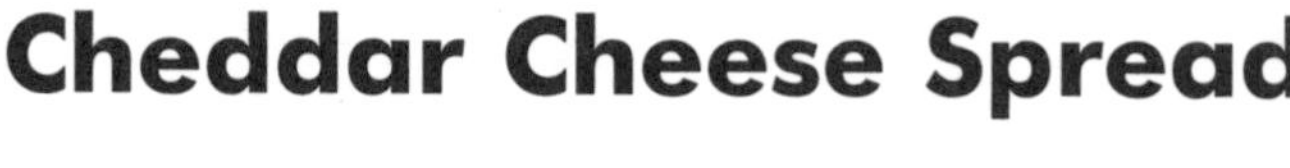

# Cheddar Cheese Spread

**Makes 1 cup (250 mL)**

*You can buy commercially prepared cheese spreads – but when this tasty homemade version is so quick and easy to prepare, why bother?*

| | | |
|---|---|---|
| 1 cup | shredded Cheddar cheese | 250 mL |
| 1/4 cup | cream cheese | 50 mL |
| 1/4 cup | mayonnaise | 50 mL |
| Pinch | dry mustard | Pinch |
| Pinch | Worcestershire sauce | Pinch |

1. In a food processor or in a bowl with an electric mixer, combine Cheddar, cream cheese, mayonnaise, mustard and Worcestershire sauce; process until very smooth. Cover and refrigerate for up to 2 weeks or freeze for longer storage.

**Kitchen Tip**

Vary the strength of flavor by using mild, medium or old Cheddar cheese – or, for a completely different taste, use mozzarella or Swiss.

| Nutritional Analysis | Energy | Protein | Carbohydrate | Fat | Calcium | Iron |
|---|---|---|---|---|---|---|
| per 1-tbsp (15 mL) serving | 62 kcal | 2.1 g | 0.2 g | 5.8 g | 7 % CDV | 1 % CDV |

# Pita Crisps

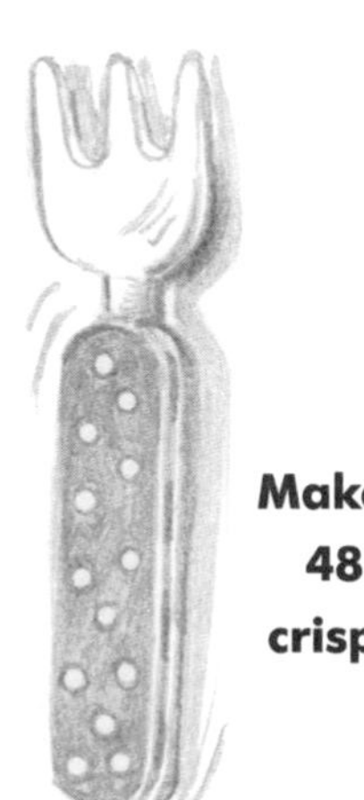

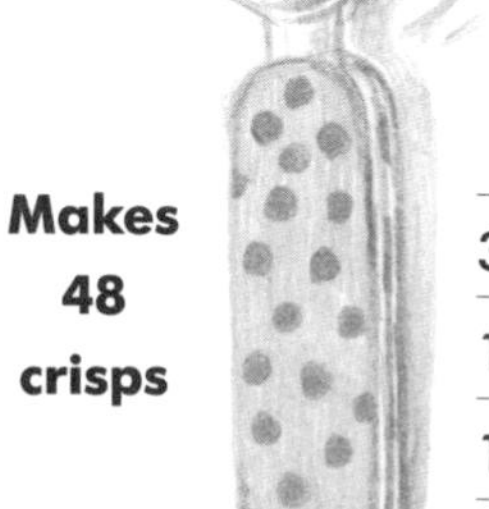

**Makes 48 crisps**

*Everyone loves these crisp crackers. They're easy and economical to make – and taste great, whether on their own or with a dip. Vary the seasonings to suit your family's preferences*

*Preheat oven to 350° F (180° C)*
*Baking sheet, ungreased*

| | | |
|---|---|---|
| 3 tbsp | olive oil | 45 mL |
| 1 | clove garlic, minced | 1 |
| 1/2 tsp | dried basil | 2 mL |
| 1/2 tsp | dried oregano | 2 mL |
| Pinch | salt | Pinch |
| Pinch | freshly ground black pepper | Pinch |
| 3 | 5-inch (12.5 cm) whole wheat pitas, each cut into 8 wedges, then separated to make 16 triangles | 3 |

1. In small bowl, combine oil, garlic, basil, oregano, salt and pepper. Brush mixture lightly over "inside" surface of each triangle and place, brushed-side up, on baking sheet. Bake in preheated oven for 12 minutes or until crisp and golden brown.
2. Remove from oven to wire rack. Allow to cool before storing in airtight container.

| NUTRITIONAL ANALYSIS | Energy | Protein | Carbohydrate | Fat | Calcium | Iron |
|---|---|---|---|---|---|---|
| per 6-crisp serving | 100 kcal | 2.5 g | 11.8 g | 5.2 g | <1 % CDV | 1 % CDV |

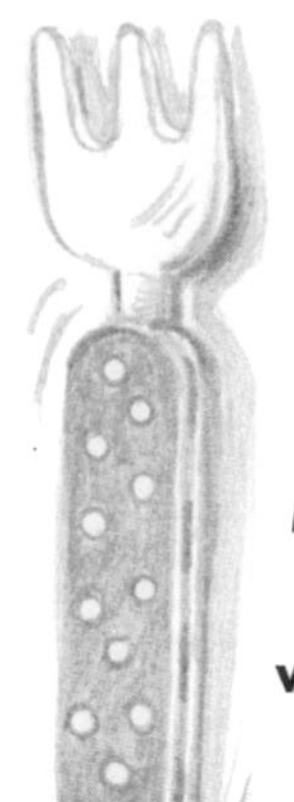
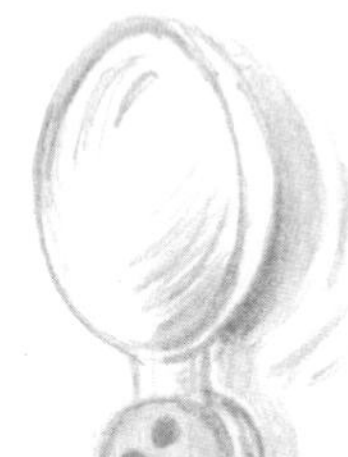

# Cheese Quesadillas

**Makes 12 wedges**

*Tired of plain old cheese and crackers? Try this quick and easy treat.*

| | | |
|---|---|---|
| 2 tsp | vegetable oil, divided | 10 mL |
| 4 | medium (8-inch [20 cm]) tortillas | 4 |
| 1 cup | shredded Cheddar cheese, divided | 250 mL |

1. In a nonstick skillet, heat half of the oil over medium-high heat. Place tortilla in skillet and sprinkle half of the cheese evenly over tortilla. Cover with second tortilla shell and press down firmly. Heat for about 1 1/2 minutes, then flip tortilla over and cook for another minute or until light brown, and cheese has melted. Transfer to a rack and let cool slightly (so little hands are not burned) before cutting into 6 wedges. Repeat procedure with remaining ingredients.

**Kitchen Tip**

For a little more zest, add layers of sour cream and salsa to cheese layer. Or reduce quantity of cheese to 1/4 cup (50 mL) and add a combination of 1/4 cup (50 mL) diced cooked chicken and 1/4 cup (50 mL) diced cooked vegetables.

| Nutritional Analysis | Energy | Protein | Carbohydrate | Fat | Calcium | Iron |
|---|---|---|---|---|---|---|
| per quesadilla wedge | 77 kcal | 3.5 g | 5.8 g | 4.6 g | 11 % CDV | 3 % CDV |

# Stovetop Cereal Snack

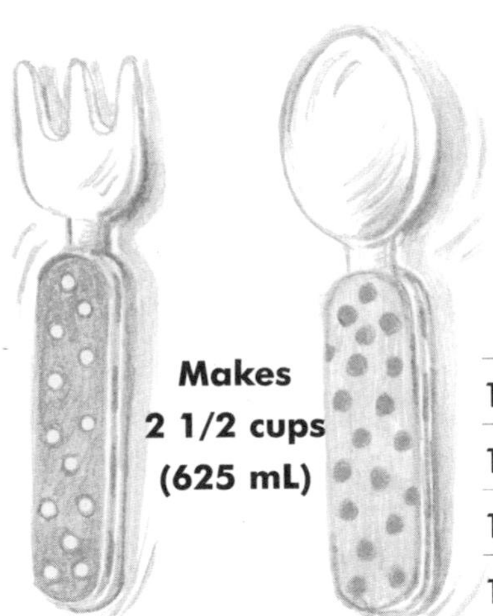

**Makes 2 1/2 cups (625 mL)**

*Here's a great alternative to commercially prepared cereal-based snacks. It's quick to make and provides more food energy than the cereal alone. Young children love to feed themselves the small, easily handled bits and pieces.*

| | | |
|---|---|---|
| 1 tbsp | butter or margarine | 15 mL |
| 1 tsp | Worcestershire sauce | 5 mL |
| 1 1/2 cups | "o-shaped" oat cereal | 375 mL |
| 1/2 cup | shredded wheat squares | 125 mL |
| 1/2 cup | stick pretzels, broken | 125 mL |

1. In a large nonstick skillet, melt butter over medium-low heat. Stir in Worcestershire sauce, cereal and squares; cook, stirring constantly, for 5 minutes or until brown. Remove from heat and allow to cool before adding pretzel sticks. Toss lightly and transfer to an airtight container.

| Nutritional Analysis | Energy | Protein | Carbohydrate | Fat | Calcium | Iron |
|---|---|---|---|---|---|---|
| per 1/2-cup (125 mL) serving | 113 kcal | 2.6 g | 18.3 g | 3.4 g | 2 % CDV | 19 % CDV |

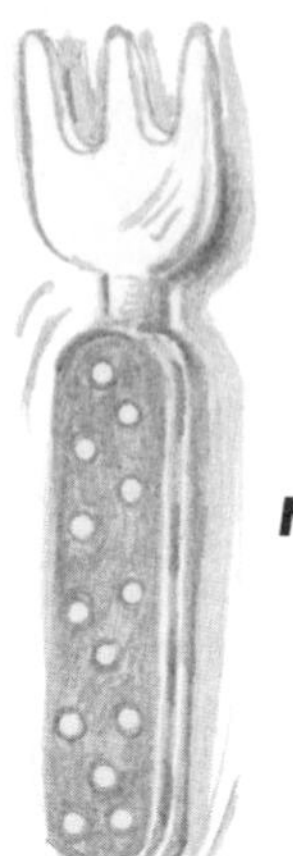
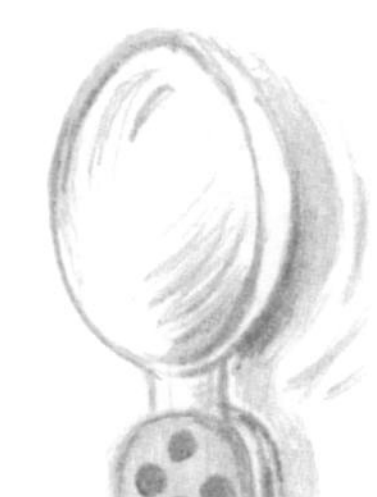

# Frozen Yogurt Pops

**Makes 8 pops**

*Try this nutritious alternative to sugary frozen treats.*

**KITCHEN TIP**

Use a variety of puréed fruits to create different flavors.

| | | |
|---|---|---|
| 1 cup | plain yogurt | 250 mL |
| 3/4 cup | frozen fruit juice concentrate, thawed or puréed fruit | 175 mL |
| 3/4 cup | 2% milk | 175 mL |

1. In a bowl combine yogurt, fruit juice concentrate and milk; stir to mix well. Pour into 8 small paper cups; freeze until partially frozen. Insert a wooden stick into center of each; freeze until firm. To serve, peel away paper cups. (Alternatively, pour mixture into an 8-compartment plastic popsicle mold; place handles on top and freeze.)

| NUTRITIONAL ANALYSIS | Energy | Protein | Carbohydrate | Fat | Calcium | Iron |
|---|---|---|---|---|---|---|
| per yogurt pop | 73 kcal | 2.5 g | 12.6 g | 1.5 g | 9 % CDV | 1 % CDV |

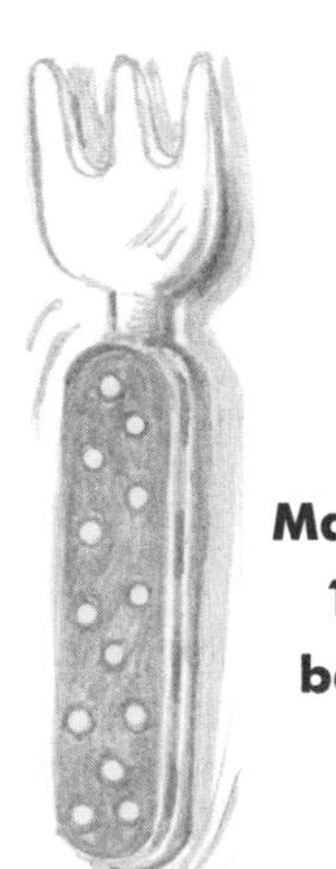

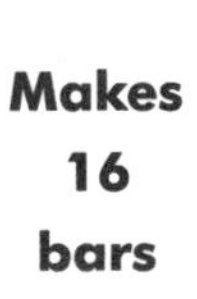

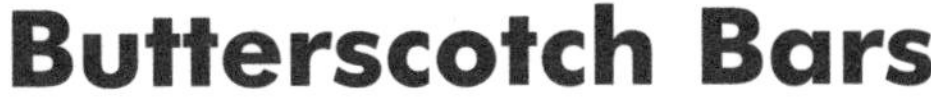

# Butterscotch Bars

*Preheat oven to 350° F (180° C)*
*8-inch (2 L) square baking pan, greased*

**Makes 16 bars**

*Dense and chewy, these bars are a classic combination of rolled oats and butterscotch chips.*

| | | |
|---|---|---|
| 1 cup | graham cracker crumbs | 250 mL |
| 2/3 cup | lightly packed brown sugar | 150 mL |
| 1/2 cup | all-purpose flour | 125 mL |
| 1/3 cup | quick-cooking oats | 75 mL |
| 1/2 cup | butterscotch chips | 125 mL |
| 1 tsp | baking powder | 5 mL |
| 2 tbsp | vegetable oil | 25 mL |
| 1 | egg | 1 |
| 1 1/2 tsp | vanilla extract | 7 mL |

### Kitchen Tip

To prevent mixture from sticking to your hands when pressing into pan, lightly coat your fingers with vegetable oil.

1. In a bowl combine graham crumbs, brown sugar, flour, oats, butterscotch chips and baking powder.
2. In a measuring cup, whisk together oil, egg and vanilla. Add to flour mixture; stir until just combined.
3. Press mixture evenly into prepared pan. Bake in preheated oven for 18 minutes or until tester inserted in center comes out clean. Remove from oven to wire rack and allow to cool before cutting into squares.

| Nutritional Analysis | Energy | Protein | Carbohydrate | Fat | Calcium | Iron |
|---|---|---|---|---|---|---|
| per bar | 129 kcal | 1.8 g | 20.2g | 2.5 g | 2 % CDV | 8 % CDV |

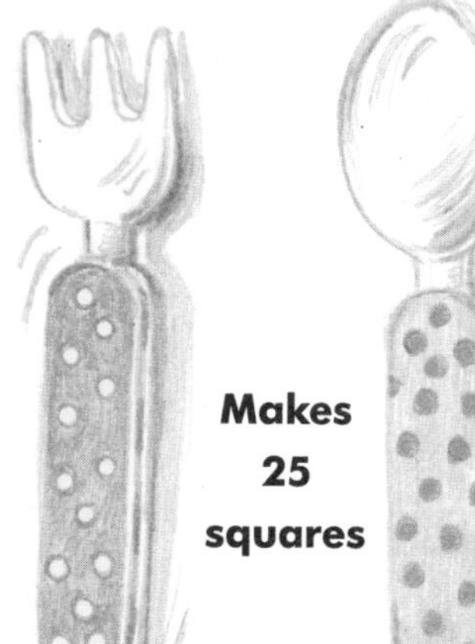

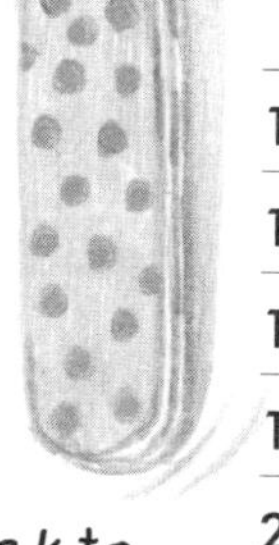

**Makes 25 squares**

# Chocolate Oatmeal Squares

*Preheat oven to 375° F (190° C)*
*8-inch (2 L) square baking pan, greased*

| | | |
|---|---|---|
| 1 1/4 cups | all-purpose flour | 300 mL |
| 1 cup | large-flake rolled oats | 250 mL |
| 1/2 cup | packed brown sugar | 125 mL |
| 1/2 tsp | ground cinnamon | 2 mL |
| 2/3 cup | butter or margarine | 150 mL |
| 1 cup | chocolate chips | 250 mL |

*Easy and quick to make (no more than 10 minutes), these squares combine the great flavors of oatmeal and chocolate.*

1. In a food processor, combine flour, oats, sugar and cinnamon. Add butter and process with on/off turns until mixture resembles coarse crumbs. Set aside 1/2 cup (125 mL) of mixture; press remainder into bottom of prepared pan.
2. Bake in preheated oven for 10 minutes or until golden brown. Remove from oven and sprinkle chips over surface. Sprinkle with reserved crumbs. Return to oven and bake for 25 minutes or until chocolate has melted and surface is golden brown. Cut into squares while still warm.

**KITCHEN TIP**

For a change, try using butterscotch chips instead of chocolate.

| NUTRITIONAL ANALYSIS | Energy | Protein | Carbohydrate | Fat | Calcium | Iron |
|---|---|---|---|---|---|---|
| per square | 131 kcal | 1.6 g | 15.6 g | 7.5 g | 1 % CDV | 8 % CDV |

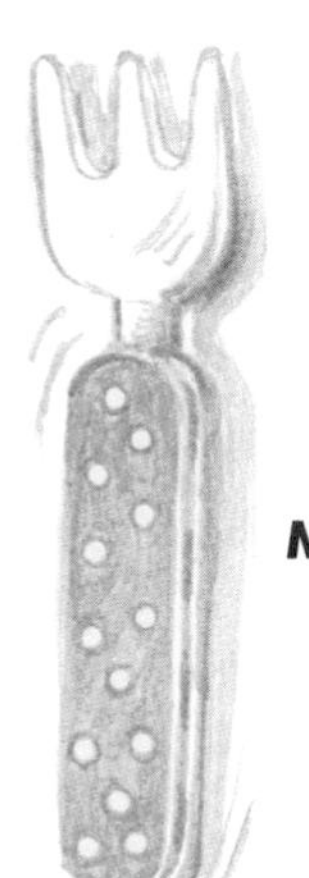
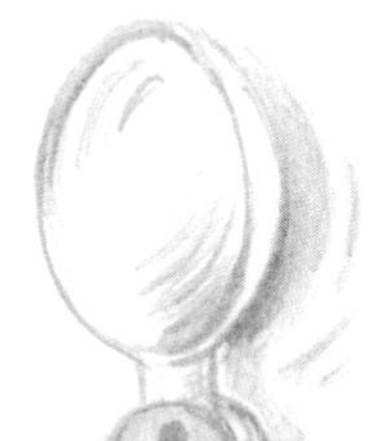
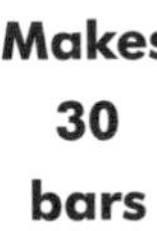
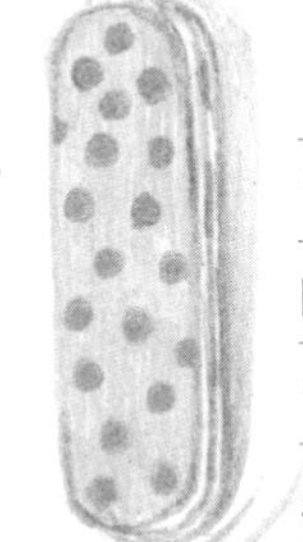

# Fruit Rice Crisp Bars

*13- by 9-inch (3 L) baking dish, greased*

**Makes 30 bars**

*Adding dried fruit to classic rice crisp squares gives them extra fiber and nutrients. The cranberries also give them a nice festive look.*

| | | |
|---|---|---|
| 1/4 cup | butter or margarine | 50 mL |
| Half | pkg (8 oz [250 g]) marshmallows | Half |
| 1 tsp | vanilla extract | 5 mL |
| 5 cups | crisp rice cereal | 1.25 L |
| 1/2 cup | dried cranberries or raisins | 125 mL |

1. In a large saucepan, melt butter over low heat. Stir in marshmallows and vanilla; blend until smooth. Remove from heat. Add rice cereal and dried fruit; stir until well combined. Press into prepared baking dish. Allow to cool completely before cutting into bars.

### Kitchen Tip

To prevent marshmallow mixture from sticking to your hands when pressing into pan, lightly coat your fingers with margarine.

If your kids are accustomed to regular rice crisp treats, they may view any change with suspicion. Try making this recipe with fruit added to only half of the bars, and let the children became used to it gradually.

| Nutritional Analysis | Energy | Protein | Carbohydrate | Fat | Calcium | Iron |
|---|---|---|---|---|---|---|
| per bar | 51 kcal | 0.5 g | 9.7 g | 1.3 g | <1 % CDV | 8 % CDV |

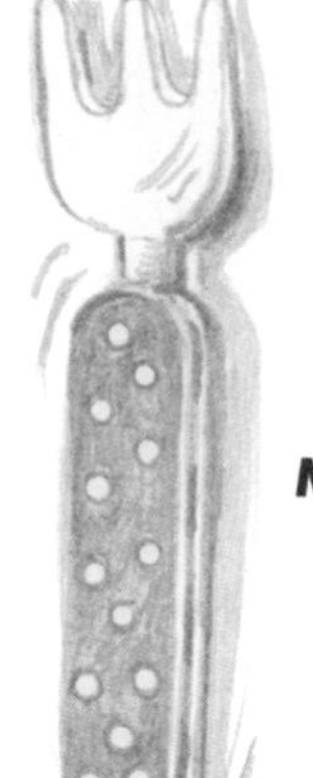
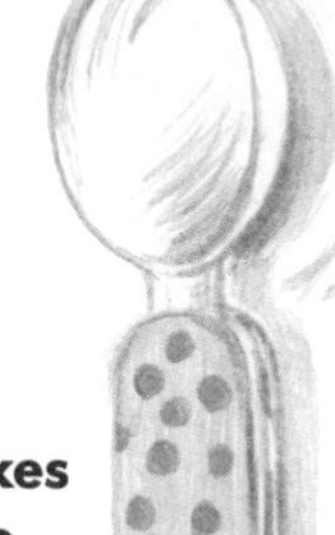

# Raspberry Granola Bars

**Makes 20 bars**

*This snack is also good for breakfast, combining cereal and jam in one bite.*

**Kitchen Tip**

Try making this recipe with other types of jam – strawberry, cherry, blueberry or your favorite.

*Preheat oven to 375° F (190° C)*
*8-inch (2 L) square baking pan, greased*

| | | |
|---|---|---|
| 3/4 cup | Homemade Microwave Granola (see recipe, page 132) | 175 mL |
| 1/2 cup | graham wafer crumbs | 125 mL |
| 1/4 cup | butter or margarine, melted | 50 mL |
| 1 | egg white | 1 |
| 1 1/2 cups | raspberry jam | 375 mL |

1. In a bowl combine granola, graham wafer crumbs, melted butter and egg white; stir until well mixed. Reserve 1/4 cup (50 mL) of mixture; press remainder into bottom of prepared pan. Bake in preheated oven for 7 minutes.
2. Spread jam evenly over baked crust. Top with reserved crumbs, return to oven and bake for 30 minutes or until bubbly. Remove from oven and run a sharp knife around edge of pan. Allow to cool completely before cutting into bars.

| Nutritional Analysis | Energy | Protein | Carbohydrate | Fat | Calcium | Iron |
|---|---|---|---|---|---|---|
| per bar | 113 kcal | 0.9 g | 21.9 g | 3.0 g | 1 % CDV | 6 % CDV |

# Hot Cheese Bread Ring

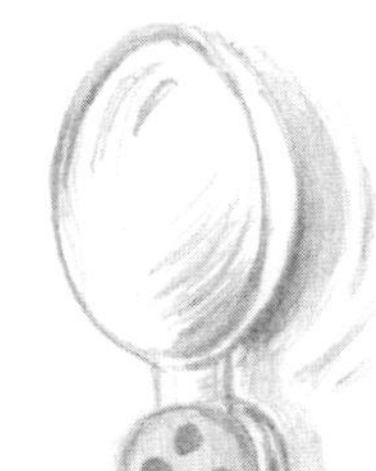

**Serves 8**

*This quickie hot bread makes an excellent accompaniment to soup or a salad.*

*Preheat oven to 375° F (190° C)*
*Tube pan, greased*

| | | |
|---|---|---|
| 1/2 cup | mayonnaise | 125 mL |
| 1/2 cup | grated Cheddar cheese | 125 mL |
| 1/4 tsp | dried oregano | 2 mL |
| 1/4 tsp | garlic powder | 2 mL |
| 2 | pkgs (11 oz [340 g]) buttermilk refrigerator biscuits | 2 |
| | Chopped fresh parsley | |

1. In a bowl combine mayonnaise, cheese, oregano and garlic powder.
2. Separate biscuits into individual pieces of dough and form each into a ball. Roll dough in mayonnaise mixture to coat well. Place in bottom of prepared tube pan, layering if necessary. Bake in preheated oven for 30 minutes or until puffed and golden brown. Turn bread ring out onto a plate and serve warm.

| Nutritional Analysis | Energy | Protein | Carbohydrate | Fat | Calcium | Iron |
|---|---|---|---|---|---|---|
| per serving | 315 kcal | 6.4 g | 36.4 g | 16.1 g | n/a | n/a |

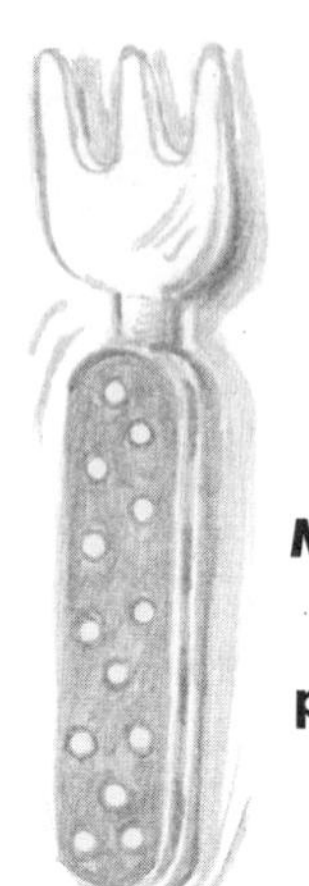
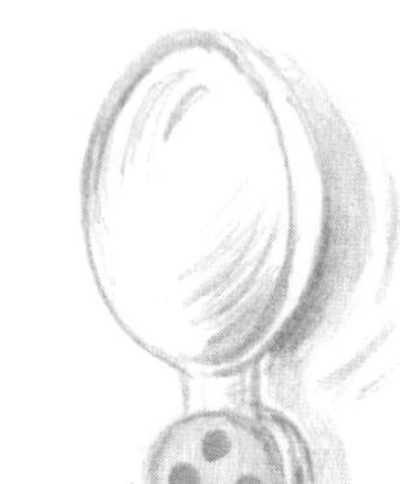

# Apple Gingerbread

*Preheat oven to 350° F (180° C)*
*13- by 9-inch (3.5 L) baking pan, greased*

**Makes 15 pieces**

*Gingerbread is one of the ultimate comfort foods, appealing to young and old alike. The addition of apple gives this gingerbread extra moisture and a fresh flavor. It's the molasses that gives this recipe its boost of iron. Serve as a snack or a dessert.*

| | | |
|---|---|---|
| 2 cups | all-purpose flour | 500 mL |
| 1/4 cup | granulated sugar | 50 mL |
| 2 tsp | baking powder | 10 mL |
| 1 tsp | baking soda | 5 mL |
| 1 tsp | ground ginger | 5 mL |
| 1/2 tsp | ground cinnamon | 2 mL |
| 1/2 tsp | ground nutmeg | 2 mL |
| 1/2 tsp | salt | 2 mL |
| 1/2 cup | butter or margarine | 125 mL |
| 2 | eggs | 2 |
| 1/2 cup | molasses | 125 mL |
| 1/3 cup | 2% milk | 75 mL |
| 1 | medium apple, peeled and grated | 1 |

1. In a bowl combine flour, sugar, baking powder, baking soda, spices, and salt. Set aside.
2. In a large bowl with an electric mixer, cream together butter, eggs and molasses. Stir in dry ingredients, a little at a time, alternating with small additions of milk. Fold in apples. Pour into prepared baking pan.
3. Bake in oven for 35 minutes or until cake tester inserted in center comes out clean. Cool on a wire rack before cutting into 15 pieces.

**KITCHEN TIP**

Serve this gingerbread with applesauce, sweetened whipped cream or Caramel Sauce (see recipe, page 267).

| NUTRITIONAL ANALYSIS | Energy | Protein | Carbohydrate | Fat | Calcium | Iron |
|---|---|---|---|---|---|---|
| per piece | 173 kcal | 2.9 g | 23.7 g | 7.6 g | 12 % CDV | 27 % CDV |

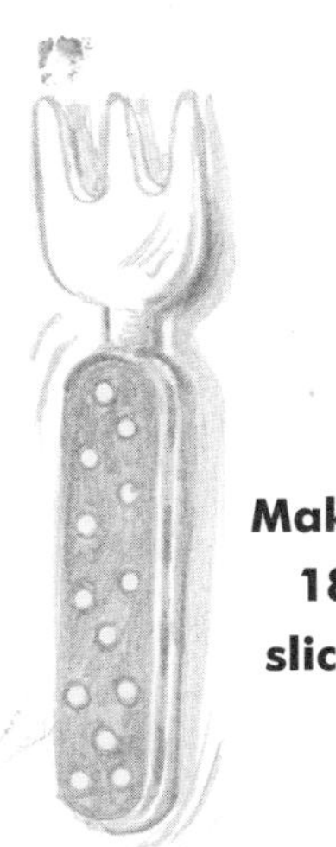

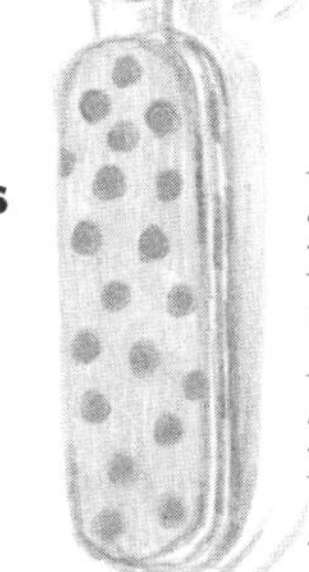

# Applesauce Cake

*Preheat oven to 350° F (180° C)*
*9-inch (2.5 L) tube pan, greased and floured*

**Makes 18 slices**

*This is a wonderfully moist snacking cake. And because it's egg-free, it is also a terrific choice for children with an egg allergy.*

| | | |
|---|---|---|
| 2 cups | lightly packed brown sugar | 500 mL |
| 1 cup | butter or margarine, softened | 250 mL |
| 2 1/2 cups | applesauce | 625 mL |
| 4 cups | all-purpose flour | 1 L |
| 1 tsp | ground cloves | 5 mL |
| 1 tsp | ground cinnamon | 5 mL |
| 1 tbsp | baking soda | 15 mL |

1. In a large bowl with an electric mixer, cream together brown sugar and butter. Stir in applesauce.
2. In another bowl, sift together flour, cloves, cinnamon and baking soda. Add sifted ingredients a little at a time to applesauce mixture, beating after each addition until just combined. Pour into prepared tube pan. Bake in preheated oven for 1 hour or until toothpick inserted in cake comes out clean.

### Kitchen Tip

This cake also tastes great with added raisins. Just combine 2 cups (500 mL) raisins with 1/2 cup (125 mL) of the flour called for in the recipe; toss until well coated (this keeps raisins from sinking to the bottom of the cake); set aside. Proceed with recipe and stir coated raisins into batter just before pouring into the pan.

| Nutritional Analysis | Energy | Protein | Carbohydrate | Fat | Calcium | Iron |
|---|---|---|---|---|---|---|
| per slice | 296 kcal | 3.2 g | 46.8 g | 11.1 g | 4 % CDV | 20 % CDV |

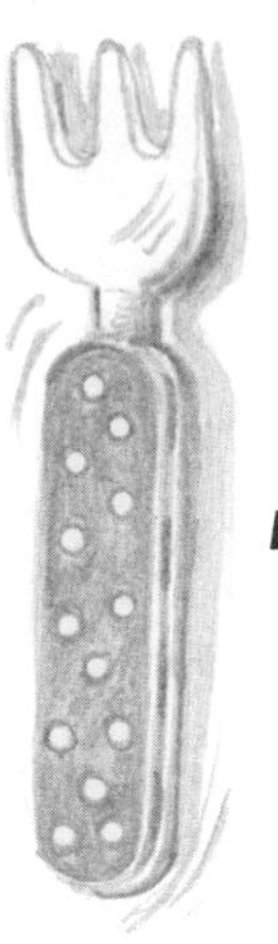

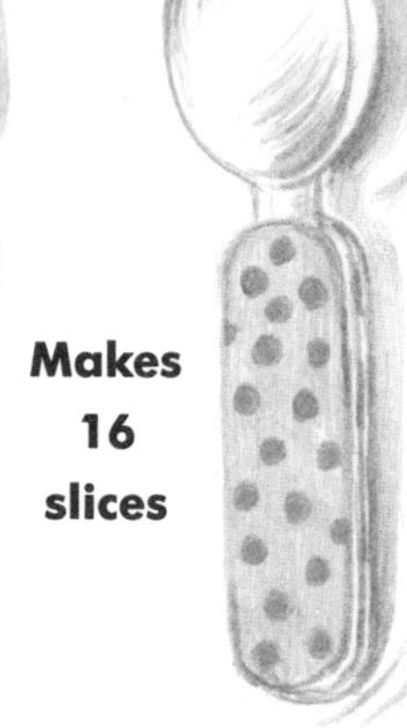

# Lemon Pound Cake

**Makes 16 slices**

*Preheat oven to 300° F (150° C)*
*8-inch (2 L) square baking pan*

| | | |
|---|---|---|
| 3 | egg whites | 3 |
| 1 1/2 cups | granulated sugar, divided | 375 mL |
| 1/2 cup | sour cream | 125 mL |
| 1/2 tsp | baking soda | 2 mL |
| 1/2 cup | butter or margarine, softened | 125 mL |
| 3 | egg yolks | 3 |
| | Juice of 1 lemon | |
| 2 cups | all-purpose flour | 500 mL |
| 3/4 tsp | baking powder | 4 mL |

1. In a small bowl with an electric mixer, beat egg whites until soft peaks form. Gradually beat in 3/4 cup (175 mL) of the sugar. Set aside.
2. In a measuring cup, stir together sour cream and baking soda. Set aside.
3. In a large bowl with an electric mixer, cream together butter and remaining sugar. Blend in egg yolks and lemon juice. Add flour and baking powder a little at a time, alternating with additions of sour cream mixture; beating after each addition until just combined.
4. Gently fold in beaten egg whites. Pour batter into prepared pan and bake for 50 minutes or until a toothpick inserted in the cake comes out clean. Allow to cool before serving.

| Nutritional Analysis | Energy | Protein | Carbohydrate | Fat | Calcium | Iron |
|---|---|---|---|---|---|---|
| per slice | 217 kcal | 3.2 g | 32.9 g | 8.4 g | 3 % CDV | 9 % CDV |

# Apple Snacking Cupcakes

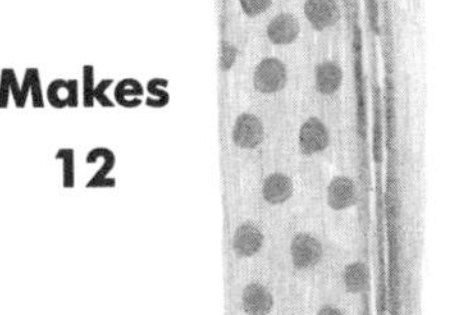

**Makes 12**

*Here's the great flavor of cake in the handy shape of a muffin – a real treat for younger children.*

*Preheat oven to 400° F (200° C)*
*12-cup muffin tin, greased or paper-lined*

| | | |
|---|---|---|
| 1/2 cup | butter or margarine | 125 mL |
| 1 cup | granulated sugar | 250 mL |
| 2 | eggs | 2 |
| 1 tsp | vanilla extract | 5 mL |
| 1 cup | all-purpose flour | 250 mL |
| 1 cup | whole wheat flour | 250 mL |
| 1 tbsp | baking powder | 15 mL |
| 1 tsp | baking soda | 5 mL |
| 1/2 tsp | ground cinnamon | 2 mL |
| 1/2 tsp | ground nutmeg | 2 mL |
| 2 cups | unsweetened applesauce | 500 mL |

1. In a large bowl with an electric mixer, cream butter and sugar. Blend in eggs and vanilla; beat until light and fluffy.
2. In another bowl, combine all-purpose flour, whole wheat flour, baking powder, baking soda, cinnamon and nutmeg. Add to butter mixture, a little at a time, alternating with applesauce; mix well after each addition.
3. Spoon batter into prepared muffin cups. Bake in preheated oven for 20 minutes, or until muffins are firm to the touch. Allow to cool for 10 minutes before removing from pan to wire rack.

| Nutritional Analysis | Energy | Protein | Carbohydrate | Fat | Calcium | Iron |
|---|---|---|---|---|---|---|
| per cupcake | 249 kcal | 3.7 g | 38.8 g | 9.4 g | 3 % CDV | 11 % CDV |

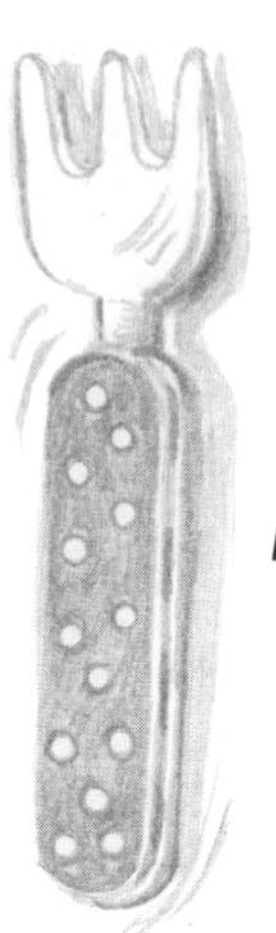

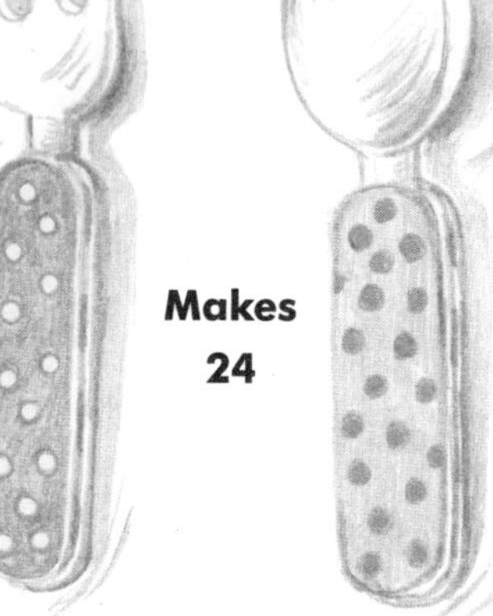

# Apple Scotch Muffins

**Makes 24**

*Preheat oven to 400° F (200° C)*
*Two 12-cup muffin tins, greased or paper-lined*

| | | |
|---|---|---|
| 2 1/2 cups | all-purpose flour | 625 mL |
| 1 | pkg (300 g [10 oz]) butterscotch chips | 1 |
| 2 cups | quick-cooking rolled oats | 500 mL |
| 1 cup | lightly packed brown sugar | 250 mL |
| 2 tsp | baking soda | 10 mL |
| 2 tsp | ground cinnamon | 10 mL |
| 3 cups | coarsely chopped apples | 750 mL |
| 1 1/2 cups | plain yogurt | 375 mL |
| 1 cup | vegetable oil | 250 mL |
| 4 | eggs | 4 |

1. In a large bowl, combine flour, butterscotch chips, oats, brown sugar, baking soda and cinnamon; mix well.
2. In another bowl, combine apples, yogurt, oil and eggs; mix well. Add to dry ingredients, stirring just until moistened. (Do not overmix.) Spoon batter into prepared muffin cups and bake for 18 minutes or until muffins are firm to the touch.

| Nutritional Analysis | Energy | Protein | Carbohydrate | Fat | Calcium | Iron |
|---|---|---|---|---|---|---|
| per muffin | 296 kcal | 4.7 g | 35.1 g | 15.5 g | 5 % CDV | 14 % CDV |

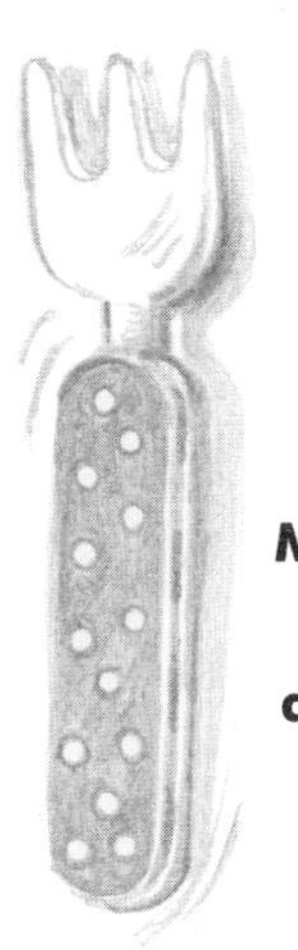

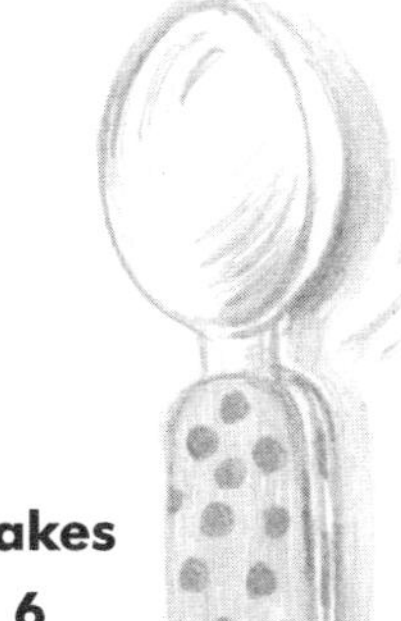

# Oatmeal Raisin Cookies

**Makes 6 dozen**

*Preheat oven to 375° F (190° C)*
*Large baking sheet, ungreased*

| | | |
|---|---|---|
| 1 cup | butter or margarine | 250 mL |
| 1 cup | lightly packed brown sugar | 250 mL |
| 2 cups | all-purpose flour | 500 mL |
| 2 cups | quick-cooking rolled oats | 500 mL |
| 1/2 cup | hot water | 125 mL |
| 1 tsp | baking soda | 5 mL |
| 1 tsp | baking powder | 5 mL |
| 1 tsp | vanilla extract | 5 mL |
| 1/2 tsp | salt | 2 mL |
| 1 cup | raisins or currants | 250 mL |

1. In a large bowl with an electric mixer, cream together butter and sugar. Add flour, oats, water, baking soda, baking powder, vanilla and salt; mix well. Fold in raisins.
2. Form dough into balls and place on cookie sheet. Flatten each ball with a fork and bake for 10 minutes or until golden brown.

| Nutritional Analysis | Energy | Protein | Carbohydrate | Fat | Calcium | Iron |
|---|---|---|---|---|---|---|
| per cookie | 63 kcal | 0.9 g | 8.6 g | 2.9 g | 1 % CDV | 1 % CDV |

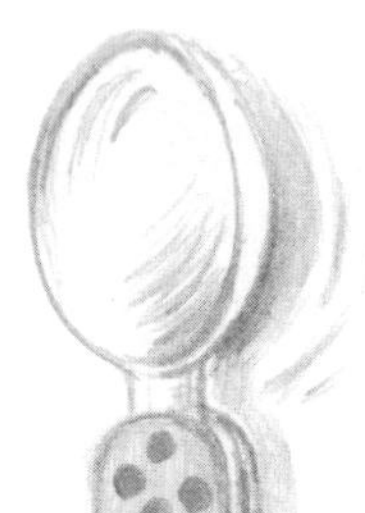

# Peanut Butter Cookies

*Preheat oven to 375° F (190° C)*
*Baking sheet, greased*

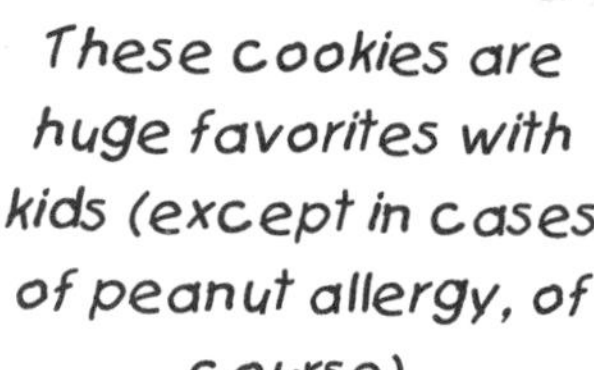

**Makes 3 dozen**

*These cookies are huge favorites with kids (except in cases of peanut allergy, of course).*

| | | |
|---|---|---|
| 1 cup | creamy peanut butter | 250 mL |
| 1/2 cup | butter or margarine | 125 mL |
| 3/4 cup | packed brown sugar | 175 mL |
| 1/2 cup | granulated sugar | 125 mL |
| 1 | egg | 1 |
| 1 tsp | vanilla extract | 5 mL |
| 1 cup | all purpose flour | 250 mL |
| 1 tsp | baking soda | 5 mL |
| 1/4 tsp | salt | 1 mL |

1. In a bowl with an electric mixer, cream together peanut butter, butter, brown sugar and granulated sugar; beat until light and fluffy. Beat in egg and vanilla.
2. In another bowl, combine flour, baking soda and salt. Gradually stir into peanut butter mixture; blend well.
3. Drop spoonfuls of batter 2 inches (5 cm) apart on prepared baking sheet. Press down with fork. (Dip fork in water, if necessary, to prevent dough from sticking.) Bake in preheated oven for 10 minutes or until golden brown.

| Nutritional Analysis | Energy | Protein | Carbohydrate | Fat | Calcium | Iron |
|---|---|---|---|---|---|---|
| per cookie | 109 kcal | 2.4 g | 10.9 g | 6.7 g | 1 % CDV | 4 % CDV |

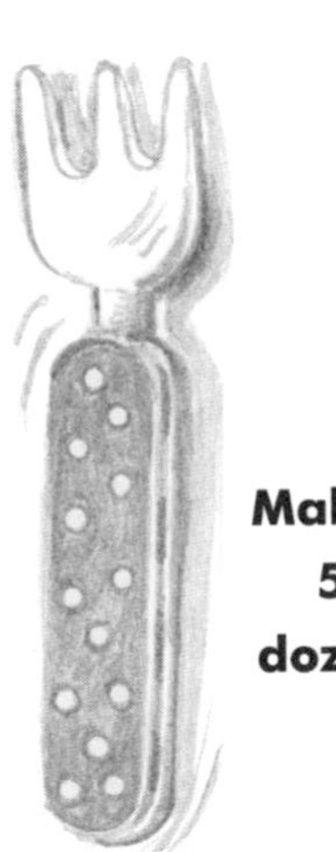

Makes 5 dozen

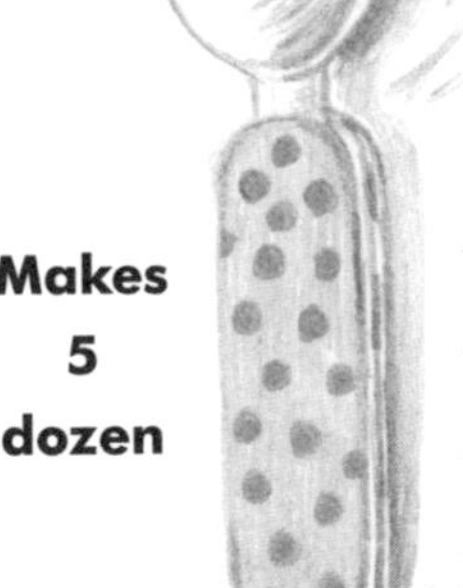

# Raisin Spice Cookies

*Preheat oven to 375° F (190° C)*
*Baking sheet, lightly greased*

| | | |
|---|---|---|
| 1/2 cup | shortening | 125 mL |
| 1/4 cup | butter, softened | 50 mL |
| 1 cup | packed brown sugar | 250 mL |
| 1 | egg | 1 |
| 1/3 cup | molasses | 75 mL |
| 2 1/4 cups | all-purpose flour | 550 mL |
| 1 tsp | baking soda | 5 mL |
| 1/2 tsp | salt | 2 mL |
| 1/2 tsp | ground cinnamon | 2 mL |
| 1/4 tsp | ground ginger | 1 mL |
| Pinch | ground allspice | Pinch |
| 1 1/2 cups | raisins | 375 mL |
| | Granulated sugar for coating | |

1. In a bowl with an electric mixer, cream together shortening and butter; beat until fluffy. Blend in brown sugar, egg and molasses.
2. In another bowl, sift together flour, baking soda, salt, cinnamon, ginger and allspice. Gradually stir into butter mixture. Add raisins and mix well. Cover and refrigerate for about 30 minutes or until dough is firm enough to handle.
3. With your hands, roll 1 to 2 tsp (5 to 10 mL) dough into balls. Roll in sugar to coat and place on prepared baking sheet. Bake for 10 minutes or until browned.

| Nutritional Analysis | Energy | Protein | Carbohydrate | Fat | Calcium | Iron |
|---|---|---|---|---|---|---|
| per cookie | 68 kcal | 0.7 g | 10.7 g | 2.6 g | 2 % CDV | 7 % CDV |

# Soft Banana and Oatmeal Cookies

*Preheat oven to 350° F (180° C)*
*Baking sheet, ungreased*

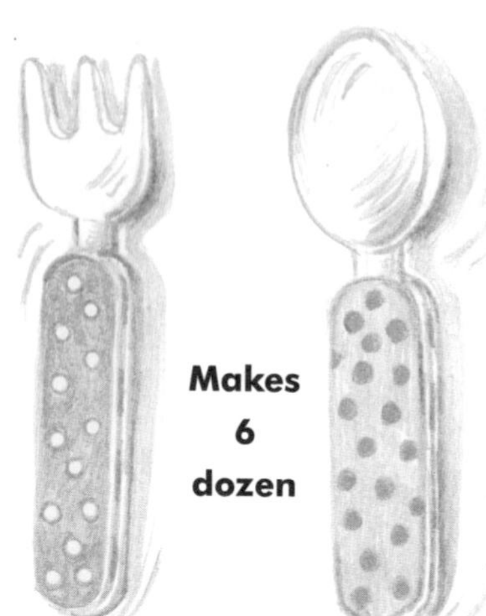

**Makes 6 dozen**

*These banana-bread bites are the perfect size for little mouths!*

**Kitchen Tip**

Try replacing raisins with other dried fruit, such as chopped dried apricots. Or, for those with a serious sweet tooth, try using chocolate chips!

| | | |
|---|---|---|
| 1 cup | packed brown sugar | 250 mL |
| 1 cup | granulated sugar | 250 mL |
| 1 cup | shortening | 250 mL |
| 1 cup | mashed ripe bananas | 250 mL |
| 3 | eggs, lightly beaten | 3 |
| 1 tsp | vanilla extract | 5 mL |
| 2 cups | all-purpose flour | 500 mL |
| 1 tsp | baking soda | 5 mL |
| 1/2 tsp | salt | 2 mL |
| 2 cups | quick-cooking rolled oats | 500 mL |
| 1 cup | raisins, rinsed and patted dry | 250 mL |

1. In a bowl with an electric mixer, cream together brown sugar, granulated sugar and shortening; beat until light and fluffy. Beat in bananas, eggs and vanilla.
2. In another bowl, combine flour, baking soda and salt. Gradually stir into banana butter mixture; blend well. Stir in rolled oats and raisins.
3. Drop spoonfuls of batter onto prepared baking sheet. Bake in preheated oven for 15 minutes or until golden brown.

| Nutritional Analysis | Energy | Protein | Carbohydrate | Fat | Calcium | Iron |
|---|---|---|---|---|---|---|
| per cookie | 85 kcal | 1.1 g | 12.9 g | 3.5 g | 1 % CDV | 5 % CDV |

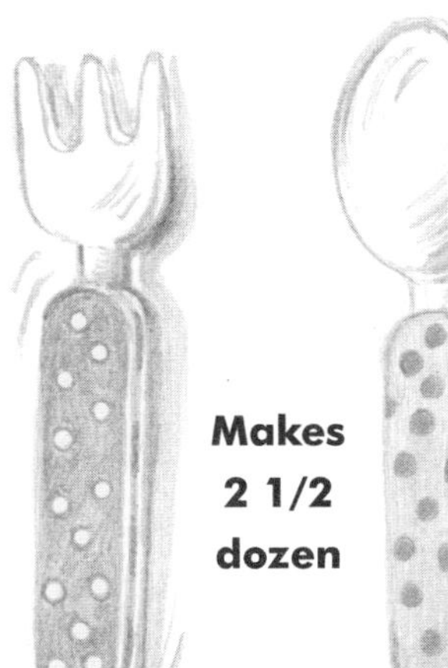

**Makes 2 1/2 dozen**

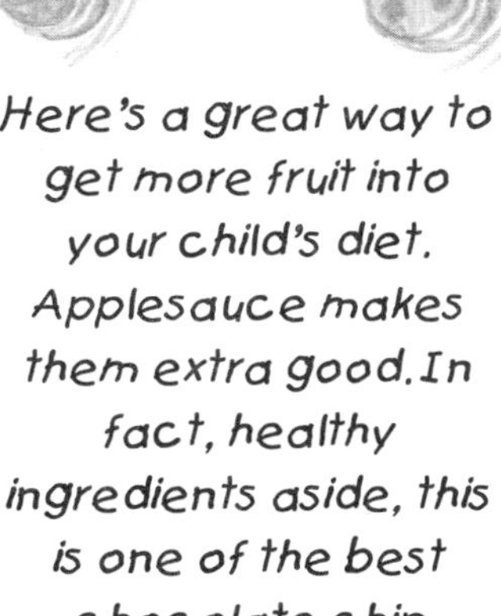

# Soft Chocolate Chip Cookies

*Preheat oven to 375° F (190° C)*
*Baking sheet, greased*

| | | |
|---|---|---|
| 1 cup | loosely packed brown sugar | 250 mL |
| 1/2 cup | unsweetened applesauce | 125 mL |
| 1/4 cup | butter or margarine, softened | 50 mL |
| 1 | egg | 1 |
| 1 tbsp | vanilla extract | 15 mL |
| 1 1/3 cups | all-purpose flour | 325 mL |
| 1 1/2 tsp | baking powder | 7 mL |
| 1/2 tsp | salt | 2 mL |
| 1 cup | miniature chocolate chips | 250 mL |

*Here's a great way to get more fruit into your child's diet. Applesauce makes them extra good. In fact, healthy ingredients aside, this is one of the best chocolate chip cookies we've ever tasted!*

1. In a bowl with an electric mixer, cream together brown sugar, applesauce, margarine, egg and vanilla; beat until light and fluffy.
2. In another bowl, combine flour, baking powder and salt. Gradually stir into applesauce mixture; blend well. Fold in chocolate chips.
3. Drop spoonfuls of batter onto prepared baking sheet 2 inches (5 cm) apart. Bake in preheated oven for 10 minutes or until golden brown. Place sheet on a wire rack and allow to cool for 3 minutes before removing.

| Nutritional Analysis | Energy | Protein | Carbohydrate | Fat | Calcium | Iron |
|---|---|---|---|---|---|---|
| per cookie | 88 kcal | 1.1 g | 13.3 g | 3.7 g | 1 % CDV | 6 % CDV |

# Soft Pumpkin Cookies

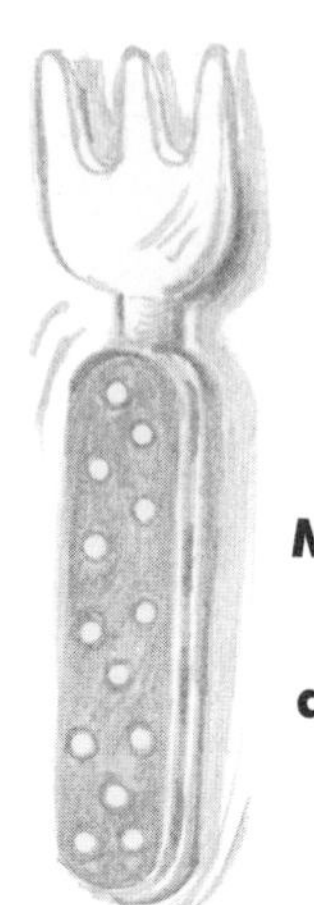
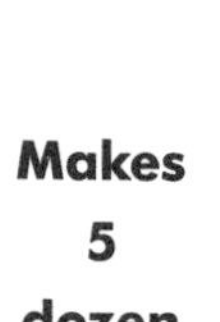
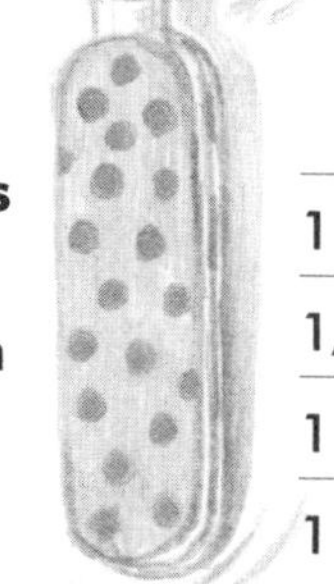

**Makes 5 dozen**

*These soft cookies are as delicious as they are unusual. Kids love them.*

*Preheat oven to 350° F (180° C)*
*Baking sheet, ungreased*

| | | |
|---|---|---|
| 1 1/2 cups | raisins | 375 mL |
| 1/2 cup | butter or margarine, softened | 125 mL |
| 1 1/4 cups | packed brown sugar | 300 mL |
| 1 cup | canned pumpkin purée (not pie filling) | 250 mL |
| 2 tbsp | applesauce | 25 mL |
| 1 | egg | 1 |
| 1 tsp | vanilla extract | 5 mL |
| 1/2 tsp | ground ginger | 2 mL |
| 1/2 tsp | ground cinnamon | 2 mL |
| 2 1/4 cups | all-purpose flour | 550 mL |
| 1 tsp | baking soda | 5 mL |
| 1 tsp | baking powder | 5 mL |

1. In a small bowl, soak raisins in hot water for 5 minutes, then rinse and pat dry with a paper towel. Set aside.
2. In a large bowl, cream together butter and sugar until fluffy. Add pumpkin purée, applesauce, egg, vanilla, ginger and cinnamon; beat until well mixed.
3. In another bowl, sift together flour, baking soda and baking powder. Gradually add to pumpkin mixture, stirring until just combined. Stir in raisins.
4. Drop spoonfuls of batter onto baking sheet. Bake in preheated oven for 12 minutes or until golden brown.

### Kitchen Tip

If you have the time, try making your own pumpkin purée instead of using the canned variety for this recipe. With a sharp knife, cut a sugar pumpkin in half and scoop out the seeds. Cut pumpkin into 1-inch (2 cm) squares (flesh and rind) and transfer to a large pot of boiling water. Cook for about 20 minutes or until tender. Drain and cool. Remove flesh from rind and transfer to a food processor; purée until smooth. Freeze in batches for use in recipes throughout the year.

| Nutritional Analysis | Energy | Protein | Carbohydrate | Fat | Calcium | Iron |
|---|---|---|---|---|---|---|
| per cookie | 64 kcal | 0.8 g | 11.6 g | 1.8 g | 1 % CDV | 5 % CDV |

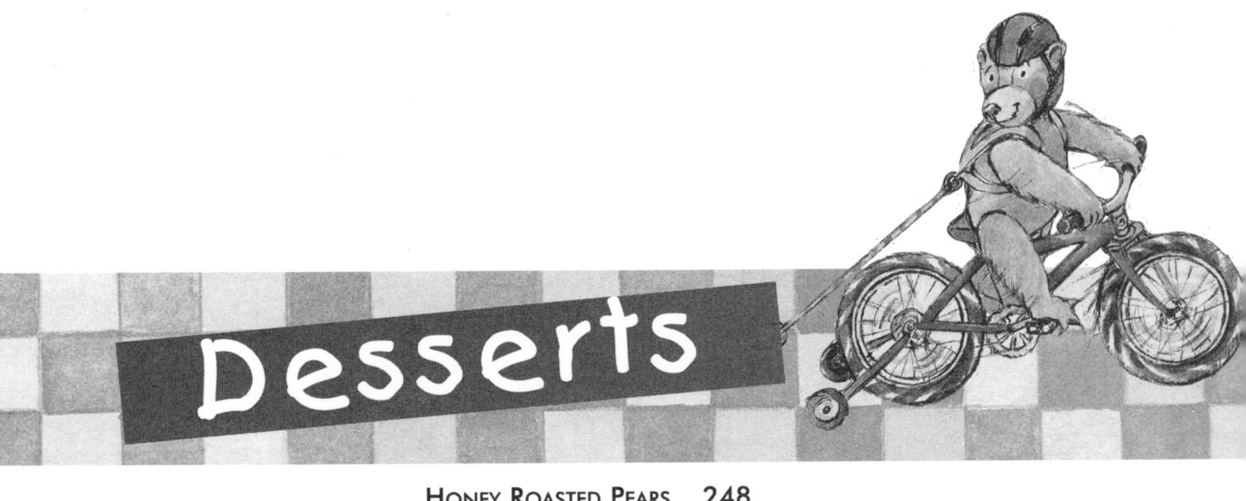


# Desserts

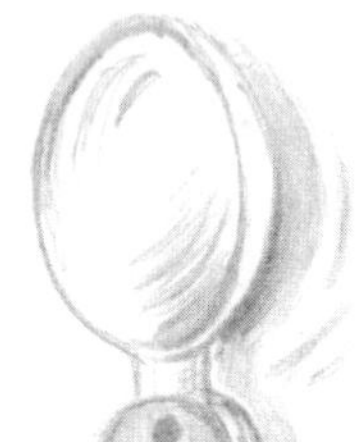

# Honey Roasted Pears

*Preheat oven to 400° F (200° C)*
*13- by 9-inch (3.5 L) baking dish, greased*

**Serves 8**

*Here's the perfect fruit to serve with vanilla ice cream or yogurt.*

| | | |
|---|---|---|
| 8 | firm Bosc pears, cut into quarters | 8 |
| 3 tbsp | butter *or* margarine | 45 mL |
| 3/4 cup | apple cider | 175 mL |
| 1/3 cup | liquid honey | 75 mL |
| 1 tbsp | lemon juice | 15 mL |
| 2 tsp | vanilla extract | 10 mL |

1. Place pears in prepared baking dish. Dot with butter.
2. In a small saucepan, combine cider, honey, lemon juice and vanilla. Bring to a boil. Pour over pears. Cover and bake in preheated oven for 20 minutes. Uncover and bake for another 30 minutes or until pears are tender. Let stand for 10 minutes before serving.

### Kitchen Tip

For this recipe, pears should be a bit on the firm side. Leave them unpeeled; the skins will turn an attractive deep amber color when roasted.

| Nutritional Analysis | Energy | Protein | Carbohydrate | Fat | Calcium | Iron |
|---|---|---|---|---|---|---|
| per serving | 195 kcal | 0.8 g | 40.2 g | 5.1 g | 3 % CDV | 6 % CDV |

# Apple 'n' Maple Dessert

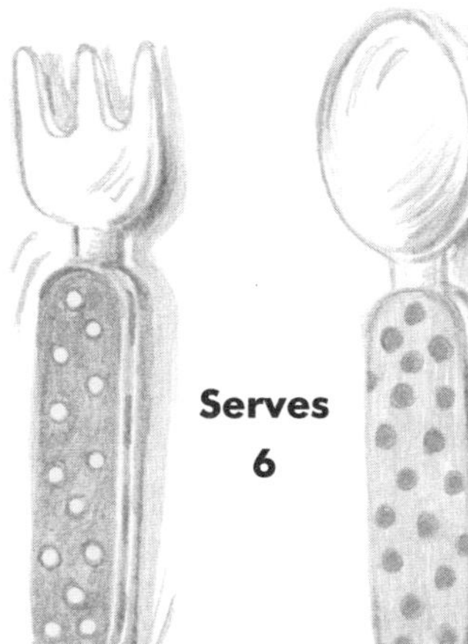

**Serves 6**

*A combination of popular flavors creates a winning effect in this dessert.*

**Kitchen Tip**

To add an extra-special touch, serve with whipped cream or ice cream.

*Preheat oven to 375° F (190° C)*
*8-inch (2 L) square baking pan, greased*

| | | |
|---|---|---|
| 4 | large apples, peeled and thinly sliced | 4 |
| 1/2 cup | dried cranberries | 125 mL |
| 1/2 cup | maple syrup, divided | 125 mL |
| 2 | eggs | 2 |
| 2 tbsp | melted butter or margarine | 25 mL |
| 1/4 cup | 2% milk | 50 mL |
| 2 tsp | vanilla extract | 10 mL |
| 1/2 cup | all-purpose flour | 125 mL |
| 2 tsp | baking powder | 10 mL |
| | Ground cinnamon | |

1. In a bowl toss together apple slices and cranberries. Transfer to prepared pan and drizzle with 1/4 cup (50 mL) of the maple syrup.
2. In a bowl with an electric mixer, beat eggs until fluffy. Beat in butter, milk, vanilla and remaining maple syrup.
3. In another bowl, stir together flour and baking powder. Add to egg mixture and blend until smooth.
4. Spoon batter evenly over fruit. Sprinkle batter with cinnamon. Bake in preheated oven for 40 minutes or until apples are tender and batter is golden brown.

| Nutritional Analysis | Energy | Protein | Carbohydrate | Fat | Calcium | Iron |
|---|---|---|---|---|---|---|
| per serving | 276 kcal | 3.7 g | 48.8 g | 5.9 g | 8 % CDV | 15 % CDV |

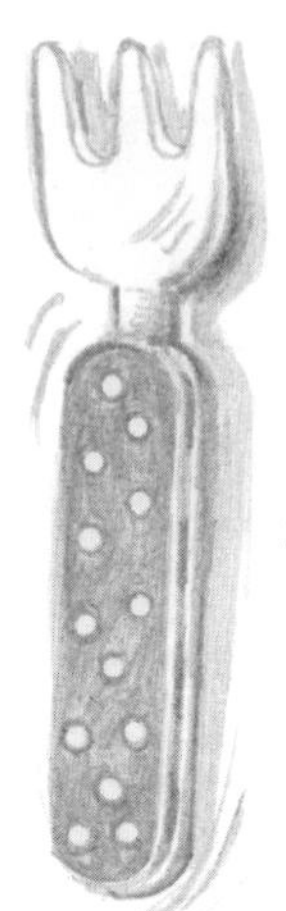

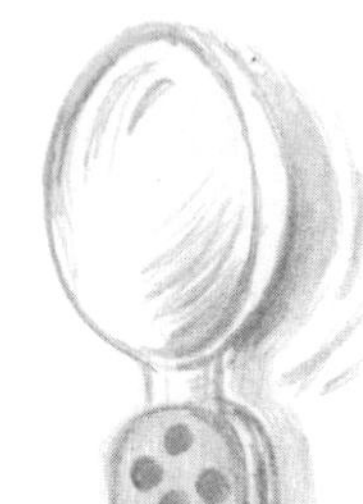

# Scotch Custard Apple Pudding

**Serves 6**

*Preheat oven to 350° F (180° C)*
*8-inch (1.5 L) shallow baking pan, greased*

| | | |
|---|---|---|
| 4 cups | sliced peeled apples or pears (about 4 medium) | 1 L |
| 3/4 cup | packed brown sugar | 175 mL |
| 1/2 cup | rolled oats | 125 mL |
| 1/2 cup | all-purpose flour | 125 mL |
| 1/3 cup | butter or margarine | 75 mL |
| 2/3 cup | 2% milk | 150 mL |
| 1 | egg | 1 |
| 1 tsp | vanilla extract | 5 mL |
| | Ground cinnamon | |

*Here's a sensational variation on apple crisp – one of our all-time favorites. The "Scotch" in the title refers to the oatmeal crisp topping.*

**Kitchen Tip**

Use apples or pears – or a combination. For added color, try adding a few cranberries.

1. Arrange fruit in prepared pan.
2. In a food processor or blender, combine brown sugar, oats, flour and butter. Process with on/off turns until mixture resembles coarse crumbs. Sprinkle over fruit.
3. In a small bowl, whisk together milk, egg and vanilla. Pour over crumb mixture. Sprinkle lightly with cinnamon. Bake in a preheated oven for 45 minutes or until bubbly and top is golden brown. Serve warm or at room temperature.

| Nutritional Analysis | Energy | Protein | Carbohydrate | Fat | Calcium | Iron |
|---|---|---|---|---|---|---|
| per serving | 324 kcal | 4.1 g | 51.7 g | 12.0 g | 9 % CDV | 25 % CDV |

# Fruit Crisp

*Preheat oven to 350° F (180° C)*
*7- by 11-inch (2 L) baking pan*

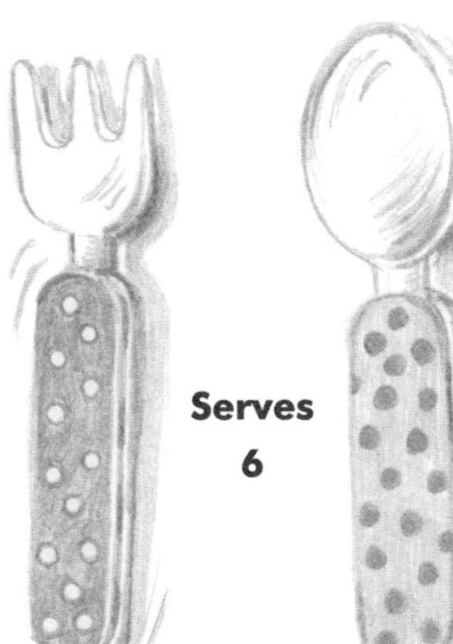

**Serves 6**

*This old-fashioned dessert is a natural candidate for adding to your "all-time favorites" recipe file.*

**KITCHEN TIP**

Choose from a wide variety of fruits, including peaches, apples, berries, rhubarb and pitted sour cherries. See chart (below, right) for preparation instructions.

| | | |
|---|---|---|
| 5 cups | prepared fruit (see Tip, at left) | 1.25 L |
| 1 cup | packed brown sugar | 250 mL |
| 1 cup | all-purpose flour | 250 mL |
| 3/4 cup | quick-cooking rolled oats | 175 mL |
| 1 tsp | ground cinnamon | 5 mL |
| 1/2 tsp | ground nutmeg | 2 mL |
| 1/2 cup | butter or margarine | 125 mL |

1. Arrange prepared fruit in baking pan.
2. In a bowl combine sugar, flour, rolled oats, cinnamon and nutmeg. Cut in butter until crumbly. Sprinkle mixture over fruit. Bake in preheated oven for 40 minutes or until fruit is cooked and topping is golden brown.

**PREPARING FRUIT FOR CRISPS AND COBBLERS**

**Apples and Peaches.** Peel, core and cut into slices.

**Blueberries.** Pick over. Remove and discard stems. Wash.

**Rhubarb.** Cut into small pieces and toss with 2/3 cup (150 mL) granulated sugar.

**Sour cherries.** Wash, pit and toss with 3/4 cup (175 mL) granulated sugar.

**Strawberry-Rhubarb combination.** Hull and slice strawberries. Cut rhubarb into small pieces and toss with 3/4 cup (175 mL) granulated sugar.

| NUTRITIONAL ANALYSIS | Energy | Protein | Carbohydrate | Fat | Calcium | Iron |
|---|---|---|---|---|---|---|
| per serving | 543 kcal | 4.9 g | 95.6 g | 17.5 g | 10 % CDV | 31 % CDV |

# Fruit Cobbler

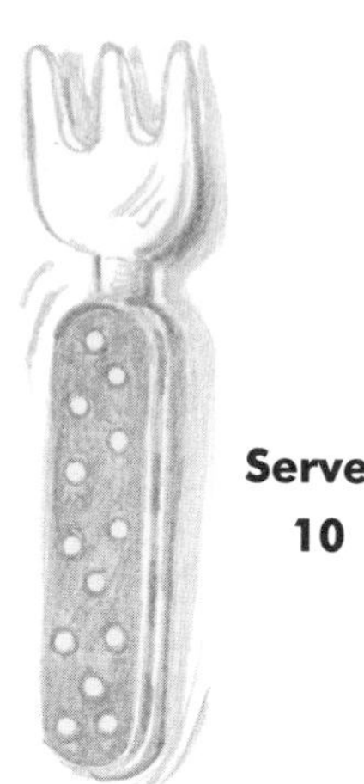
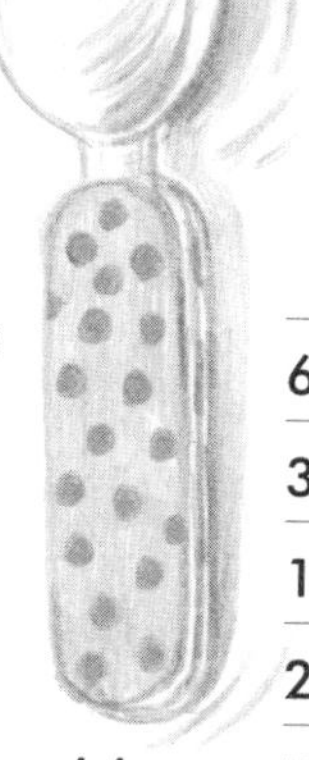

**Serves 10**

*This versatile cobbler recipe combines your favorite fruit with a thick biscuit crust. Delicious served hot or cold!*

### Kitchen Tip

This recipe works well with sliced apples or peaches, pears, blueberries, pitted cherries or plums. See page 251 for preparation instructions.

For a special treat, serve with a scoop of ice cream or frozen vanilla yogurt.

*Preheat oven to 350° F (180° C)*
*13- by 9-inch (3.5 L) baking pan, greased*

| | | |
|---|---|---|
| 6 cups | prepared fruit (see Tip, at left) | 1.5 L |
| 3/4 cup | granulated sugar | 175 mL |
| 1 tbsp | tapioca | 15 mL |
| 2 tsp | grated lemon zest | 10 mL |
| **Batter** | | |
| 1 1/4 cups | all-purpose flour | 300 mL |
| 1/3 cup | cornmeal | 75 mL |
| 1/3 cup | granulated sugar | 75 mL |
| 2 1/2 tsp | baking powder | 12 mL |
| 1/4 tsp | baking soda | 1 mL |
| 1/4 tsp | salt | 1 mL |
| 1/3 cup | butter or margarine | 75 mL |
| 1 1/3 cups | buttermilk | 325 mL |
| 1 tbsp | granulated sugar | 15 mL |
| 1 tsp | ground cinnamon | 5 mL |

1. In a bowl combine fruit, sugar, tapioca and zest. Transfer to prepared pan. Allow to stand for 15 minutes.
2. Meanwhile, in a food processor or blender, combine flour, cornmeal, sugar, baking powder, baking soda and salt; process until mixed. Add butter and process with on/off turns until mixture resembles coarse crumbs.
3. In a large bowl, combine flour-butter mixture and buttermilk; stir just until moistened. Spoon batter over fruit. Sprinkle with sugar and cinnamon. Bake in preheated oven for 30 minutes or until topping is golden and fruit bubbles around sides. Serve warm or cold.

| Nutritional Analysis | Energy | Protein | Carbohydrate | Fat | Calcium | Iron |
|---|---|---|---|---|---|---|
| per serving | 267 kcal | 3.3 g | 50.4 g | 6.7 g | 7 % CDV | 9 % CDV |

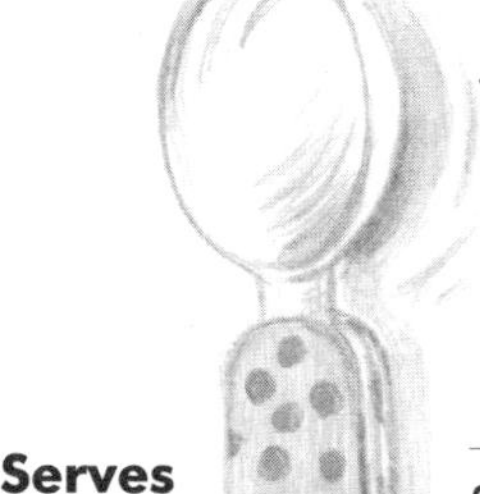

# Speedy Rice Pudding with Golden Raisins

*8-cup (2 L) microwave-safe casserole with lid*

**Serves 6**

*Traditional rice pudding takes a long time to prepare. But this version is ready in just a fraction of the time. What's more, it provides extra nutrition (from both brown and white long grain rice) and plenty of juicy raisins.*

| | | |
|---|---|---|
| 3 1/2 cups | 2% milk | 875 mL |
| 1/4 cup | long grain white rice | 50 mL |
| 1/4 cup | long grain brown rice | 50 mL |
| 1/2 cup | granulated sugar | 125 mL |
| 1 | cinnamon stick | 1 |
| 1 | egg | 1 |
| 1/3 cup | golden raisins | 75 mL |
| 1 tsp | vanilla extract | 5 mL |

1. In casserole, combine milk, white rice, brown rice, sugar and cinnamon stick. Cook, uncovered, on High for 7 minutes or until boiling. Cook, stirring every 5 minutes, on Medium-High for another 20 minutes or until rice is tender.
2. In a small bowl, whisk together egg with 1/4 cup (50 mL) of the hot rice mixture. Return egg mixture to casserole and stir well
3. Stir in raisins and cook on Medium for 3 minutes or until slightly thickened. Remove and discard cinnamon stick; stir in vanilla. Let pudding stand for 5 minutes before serving. Serve warm or cover and refrigerate.

| NUTRITIONAL ANALYSIS | Energy | Protein | Carbohydrate | Fat | Calcium | Iron |
|---|---|---|---|---|---|---|
| per serving | 228 kcal | 7.2 g | 41.5 g | 4.0 g | 24 % CDV | 6 % CDV |

# Creamy Delight

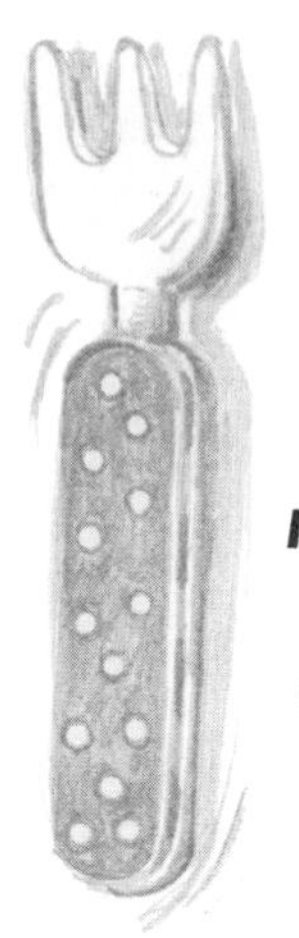

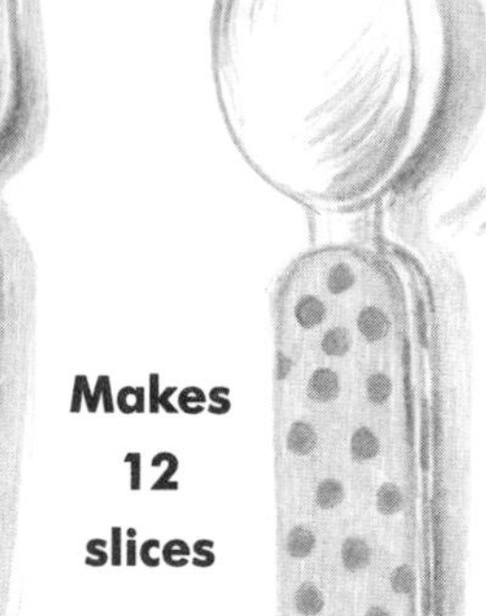

**Makes 12 slices**

*This simple dessert is a snap to prepare. Bring along your sweet tooth for this one!*

**KITCHEN TIP**

For a simpler version of this recipe, eliminate the jam and chocolate. It still tastes delicious!

*Preheat oven to 350° F (180° C)*
*9-inch (23 cm) pie plate, lightly greased*

| | | |
|---|---|---|
| 2 1/2 cups | 2% milk | 625 mL |
| 3 | eggs | 3 |
| 1/4 cup | granulated sugar | 50 mL |
| 1/2 tsp | vanilla extract | 2 mL |
| 1/2 cup | apricot or peach jam | 125 mL |
| 1 1/4 cups | whipped cream | 300 mL |
| | Grated chocolate for garnish | |

1. In a large bowl, combine milk, eggs, sugar and vanilla. Beat until the sugar is dissolved. Pour into prepared pie plate. Bake for 20 minutes or until set. Cool.
2. When custard is cool, spread jam over and cover with whipped cream. Garnish with grated chocolate.

| NUTRITIONAL ANALYSIS | Energy | Protein | Carbohydrate | Fat | Calcium | Iron |
|---|---|---|---|---|---|---|
| per slice | 207 kcal | 4.1 g | 19.8 g | 13.0 g | 12 % CDV | 6 % CDV |

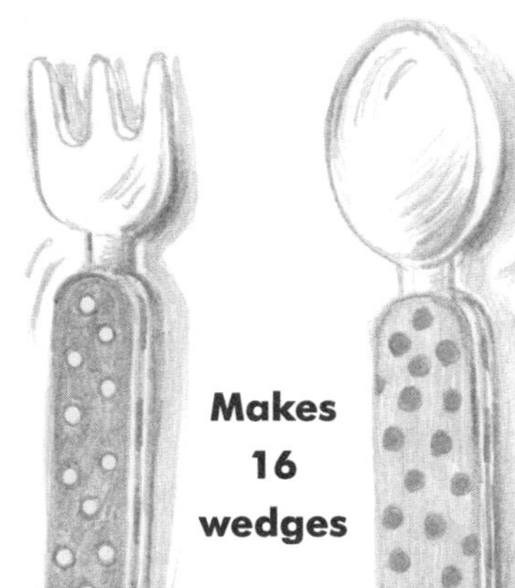

# Chocolate Chip Pizza Cookie

*Preheat oven to 350° F (180° C)*
*Baking sheet, greased*

**Makes 16 wedges**

*Instead of a birthday cake, why not try a birthday cookie? This one is always a favorite at kids' birthday parties.*

| | | |
|---|---|---|
| 1/3 cup | butter or margarine | 75 mL |
| 1/2 cup | packed brown sugar (preferably golden brown) | 125 mL |
| 1/4 cup | granulated sugar | 50 mL |
| 1 | egg | 1 |
| 1 tsp | vanilla extract | 5 mL |
| 1 1/2 cups | all-purpose flour | 375 mL |
| 1/2 tsp | baking soda | 2 mL |
| 1/4 tsp | salt | 1 mL |
| 1 1/2 cups | chocolate chips | 375 mL |

1. In a bowl with an electric mixer, cream together butter, brown sugar, granulated sugar, egg and vanilla. Blend in flour, baking soda and salt. Stir in chocolate chips.
2. Place dough on baking sheet and roll or pat into large round circle (like a pizza). Bake in preheated oven for 8 minutes or until golden brown. Cut into 16 pizza wedges and serve.

| Nutritional Analysis | Energy | Protein | Carbohydrate | Fat | Calcium | Iron |
|---|---|---|---|---|---|---|
| per wedge | 200 kcal | 2.4 g | 27.4 g | 10.1 g | 2 % CDV | 12 % CDV |

# Peanut Butter Brownies

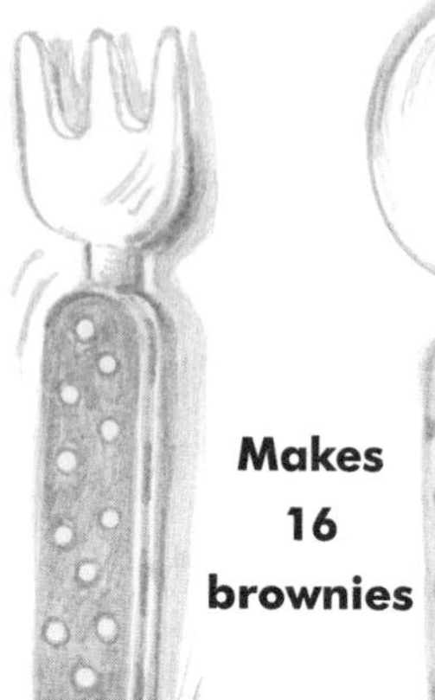
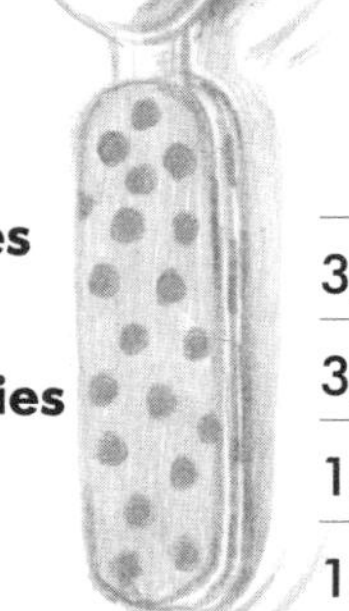

**Makes 16 brownies**

*No fuss, no muss – these scrumptious treats require only one bowl for mixing.*

*Preheat oven to 350° F (180° C)*
*8-inch (2 L) square baking pan, greased*

| | | |
|---|---|---|
| 3/4 cup | cake-and-pastry flour | 175 mL |
| 3/4 cup | granulated sugar | 175 mL |
| 1/3 cup | unsweetened cocoa | 75 mL |
| 1/2 tsp | baking powder | 2 mL |
| 1/2 tsp | salt | 2 mL |
| 1/4 cup | butter or margarine, softened | 50 mL |
| 1/4 cup | creamy peanut butter (see Tip, at left) | 50 mL |
| 1 | egg | 1 |
| 1 tsp | vanilla extract | 5 mL |

1. In a large bowl, combine flour, sugar, cocoa, baking powder and salt. Make a hole in center and stir in butter, peanut butter, egg and vanilla. Stir until fairly smooth. Press batter into prepared pan. Bake in preheated oven for 25 minutes or until cake tester inserted in center comes out clean. Cool on wire rack before cutting into 16 squares.

### Kitchen Tip

To make a peanut-free version of this recipe (in cases of peanut allergy, for example), replace peanut butter with an equal amount of butter or margarine.

To prevent batter from sticking when pressing it into the baking pan, lightly coat your hands with oil.

| Nutritional Analysis | Energy | Protein | Carbohydrate | Fat | Calcium | Iron |
|---|---|---|---|---|---|---|
| per brownie | 110 kcal | 2.1 g | 15.5 g | 5.2 g | 1 % CDV | 6 % CDV |

# Date Squares

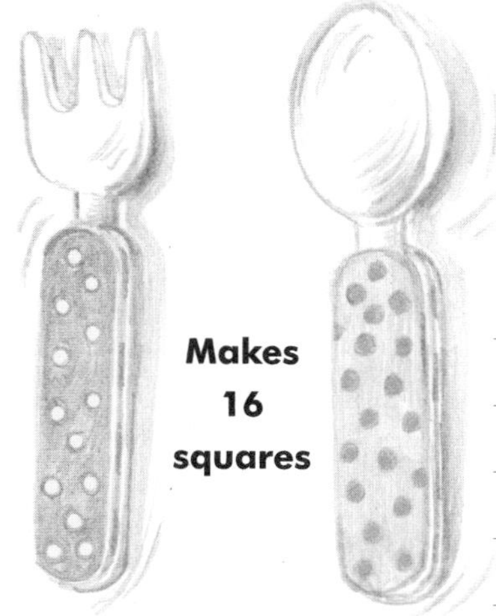

**Makes 16 squares**

*Also known as "matrimonial squares," these delicious date squares are a terrific source of iron!*

*Preheat oven to 350° F (180° C)*
*8-inch (2 L) square baking dish, ungreased*

| | | |
|---|---|---|
| 1 1/2 cups | rolled oats | 375 mL |
| 1 1/2 cups | all-purpose flour | 375 mL |
| 1 1/3 cups | packed brown sugar, divided | 325 mL |
| 1/4 tsp | salt | 1 mL |
| 1/2 tsp | baking soda | 2 mL |
| 3/4 cup | butter, softened | 200 mL |
| 1 lb | pitted dates, chopped | 500 g |
| 1 1/4 cups | water | 300 mL |
| 1 tsp | lemon juice | 5 mL |

1. In a large bowl, combine rolled oats, flour, 1 cup (250 mL) of the brown sugar, salt and baking soda. With pastry blender or with a pair of knives, cut butter into dry ingredients until mixture resembles coarse crumbs. Set aside.
2. In a saucepan over medium heat, combine dates, water and remaining brown sugar. Bring to a boil and cook for 5 minutes or until thickened. Remove from heat and stir in lemon juice.
3. Assembly: Lightly press one-half oat mixture into baking dish. Spread filling over base then crumble remaining oat mixture on top. Bake in preheated oven for 20 minutes or until golden brown. Cool on wire rack before cutting into 16 squares.

| Nutritional Analysis | Energy | Protein | Carbohydrate | Fat | Calcium | Iron |
|---|---|---|---|---|---|---|
| per square | 305 kcal | 3.3 g | 52.7 g | 10.5 g | 4 % CDV | 17 % CDV |

# Apple Cake

*Preheat oven to 400° F (200° C)*
*8-inch (2 L) square baking pan, greased*

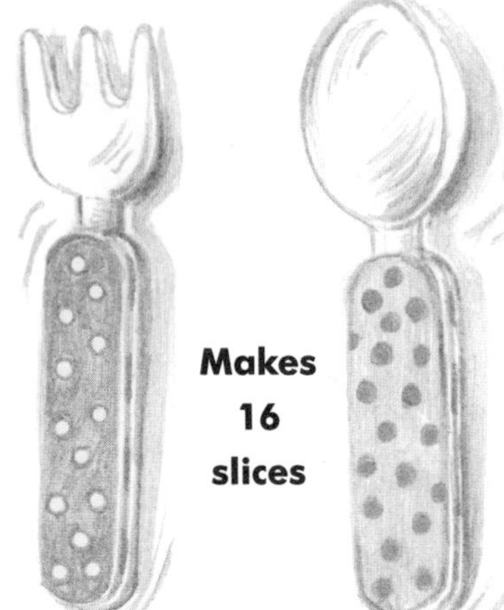

**Makes 16 slices**

*This moist and delicious cake is even better when drizzled with Caramel Sauce (see recipe, page 267).*

| | | |
|---|---|---|
| 1 cup | all-purpose flour | 250 mL |
| 1 tsp | baking soda | 5 mL |
| 1 tsp | ground cinnamon | 5 mL |
| 3/4 tsp | ground nutmeg | 4 mL |
| 1/4 tsp | salt | 1 mL |
| 1/4 cup | butter or margarine, softened | 50 mL |
| 1 cup | granulated sugar | 250 mL |
| 1 | egg | 1 |
| 2 cups | sliced peeled apples | 500 mL |

1. In a bowl combine flour, baking soda, cinnamon, nutmeg and salt; stir to mix well.
2. In a bowl with an electric mixer, cream together butter and sugar. Blend in egg. Fold in apple slices. Gradually add flour mixture, stirring after each addition. Pour batter into prepared pan. Bake in preheated oven for 30 minutes or until toothpick inserted in center comes out clean. Cool on a wire rack before serving.

| NUTRITIONAL ANALYSIS | Energy | Protein | Carbohydrate | Fat | Calcium | Iron |
|---|---|---|---|---|---|---|
| per slice | 116 kcal | 1.3 g | 21.7 g | 3.0 g | 1 % CDV | 5 % CDV |

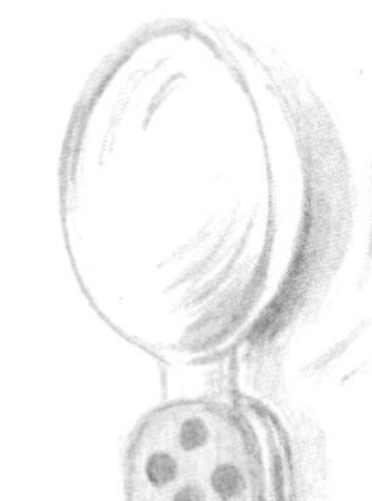

# Chocolate Surprise Cake

**Serves 12**

*What's the "surprise" in this cake? Well, how about beets? Seriously! They add great flavor and texture, as well as good nutrition (they're a good source of iron and folate). And this cake is so moist, you don't need any icing.*

*Preheat oven to 325° F (160° C)*
*8-inch (2 L) square baking pan, greased*

| | | |
|---|---|---|
| 1 3/4 cups | all-purpose flour | 425 mL |
| 6 tbsp | cocoa powder | 90 mL |
| 1 1/2 tsp | baking powder | 7 mL |
| 1/4 tsp | salt | 1 mL |
| 1 | can (19 oz [570 g]) beets, drained and puréed | 1 |
| 1 cup | granulated sugar | 250 mL |
| 1/2 cup | packed brown sugar | 125 mL |
| 3/4 cup | vegetable oil | 175 mL |
| 1/4 cup | butter or margarine, softened | 50 mL |
| 2 | eggs | 2 |
| 1 tsp | vanilla extract | 5 mL |

1. In a bowl sift together flour, cocoa powder, baking powder and salt.
2. In a bowl with an electric mixer, combine beets, granulated sugar, brown sugar, oil, butter, eggs and vanilla. Beat slowly until blended, then on high for 1 to 2 minutes or until thoroughly mixed. Gradually blend in flour-cocoa mixture.
3. Transfer batter to prepared baking pan and bake for 40 minutes or until toothpick inserted in center comes out clean. Cool on a wire rack before serving.

### Kitchen Tip

For a chocolate-mint flavor, add 3/4 tsp (4 mL) peppermint extract.

If making a cake with beets is just a little too "surprising" for you, replace them with 4 bananas, mashed, and 1/2 cup (125 mL) milk.

| Nutritional Analysis | Energy | Protein | Carbohydrate | Fat | Calcium | Iron |
|---|---|---|---|---|---|---|
| per serving | 355 kcal | 4.1 g | 45.1 g | 18.9 g | 4 % CDV | 25 % CDV |

# Chocolate Chip and Banana Cake

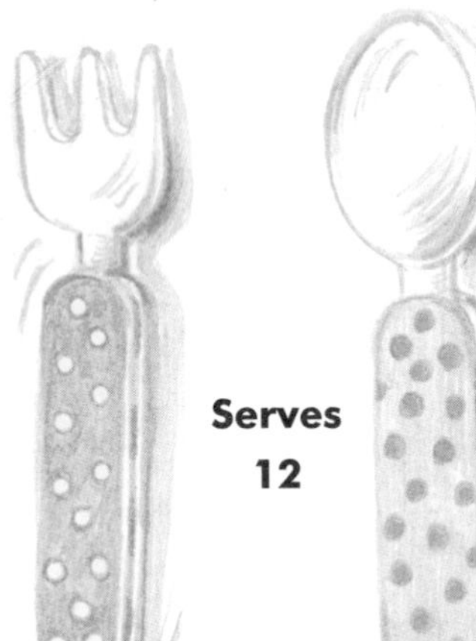

**Serves 12**

*Most kids love chocolate and bananas. No wonder this cake is so popular!*

**Kitchen Tip**

This recipe is a great use for any overripe bananas that have been lurking in the freezer waiting to be used.

*Preheat oven to 350° F (180° C)*
*13- by 9-inch (3.5 L) baking pan, greased*

| | | |
|---|---|---|
| 1/3 cup | butter or margarine, softened | 75 mL |
| 1/2 cup | granulated sugar | 125 mL |
| 1/2 cup | lightly packed brown sugar | 125 mL |
| 3 | eggs | 3 |
| 3 | mashed ripe bananas (see Tip, at left) | 3 |
| 2 tsp | vanilla extract | 10 mL |
| 1 1/2 cups | all-purpose flour | 375 mL |
| 1/2 cup | whole wheat flour | 125 mL |
| 1 tbsp | baking powder | 15 mL |
| 1/2 tsp | baking soda | 2 mL |
| 1/2 tsp | salt | 2 mL |
| 1 cup | 2% milk | 250 mL |
| 1 | pkg (12 oz [300 g]) chocolate chips | 1 |

1. In a bowl with an electric mixer, cream together butter, granulated sugar and brown sugar; beat until light and fluffy. Beat in eggs, one at a time. Blend in bananas and vanilla.
2. In another bowl, combine all-purpose flour, whole wheat flour, baking powder, baking soda and salt. Stir into egg mixture, a little at a time, alternately with milk. Stir in chocolate chips.
3. Transfer batter to prepared pan and bake in preheated for about 35 minutes or until tester inserted in center comes out clean. Cool on a wire rack before slicing.

| Nutritional Analysis | Energy | Protein | Carbohydrate | Fat | Calcium | Iron |
|---|---|---|---|---|---|---|
| per serving | 371 kcal | 6.0 g | 55.4 g | 16.0 g | 8 % CDV | 21 % CDV |

# Citrus Orange Bundt Cake

**Serves 12**

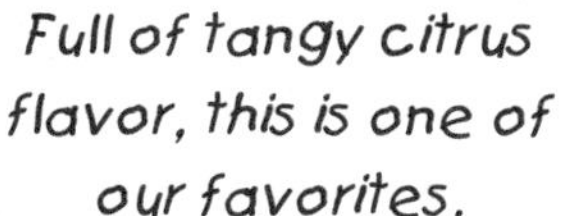

*Full of tangy citrus flavor, this is one of our favorites.*

### Kitchen Tip

This cake is excellent when served with your choice of seasonal fresh fruit. Try sliced strawberries, peaches, nectarines or apricots.

*Preheat oven to 350° F (180° C)*
*10-inch (3 L) bundt pan, greased and floured*

| | | |
|---|---|---|
| 1/2 cup | butter or margarine | 125 mL |
| 2 1/2 cups | granulated sugar, divided | 625 mL |
| 2 | eggs | 2 |
| 1 1/4 cups | plain yogurt | 300 mL |
| | Zest of 1 orange | |
| 2 cups | all-purpose flour | 500 mL |
| 2 tsp | baking powder | 10 mL |
| 1/2 cup | freshly squeezed orange juice | 125 mL |

1. In a bowl with an electric mixer, cream together butter and 2 cups (500 mL) of the sugar; beat until light and fluffy. Beat in eggs until blended.
2. In a small bowl, combine yogurt and orange zest; set aside.
3. In another bowl, combine flour and baking powder. Stir into butter mixture, a little at a time, alternating with yogurt mixture.
4. Spoon batter into prepared pan. Bake in preheated oven for 50 minutes or until tester inserted in center comes out clean. Remove from oven to rack and cool for 5 minutes. Invert cake onto a plate with a rim. Insert a toothpick, 1-inch (2.5 cm) deep, several times into surface of cake.
5. In a measuring cup, whisk together orange juice and remaining 1/2 cup (125 mL) sugar. Drizzle mixture over warm cake. Allow to cool before serving.

| Nutritional Analysis | Energy | Protein | Carbohydrate | Fat | Calcium | Iron |
|---|---|---|---|---|---|---|
| per serving | 355 kcal | 4.4 g | 63.8 g | 10.1 g | 7 % CDV | 12 % CDV |

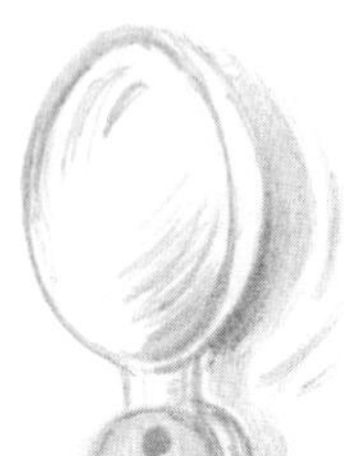

# Molded Orange Angel Cake Dessert

**Serves 10**

*For a special dinner or a birthday party, this dessert is a real show-stopper.*

| | | |
|---|---|---|
| 1 | pkg (7 g) unflavored gelatin | 1 |
| 1/4 cup | granulated sugar | 50 mL |
| 2/3 cup | frozen orange juice concentrate, thawed | 175 mL |
| 1/2 cup | water | 125 mL |
| 1 cup | whipping (35%) cream | 250 mL |
| 1 | angel food cake (10 oz [300 g]), torn into 1-inch (2.5 cm) cubes | 1 |
| 1 | can (10 oz [284 mL]) mandarin orange sections, drained | 1 |
| 1/3 cup | frozen orange juice concentrate, thawed | 75 mL |

1. In a small saucepan, combine gelatin and sugar. Stir in orange juice and water. Bring to a boil over medium-high heat. Cook, stirring constantly, until sugar is dissolved. Remove from heat and allow to cool slightly. Refrigerate until mixture starts to set.
2. In a bowl with an electric mixer, whip cream until it forms stiff peaks. Set aside.
3. In another bowl with the electric mixer, beat gelatin mixture at high speed until light. Fold in whipped cream and orange sections.
4. Line a large bowl with plastic wrap, overlapping sides. Place one-third of cake pieces in bowl. Cover with one-third of gelatin mixture. Repeat layers twice more. Push any cake pieces down into orange mixture.
5. Cover with plastic wrap and refrigerate overnight. Remove plastic wrap. Turn cake over onto a large serving plate. Drizzle with 1/3 cup (75 mL) orange juice concentrate. Refrigerate until ready to serve.

| Nutritional Analysis | Energy | Protein | Carbohydrate | Fat | Calcium | Iron |
|---|---|---|---|---|---|---|
| per serving | 237 kcal | 4.0 g | 35.0 g | 9.7 g | 4 % CDV | 5 % CDV |

# Pineapple Sour Cream Cake

*Preheat oven to 350° F (180° C)*
*13- by 9-inch (3.5 L) baking pan, greased*

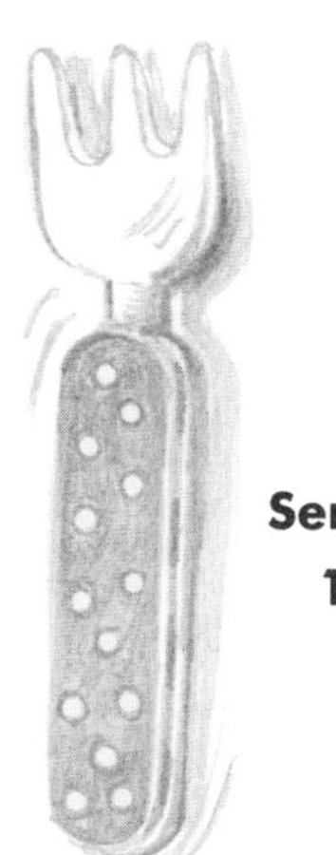
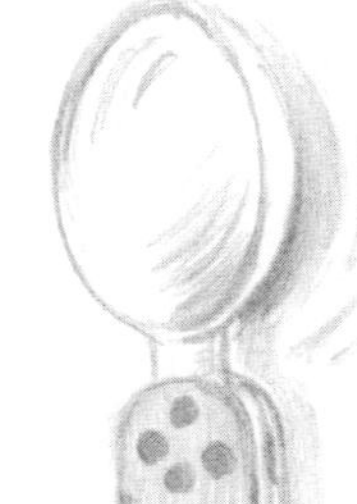
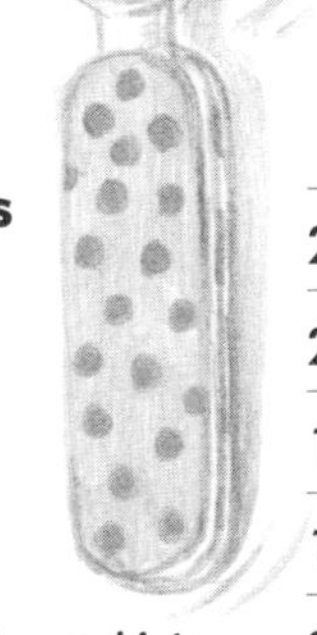

**Serves 10**

*Pineapple gives this cake its wonderful tropical flavor – and helps to keep it moist for several days.*

| | | |
|---|---|---|
| 2 cups | cake-and-pastry flour | 500 mL |
| 2 tsp | baking powder | 10 mL |
| 1 tsp | baking soda | 5 mL |
| 1/4 cup | butter or margarine | 50 mL |
| 2 | eggs | 2 |
| 1 cup | granulated sugar | 250 mL |
| 1 cup | crushed canned pineapple and juice (see Tip, at left) | 250 mL |
| 3/4 cup | sour cream | 175 mL |

1. In a bowl combine flour, baking powder and baking soda. Set aside.
2. In a bowl with an electric mixer, beat butter and eggs until frothy. Gradually add sugar, beating until very thick. Stir in pineapple. Add flour mixture alternately with sour cream, ending with flour; stir well after each addition.
3. Spread batter in prepared pan. Bake in preheated oven for 30 minutes or until tester inserted in center comes out clean. Cool completely on wire rack before cutting into pieces.

### Kitchen Tip

If you wish, use any leftover pineapple to make a frosting. (See recipe below.)

### Pineapple Frosting

In a bowl with an electric mixer, cream 1/4 cup (50 mL) butter or margarine until light and fluffy. Gradually beat in confectioner's (icing) sugar, 1/4 cup (50 mL) at a time, adding extra crushed pineapple and juice as mixture thickens. (You will probably use about 1 1/2 cups [375 mL] sugar, depending on amount of pineapple and juice added.)

| Nutritional Analysis | Energy | Protein | Carbohydrate | Fat | Calcium | Iron |
|---|---|---|---|---|---|---|
| per serving | 255 kcal | 3.6 g | 43.2 g | 7.7 g | 5 % CDV | 13 % CDV |

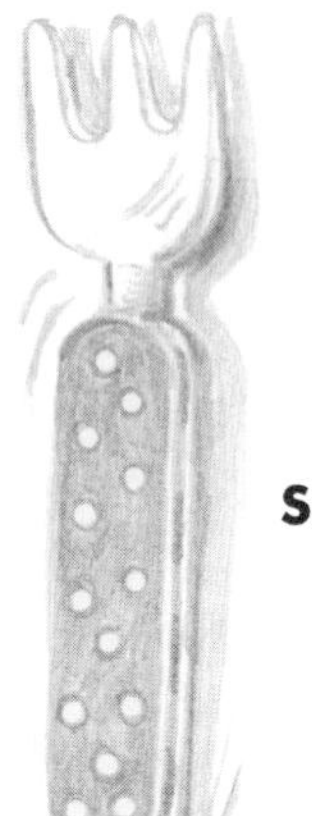
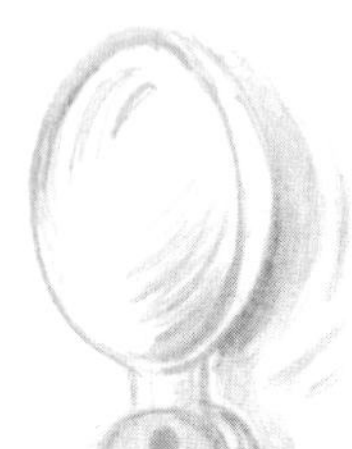
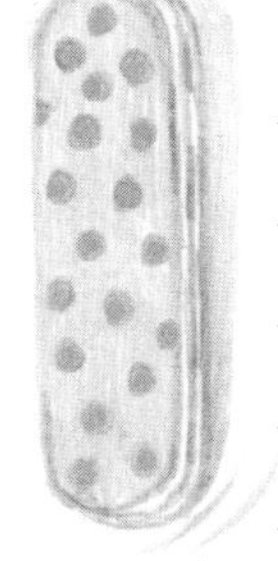

# Orange and Chocolate Marble Cake

*Preheat oven to 350° F (180° C)*
*8-inch (2 L) baking pan, greased*

**Serves 12**

*Absolutely moist and delicious – there won't be any left-overs with this cake!*

**KITCHEN TIP**

To melt chocolate, microwave on High for about 1 minute or until soft.

| | | |
|---|---|---|
| 1 cup | butter or margarine, softened | 250 mL |
| 1 cup | granulated sugar | 250 mL |
| 3 | egg yolks | 3 |
| 1 3/4 cups | all-purpose flour | 425 mL |
| 3/4 tsp | baking soda | 4 mL |
| 3/4 tsp | baking powder | 4 mL |
| 1 cup | plain yogurt | 250 mL |
| | Grated zest of 1 orange | 1 |
| 2 oz | unsweetened chocolate, melted (see Tip, at left) | 50 g |
| 3 | egg whites | 3 |
| Pinch | cream of tartar | Pinch |
| **GLAZE** | | |
| 1/2 cup | orange juice | 125 mL |
| 1/4 cup | granulated sugar | 50 mL |

1. In a bowl with an electric mixer, cream together butter and sugar. Beat in egg yolks one at a time.
2. In another bowl, sift together flour, baking soda and baking powder. Add to butter mixture a little at a time, alternating with additions of yogurt. Beat after each addition until combined.
3. Divide batter between two clean bowls. Into one bowl, stir in orange zest. Stir melted chocolate into the other.

| NUTRITIONAL ANALYSIS | Energy | Protein | Carbohydrate | Fat | Calcium | Iron |
|---|---|---|---|---|---|---|
| per slice | 369 kcal | 5.6 g | 39.9 g | 21.7 g | 5 % CDV | 1 % CDV |

4. In another bowl with an electric mixer, beat egg whites until foamy. Add cream of tartar; beat whites to form stiff peaks. Gently fold one-half of the whites into the orange batter and one-half of the whites into the chocolate batter.
5. Place batters alternately by spoonful into baking pan. Bake in preheated oven for 1 hour and 10 minutes or until tester inserted in center comes out clean. Let cool for 5 minutes.
6. Glaze: In a small bowl, whisk together orange juice and sugar. Pour glaze over cake while still in pan. Let cool completely and serve.

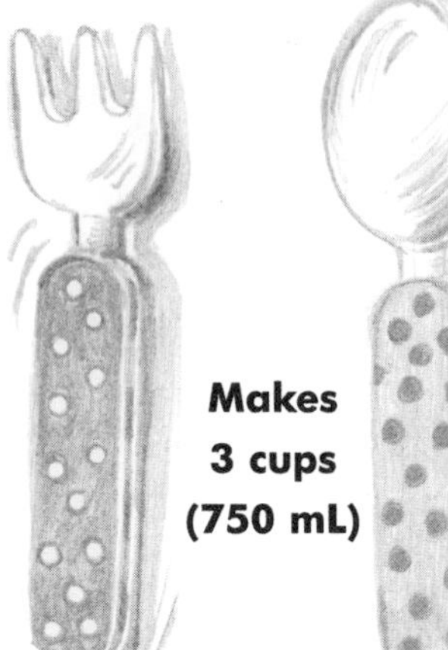


# Apple Cranberry Sauce

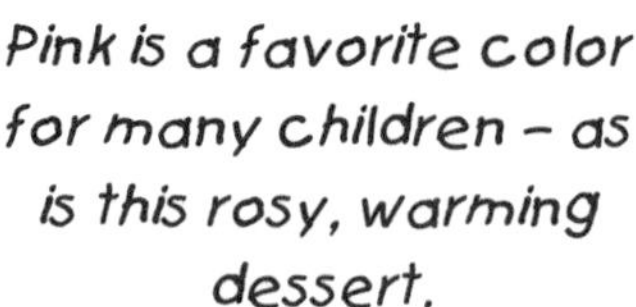


| | | |
|---|---|---|
| 1 cup | apple juice or sweet apple cider | 250 mL |
| 1/2 cup | liquid honey | 125 mL |
| 2 tbsp | brown sugar | 25 mL |
| 2 cups | fresh or frozen cranberries | 500 mL |
| 3 cups | chopped peeled apples | 750 mL |
| 1/2 tsp | ground cinnamon | 2 mL |

1. In a saucepan over medium-high heat, combine apple juice, honey and sugar. Bring to a boil. Add cranberries and apples. Reduce heat to medium and cook, uncovered, for 10 minutes or until fruit is tender and sauce has thickened.
2. Remove from heat and allow to cool. Add cinnamon and taste for seasoning. For a smoother texture (which young children may prefer), purée mixture in a food processor or blender.

| NUTRITIONAL ANALYSIS | Energy | Protein | Carbohydrate | Fat | Calcium | Iron |
|---|---|---|---|---|---|---|
| per 1/2-cup (125 mL) serving | 173 kcal | 0.3 g | 45.8 g | 0.6 g | 2 % CDV | 6 % CDV |

# Caramel Sauce

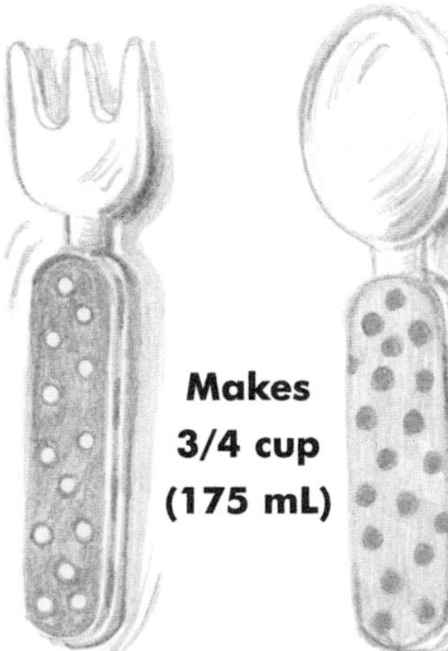

**Makes 3/4 cup (175 mL)**

*This sauce is just about the perfect accompaniment for gingerbread (see page 236). It's also excellent served over ice cream or any plain cake.*

| | | |
|---|---|---|
| 1/2 cup | butter or margarine | 125 mL |
| 1 1/4 cups | packed brown sugar | 300 mL |
| 2 tbsp | corn syrup | 25 mL |
| 1/2 cup | light (10%) cream or whipping (35%) cream | 125 mL |

1. In a saucepan melt butter over medium-high heat. Stir in sugar and corn syrup; bring to a boil. Cook, stirring constantly, until sugar dissolves. Stir in cream and return to a boil. Remove from heat; serve warm or allow to cool.

### Kitchen Tip

The sauce keeps well, covered, for up to 1 week in the refrigerator. Warm in the microwave before serving.

| Nutritional Analysis | Energy | Protein | Carbohydrate | Fat | Calcium | Iron |
|---|---|---|---|---|---|---|
| per 1 tbsp (15 mL) | 169 kcal | 0.4 g | 21.8 g | 9.4 g | 4 % CDV | 8 % CDV |

# Tangy Fruit Sauce

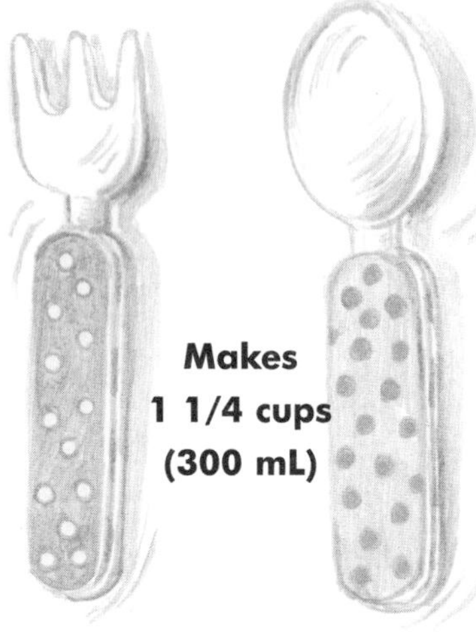

**Makes 1 1/4 cups (300 mL)**

*This sauce is wonderful served on pancakes (see page 122), as a topping for ice cream, or with angel food cake.*

| | | |
|---|---|---|
| 1/4 cup | granulated sugar | 50 mL |
| 2 tbsp | cornstarch | 25 mL |
| 1/2 cup | orange juice | 125 mL |
| 1/2 cup | water or juice from fruit (see below) | 125 mL |
| 1 cup | sliced strawberries, raspberries, blueberries or sour cherries | 250 mL |
| 1 tsp | grated lemon zest | 5 mL |
| 1 tbsp | lemon juice | 15 mL |

1. In a saucepan over medium heat, combine sugar, cornstarch, orange juice and water; bring to a boil. Reduce heat and cook, stirring constantly, until sauce has thickened. Stir in fruit, zest and lemon juice. Serve warm or cover and refrigerate until needed.

| Nutritional Analysis | Energy | Protein | Carbohydrate | Fat | Calcium | Iron |
|---|---|---|---|---|---|---|
| per 1/4 cup (50 mL) | 54 kcal | 0.3 g | 13.5 g | 0.1 g | 1 % CDV | 1 % CDV |

APPENDIX

# References

## *and resources*


### Feeding 2- to 4-year-olds

Baker, S. S.; Cochran, W. J.; Greer, F. R.; Heyman, M. B.; Jacobson, M. S.; Jaksic, T.; and Krebs, N. F. American Academy of Pediatrics. "The use and misuse of fruit juice in pediatrics." *Pediatrics* 2001;107:1210-1213.

Birch, L. L.; Johnson, S. L.; Andresen, G.; Peters, J. C.; Schulte, M. C. "The variability of young children's energy intake." *New England Journal of Medicine* 1991; 324:232-235.

Briley, M. E.; Jastrow, S.; Vickers, J.; and Roberts-Gray, C. "Dietary intake at child-care centers and away: are parents and care providers working as partners or at cross-purposes?" *Journal of the American Dietetic Association* 1999; 99:950-4.

Briley, M. E. and Roberts-Gray, C. Position of The American Dietetic Association: "Nutrition standards for child care programs." *Journal of the American Dietetic Association* 1994; 94:3223-328.

Carruth, B. R. and Skinner, J. D. "Revisiting the picky eater phenomenon: neophobic behaviors of young children." *Journal of the American College of Nutrition* 2000; 19:771-80.

Canada's Food Guide to Healthy Eating: Focus on Preschoolers. 1995; Health Canada.

Dennison, B. A. "Fruit juice consumption by infants and children: a review." *Journal of the American College of Nutrition* 1996; 15:4S-11S.

Dennison, B. A.; Rockwell, H. L.; and Baker, S. L. "Fruit and vegetable intake in young children." *Journal of the American College of Nutrition* 1998; 17:371-8.

Koivisto Hursti, U. K. "Factors influencing children's food choice." *Annals of Medicine* 1999; Suppl:26-32

Leung, A. K. and Robson, W. L. "The toddler who does not eat." *American Family Physician* 1994; 49:1789-92.

Leung, M.; Yeung, D. L.; Pennell, M. D.; and Hall, J. "Dietary intakes of preschoolers." *Journal of the American Dietetic Association* 1984; 84:551-554.

Omar, M. A.; Coleman, G.; and Hoerr, S. "Healthy eating for rural low-income toddlers: caregivers' perceptions." *Journal of Community Health and Nursing* 2001;18:93-106.

Petter L. P.; Hourihane J. O.; and Rolles C. J. "Is water out of vogue? A survey of the drinking habits of 2-7 years olds." *Archives of Disease in Children* 1995; 72:137-40.

Pollock, I. and Warner, J. O. "Effect of artificial food colours on childhood behaviour." *Archives of Disease in Childhood* 1990; 65:74-77.

Scarr, S. "American child care today." *American Psychology* 1998; 53:95-108.

Skinner, J. D.; Carruth, B. R.; Houck, K. S.; Bounds, W.; Morris, M.; Cox, D. R.; Moran, J, III; and Coletta, F. "Longitudinal study of nutrient and food intakes of white preschool children aged 24 to 60 months." *Journal of the American Dietetic Association* 1999; 99:1514-21.

Wilson, N. and Scott, A. "A double-blind assessment of additive intolerance in children using a 12 day challenge period at home." *Clinical Experimental Allergy* 1989; 19:267-72.

Wolraich, M. L.; Lindgren, S. D.; Stumbo, P. J.; Stegink, L. D.; Appelbaum, M. I.; and Kiritsy, M. C. "Effects of diets high in sucrose or aspartame on the behaviour and cognitive performance of children." *New England Journal of Medicine* 1994; 330:301-7.

## Feeding 4- to 6-year-olds

Canada's Food Guide to Healthy Eating: Focus on Preschoolers. 1995; Health Canada.

Meyers, A. F.; et al. "School breakfast program and school performance." *American Journal of Disease in Childhood* 1989; 143: 1234-1239.

Mobley, C. E. and Evashevski, J. "Evaluating health and safety knowledge of preschoolers: assessing their early start to being health smart." *Journal of Pediatric Health Care* 2000; 14:160-165.

Pollitt, E. "Does breakfast make a difference in school?" *Journal of the American Dietetic Association* 1995; 95:1134-1139.

Satter, E. *How to get your kid to eat...but not too much.* Palo Alto: Bull Publishing Co., 1987.

Worthington-Roberts, B. S. and Rodwell Williams, S. *Nutrition throughout the life-cycle.* 3rd ed. St. Louis: Mosby-Year Book, Inc., 1996.

## Nutrients, vitamins and minerals

Groff, J. L.; Gropper, S. S.; and Hunt, S. M. *Advanced Nutrition and Human Metabolism.* St.Paul: West Publishing Co. 1995,

### Fiber

American Academy of Pediatrics – Committee on Nutrition. "Plant fiber intake in the pediatric diet." *Pediatrics* 1981; 67(4):572-575.

Conference on Dietary Fiber in Childhood. "A summary of conference recommendations on dietary fiber in children." *Pediatrics* 1995; Suppl:1023-1028.

Dwyer, J. T. "Dietary fiber for children. How much?" *Pediatrics* 1995; 96:1019-1022.

Guthrie, H. A. and Picciano, M. F. *Human Nutrition.* St. Louis: Mosby-Year Book Inc., 1995.

Hampl, J. S.; Betts, N. M.; and Benes, B. A. "The 'age+5' rule: Comparisons of dietary fiber intake among 4- to 10-year old children." *Journal of the American Dietetic Association.* 1998; 98:1418-1423.

Hillemeier, C. "An overview of the effects of dietary fiber on gastrointestinal transit." *Pediatrics* 1995; 96: 997-999.

McClung, H. J.; Boyne, L.; and Heitlinger, L. "Constipation and dietary fiber intake in children." *Pediatrics* 1995; 96:999-1001.

Saldanha, L. G. "Fiber in the diet of US children: Results of national surveys." *Pediatrics* 1995; 96:994-997.

Williams, C. L. "Importance of dietary fiber in childhood." *Journal of the American Dietetic Association* 1995; 95:1140-1149.

Williams, C. L. and Bollella, M. "Is a high-fiber diet safe for children?" *Pediatrics* 1995; 96:1014-1019.

### Calcium

Baker, S. S.; Cochran, W. J.; Flores, C. A.; Georgieff, M. K.; Jacobson, M. S.; Jaksic, T.; and Krebs, N. F. American Academy of Pediatrics. Committee on Nutrition. "Calcium requirements of infants, children and adolescents." *Pediatrics* 1999; 104:1152-1157.

Carvalho, N. F.; Kenney, R. D.; Carrington, P. H.; and Hall, D. E. "Severe nutritional deficiencies in toddlers resulting from health food milk alternatives." *Pediatrics* 2001; 107:E46.

Gallo, A. M. "Building strong bones in childhood and adolescence: reducing the risk of fractures in later life." *Pediatric Nursing* 1996; 22:369-374.

Johnston, C. C.; Miller, J. Z.; and Slemenda, C. W. "Calcium supplementation and increases in bone mineral density in children." *New England Journal of Medicine* 1992; 327:82-87.

Lee, W. T.; Leung, S. S.; and Wang, S. H. "Double-blind, controlled calcium supplementation and bone mineral accretion in children accustomed to a low-calcium diet." *American Journal of Clinical Nutrition* 1994; 60:744-750.

Lee, W. T.; Leung, S. F.; Lui, S. S.; and Lau, J. "Relationship between long-term calcium intake and bone mineral content of children aged from birth to 5 years." *British Journal of Nutrition* 1993; 70:235-248.

National Institute of Health. "Optimal calcium intake." *NIH Consensus Statement* 1994; 12:1-31.

Sandstrom, B. "Micronutrient interactions: effects on absorption and bioavailability." *British Journal of Nutrition* 2001; 85:S181-S185.

### Iron

Cowin, I.; Edmond, A.; and Emmett, P. "Association between composition of the diet and haemoglobin and ferritin levels in 18-month-old children." *European Journal of Clinical Nutrition* 2001; 55:278-86.

Duggan, M. B.; Steel, G.; Elwys, G.; Harbottle, L.; and Noble, C. "Iron status, energy intake, and nutritional status of healthy young Asian children." *Archives of Disease in Children* 1991; 66:1386-9.

Fomon, S. "Infant feeding in the 20th century: formula and beikost." *Journal of Nutrition* 2001; 131:409S-20S.

Lampe, J. B. and Velez, N. "The effect of prolonged bottle feeding on cow's milk intake and iron stores at 18 months of age." *Clinical Pediatrics* 1997; 36:569-72.

Looker, A. C.; Dallman, P. R.; Carroll, M. D.; Gunter, E. W.; and Johnson, C. L. "Prevalence of iron deficiency in the United States." *Journal of the American Medical Association* 1997; 277:973-6.

Lozoff, B.; Jimenez, E.; Hagen, J.; Mollen, E; Wolf, A. W. "Poorer behavioral and developmental outcome more than 10 years after treatment for iron deficiency in infancy." *Pediatrics* 2000; 105:E51.

Olivares, M.; Walter, T.; Hertrampf, E.; and Pizarro, F. "Anaemia and iron deficiency disease in children." *British Medical Bulletin* 1999; 55:534-543.

Reeves, J. D.; Yip, R. "Lack of adverse side effects of oral ferrous sulfate therapy in 1-year-old infants." *Pediatrics* 1985; 75:352-5.

Thane, C. W.; Walmsley, C. M.; Bates, C. J.; Prentice, A.; and Cole, T. J. "Risk factors for poor iron status in British toddlers: further analysis of data from the National Diet and Nutrition Survey of children aged 1.5-4.5 years." *Public Health Nutrition* 2000; 3:433-440.

Singhal, A.; Morley, R.; Abbott, R.; Fairweather-Tait, S.; Stephenson, T.; and Lucas, A. "Clinical safety of iron-fortified formulas." *Pediatrics* 2000; 105:E38.

Zive, M. M.; Taras, H. L.; Broyles, S. L.; Frank-Spohrer, G. C.; and Nader, P. R. "Vitamin and mineral intakes of Anglo-American and Mexican-American preschoolers." *Journal of the American Dietetic Association* 1995; 95:533.

#### Vitamin C

Guthrie, H. A. and Picciano, M. F. *Human Nutrition*. St. Louis: Mosby-Year Book Inc., 1995.

#### Zinc

Briefel, R. R. et al. "Zinc intake of the US population: findings from the third national health and nutrition examination survey, 1988-1994." *Journal of Nutrition* 2000; 130:1367S-1373S.

Gibson, R. S.; Yeudall, F.; and Drost, N. "Dietary interventions to prevent zinc deficiency." *American Journal of Clinical Nutrition* 1998; 68(2suppl):48S-87S.

Gibson, R. S. "Content and bioavailability of trace elements in vegetarian diets." *American Journal of Clinical Nutrition* 1994; 59(5suppl):1223S-32S.

Guthrie, H.A. and Picciano, M. F. *Human Nutrition*. St. Louis: Mosby-Year Book Inc., 1995.

Skinner, J.D. et al. "Longitudinal study of nutrient and food intakes of white preschool children aged 24 to 60 months." *Journal of the American Dietetic Association* 1999; 99(12):1514-1521.

Sandstead, H. H. "Is zinc deficiency a public health problem?" *Nutrition* 1995; 11(1suppl):87-92.

### Vegetarian diets

American Dietetic Association. "Position of the American Dietetic Association: vegetarian diets." *Journal of the American Dietetic Association* 1993; 93(11): 1317-1319.

Haddad, E. H.; Sabate, J.; and Whitten, C. G. "Vegetarian food guide pyramid: a conceptual framework." *American Journal of Clinical Nutrition* 1999; 70(suppl):615S-619S.

Hebbelinck, M.; Clarys, P.; and DeMalsche, A. "Growth, development and physical fitness of Flemish vegetarian children, adolescents and young adults." *American Journal of Clinical Nutrition* 1999; 70(suppl):579S-585S.

Melina, V.; Davis, B.; and Harrison, V. *Becoming Vegetarian*. Toronto: Macmillan Canada, 1994.

Messina, V. and Mangels, A. R. "Considerations in planning vegan diets: children." *Journal of the American Dietetic Association* 2001; 101(6):661-669.

O'Connell, J.M. et al. "Growth of vegetarian children: the farm study." *Pediatrics* 1989; 84:475-481.

Sanders, T. A. "Growth and development of British vegan children." *American Journal of Clinical Nutrition* 1988; 48:822-825.

Truesdell, D. D. and Acosta, P. B. "Feeding the vegan infant and child." *Journal of the American Dietetic Association* 1985; 85(7):837-840.

Weaver, C. M.; Proulx, W. R.; and Heaney, R. "Choices for achieving adequate dietary calcium with a vegetarian diet." *American Journal of Clinical Nutrition* 1999; 70(suppl):543S-548S.


## Food safety


Canadian Pediatric Society Infectious Diseases and Immunization Committee. *Preventing Hamburger Disease.* Ottawa: Canadian Paediatric Society, 1995.

Guthrie, H.A. and Picciano, M. F. *Human Nutrition.* St. Louis: Mosby-Year Book Inc., 1995.

Joint Working Group of the Canadian Paediatric Society, Dietitians of Canada and Health Canada. *Nutrition for Healthy Term Infants.* Ottawa, 1998.


## Conventional vs organic foods


Calder, J.; Issenman, R.; Cawdron, R. "Health information provided by retail health food outlets." *Canadian Journal of Gastroenterology* 2000; 14:767-771.

Dietrich, K. N. "Environmental chemicals and child development." *Journal of Pediatrics* 1999; 134:7-9.

Health Canada website: "Frequently asked questions on genetically modified foods." *http://www.hc-sc.gc.ca*

Leckie, J. "Is organic food production feasible?" *Nutrition Health* 1999; 13:109-119.

Patandin, S.; Dagnelie, P. C.; Mulder, P. G.; Op de Coul, E.; van der Veen, J. E.; Weisglas-Kuperus, N.; and Sauer, P. J. "Dietary exposure to polychlorinated biphenyls and dioxins from infancy until adulthood: A comparison between breast-feeding, toddler, and long-term exposure." *Environmental Health Perspectives* 1999; 107:45-51.

Tryphonas, H. "The impact of PCB's and dioxins on children's health: immunological considerations." *Canadian Journal of Public Health* 1998; 890008-4263:S49-S52.

Schrezenmeir, J. and de Vrese, M. "Probiotics, prebiotics, and synbiotics-approaching a definition." *American Journal of Clinical Nutrition* 2001; 73(2Suppl):361S-364S.


## Food allergy and intolerance


Bock, S. A. "Prospective appraisal of complaints of adverse reactions to foods in children during the first 3 years of life." *Pediatrics* 1987; 79:683-88.

Bruno, G.; Giampietro, P. G.; Del Guerico, M. J. et. al. "Soy allergy is not common in atopic children: a multicenter study." *Pediatric Allergy and Immunology* 1997; 8:190-93.

Businoco, L. et. al. "Allergenicity and nutritional adequacy of soy protein formulas." *Journal of Pediatrics* 1992; 121:s21-s28.

Exl, B. M. and Fritsché, R. "Cow's milk protein allergy and possible means for its prevention." *Nutrition* 2001; 17:642-51.

Vickerstaff-Joneja, J. *Managing food allergy and intolerance: A practical guide.* 1995.

Wahn, U. "Aspects of nutritional management of food allergy." *Pediatric Allergy and Immunology* 2001; 12(suppl14):75-77.

## Disturbances in bowel function


Armon, K.; Stephenson, T.; MacFaul, R.; Eccleston, P.; and Werneke, U. "An evidence and consensus based guideline for acute diarrhea management." *Archives of Disease in Childhood* 2001; 85:132-142.

Baker, S. S.; Liptak, G, S.; Colletti, R. B.; Croffie, J. M.; Di Lorenzo, C.; Ector, W.; and Nurko, S. "Constipation in infants and children: evaluation and treatment." *Journal of Pediatric Gastroenterology and Nutrition* 1999; 29:612-626.

Harakka, K.; Savilahti, E.; Ponka, A.; Meurman, J. H.; Poussa, T.; Nase, L.; Saxelin, M.; and Korpela, R. "Effect of long term consumption of probiotics milk on infections in children attending day care centres: double blind, randomised trial." *British Medical Journal* 2001; 322:1327-9.

Kneepkens, C. M. and Hoekstra, J. H. "Chronic nonspecific diarrhea of childhood: pathophysiology and management." *Pediatric Clinics of North America* 1996; 43:375-90.

Loening-Baucke, V. "Constipation in early childhood: patient characteristics, treatment, and longterm follow up." *Gut* 1993; 34:1400-4.

Murphy, M. S. "Guidelines for managing acute gastroenteritis based on a systematic review of published research." *Archives of Disease in Childhood* 1998; 79:279-84.

Pashankar, D. S. and Bishop, W. P. "Efficacy and optimal dose of daily polyethylene glycol 3350 for treatment of constipation and encopresis in children." *Journal of Pediatrics* 2001; 139:428-32.

Poenaru, D.; Roblin, N.; Bird, M.; Duce, S.; Groll, A.; Pietak, D.; Spry, K.; and Thompson, J. "The pediatric bowel management clinic: initial results of multidisciplinary approach to functional constipation in children." *Journal of Pediatric Surgery* 1997; 32:843-8.

Reeves, J. D. and Yip R. "Lack of adverse side effects of oral ferrous sulfate therapy in 1-year-old infants." *Pediatrics* 1985; 75:352-355

Staiano, A.; Andreotti, M. R.; Greco, L.; Basile, P.; and Auricchio, S. "Long-term follow-up of children with chronic idiopathic constipation." *Digestive Disease and Sciences* 1994; 39:561-564.

Szajewska, H.; Kotowska, M.;, Mrukowicz, J. Z.; Armanska, M.; and Mikolajczyk, W. "Efficacy of Lactobacillus GG in prevention of nosocomial diarrhea in infants." *The Journal of Pediatrics* 2001; 138:361-5

Weaver, L. T. and Steiner, H. "The bowel habit of young children." *Archives of Disease in Childhood* 1984; 59:649-652.

Youssef, N. N. and Di Lorenzo, C. "Childhood constipation: evaluation and treatment." *Journal of Clinical Gastroenterology* 2001; 33:199-205.


## Childhood obesity


Abramovitz, B. A. and Birch, L. L. "Five-year-old girls' ideas about dieting are predicted by their mothers' dieting." *Journal of the American Dietetic Association* 2000; 100(10):1157-1163.

American Academy of Pediatrics – Committee on Nutrition. "Cholesterol in childhood." *Pediatrics* 1998; 101(1):141-147.

Birch, L. L. and Fisher, J. O. "Mothers' child-feeding practices influence daughters' eating and weight." *American Journal of Clinical Nutrition* 2000; 71(5):1054-1061.

Bundred, P.; Kitchiner, D.; and Buchan, I. "Prevalence of overweight and obese children between 1989 and 1998: population based series of cross sectional studies." *British Medical Journal* 2001; 322:326-328.

Davison, K. K. and Birch, L. L. "Weight status, parent reaction and self-concept in five-year-old girls." *Pediatrics* 2001; 107(1): 46-53.

Edmunds, L.; Waters, E.; and Elliott, E. J. "Evidence based management of childhood obesity." *British Medical Journal* 2001; 323:916-919.

Fisher, J. O. and Birch, L, L. "Restricting access to palatable foods affects children's behavioral response, food selection and intake." *American Journal of Clinical Nutrition* 1999; 69:1264-1272.

Johnson, S. L. "Improving preschoolers' self-regulation of energy intake." *Pediatrics* 2000; 106(6):1429-1435.

Johnson, S. L. and Birch, L. L. "Parents' and children's adiposity and eating style." *Pediatrics* 1994; 94(5):653-661.

Joint Working Group of the Canadian Pediatric Society and Health Canada. *Nutrition recommendations update.... dietary fat and children.* Ottawa, 1994.

MacKenzie, N. R. "Childhood obesity: strategies for prevention." *Pediatric Nursing* 2000; 26(5):527-530.

McVeagh, P. "Eating and nutritional problems in children." *Australian Family Physician* 2000; 29(8):735-740.

Stice, E.; Agras, S.; and Hammer, L. D. "Risk factors for the emergence of childhood eating disturbances: a five-year prospective study." *International Journal of Eating Disorders* 1999; 25:375-387.

Westenhoefer, J. "Establishing good dietary habits – capturing the minds of children." *Public Health Nutrition* 2001; 4(1A): 125-129.

## Dental care for kids

Canadian Dental Association: Statement on Fluoridation 2000. *www.cda-adc.ca*

Canadian Paediatric Society, Nutrition Committee. "The use of fluoride in infants and children." *Paediatrics and Child Health* 1996; 1:131-134

City of Toronto Department of Public Health. "Baby teeth are important."

City of Toronto Department of Public Health. Canadian Dental Association Fact Sheet. "Growing up: how your dental needs change."

Henderson, H. Z.; Dean, J. A.; and Hatcher, E. A. *Indiana infant-toddler dental care survey.* Indiana Dental Association 1991;70:8-13

Johnsen, D. C. "Characteristics and backgrounds of children with 'nursing caries'." *Pediatric Dentistry* 1982; 4:218-224.

Marino, R. V.; Bornze, K.; Scholl, T. O.; and Anhalt, H. "Nursing bottle caries: characteristics of children at risk." *Clinical Pediatrics* 1989:129-131.

Ophaug, R. H.; Singer, L.; and Harland, B. F. "Dietary fluoride intake of 6-month and 2-year-old children in four dietary regions of the United Sates." *American Journal of Clinical Nutrition* 1985; 42:701-7

## Resources for parents

American Food Safety
*www.foodsafety.gov*

American Academy of Pediatrics
141 Northwest Point Boulevard
Elk Grove Village, IL 60007-1098
USA
*www.aap.org*

American Dietetic Association
Headquarters
216 W. Jackson Blvd.
Chicago, IL 60606-6995
*www.eatright.org*

Anaphylaxis Network of Canada
*www.anaphylaxis.org*

Body Image
*www.bodypositive.org*

Canadian Pediatric Society
2204 Walkley Road
Suite 100
Ottawa, ON Canada
K1G 4G8
*www.cps.ca*

Canadian Organic Advisory Board
www.coab.ca

Canadian Organic Growers
*www.cog.ca*

Dietitians of Canada
480 University Avenue, Suite 604
Toronto, ON Canada
M5G 1V2
*www.dietitians.ca*

Food Allergy Network of Canada
*www.foodallergy.org*

FAO - Food and Agriculture Organization
*www.fao.org/organicag*

Health Canada
A.L. 0900C2
Ottawa, ON Canada
K1A 0K9
*www.hc-sc.gc.ca*
Food labeling
*www.hc-sc.gc.ca/hppb/nutrition/labels/e_before.html*
Canada's Food Guide to Healthy Eating
*www.hc-sc.gc.ca/hppb/nutrition/pube/foodguid/index.html*

Food and Drug Administration
U. S. Food and Drug Administration
5600 Fishers Lane, Rockville
MD, USA 20857-0001
1-888-INFO-FDA (1-888-463-6332)
*www.fda.gov*
The Food Pyramid
*www.nal.usda.gov/fnic/Fpyr/pyramid.gif*

Specialty Food Shop
The Hospital for Sick Children
555 University Ave.
Toronto, Ontario M5G 1X8
1-800-SFS-7976 or 416-977-4360
(Wide product selection. Purchase wheat free, milk free, egg free products. Dietitians available to answer questions.)
*www.specialtyfoodshop.com*

# Index

## A



## B

## C

## D



## E

# F



# G

# Q



# R

# S

## T



## U



## V

## W

## Z